Spine Imaging and Intervention

Editor

VINIL SHAH

RADIOLOGIC CLINICS
OF NORTH AMERICA

www.radiologic.theclinics.com

Consulting Editor
FRANK H. MILLER

March 2024 • Volume 62 • Number 2

ELSEVIER

1600 John F. Kennedy Boulevard • Suite 1800 • Philadelphia, Pennsylvania, 19103-2899

http://www.theclinics.com

RADIOLOGIC CLINICS OF NORTH AMERICA Volume 62, Number 2
March 2024 ISSN 0033-8389, ISBN 13: 978-0-443-13017-5

Editor: John Vassallo (j.vassallo@elsevier.com)
Developmental Editor: Isha Singh

Radiologic Clinics of North America (ISSN 0033-8389) is published bimonthly by Elsevier Inc., 360 Park Avenue South, New York, NY 10010-1710. Months of issue are January, March, May, July, September, and November. Periodicals postage paid at New York, NY and additional mailing offices. Subscription prices are USD 561 per year for US individuals, USD 100 per year for US students and residents, USD 643 per year for Canadian individuals, USD 754 per year for international individuals, USD 100 per year for Canadian students/residents, and USD 315 per year for international students/residents. For institutional access pricing please contact Customer Service via the contact information below. To receive student and resident rate, orders must be accompanied by name of affiliated institution, date of term and the signature of program/residency coordinatior on institution letterhead. Orders will be billed at individual rate until proof of status is received. Foreign air speed delivery is included in all *Clinics* subscription prices. All prices are subject to change without notice. **POSTMASTER:** Send address changes to *Radiologic Clinics of North America*, Elsevier Health Sciences Division, Subscription Customer Service, 3251 Riverport Lane, Maryland Heights, MO63043. **Customer Service: Telephone: 1-800-654-2452** (U.S. and Canada); **1-314-447-8871** (outside U.S. and Canada). **Fax: 1-314-447-8029. E-mail: journalscustomerservice-usa@ elsevier.com (for print support); journalsonlinesupport-usa@elsevier.com (for online support)**.

Reprints. For copies of 100 or more of articles in this publication, please contact the Commercial Reprints Department, Elsevier Inc., 360 Park Avenue South, New York, New York 10010-1710. Tel.: +1-212-633-3874; Fax: +1-212-633-3820; E-mail: reprints@elsevier.com.

Radiologic Clinics of North America also published in Greek Paschalidis Medical Publications, Athens, Greece.

Radiologic Clinics of North America is covered in *MEDLINE/PubMed (Index Medicus), EMBASE/Excerpta Medica, Current Contents/Life Sciences, Current Contents/Clinical Medicine, RSNA Index to Imaging Literature, BIOSIS, Science Citation Index,* and *ISI/BIOMED.*

Printed in the United States of America.

Contributors

CONSULTING EDITOR

FRANK H. MILLER, MD, FACR, FSAR, FSABI
Lee F. Rogers, MD Professor of Medical
Education, Chief, Body Imaging Section,
Medical Director, MRI, Professor, Department
of Radiology, Northwestern Memorial Hospital,
Northwestern University Feinberg School of
Medicine, Chicago, Illinois, USA

EDITOR

VINIL SHAH, MD
Associate Professor of Radiology, Department
of Radiology and Biomedical Imaging, Chief,
Neuroradiology Division, University of
California, San Francisco, San Francisco,
California, USA

AUTHORS

FREDERIK ABEL, MD
Research Fellow, Department of Radiology
and Imaging, Hospital for Special Surgery, New
York, New York, USA

FRANZISKA C.S. ALTORFER, MD
Research Fellow, Department of Spine
Surgery, Hospital for Special Surgery, New
York, New York, USA; Department of
Orthopedic Surgery, Balgrist University
Hospital, University of Zurich, Zurich,
Switzerland

TIMOTHY J. AMRHEIN, MD
Associate Professor, Department of Radiology,
Duke University Medical Center, Durham,
North Carolina, USA

GOKCE B. BELGE BILGIN, MD
Department of Radiology, Mayo Clinic,
Rochester, Minnesota, USA

UPASANA UPADHYAY BHARADWAJ, MD
Fellow, Department of Radiology and
Biomedical Imaging, University of California,
San Francisco, San Francisco, California, USA

CEM BILGIN, MD
Fellow, Department of Radiology, Mayo Clinic,
Rochester, Minnesota, USA

WALEED BRINJIKJI, MD
Assistant Professor, Departments of Radiology
and Neurologic Surgery, Mayo Clinic,
Rochester, Minnesota, USA

STEPHEN M. BROSKI, MD
Associate Professor, Department of Radiology,
Mayo Clinic, Rochester, Minnesota, USA

JOSEPH LEVI CHAZEN, MD
Associate Professor, Neuroradiology, Director,
Spine Imaging, Department of Radiology and
Imaging, Hospital for Special Surgery, New
York, New York, USA

CYNTHIA T. CHIN, MD
Professor of Radiology and Biomedical
Imaging, University of California, San
Francisco, San Francisco, California, USA

JEREMY K. CUTSFORTH-GREGORY, MD
Consultant, Department of Neurology, Mayo
Clinic, Rochester, Minnesota, USA

WILLIAM P. DILLON, MD
Elizabeth A. Guillaumin Professor of Radiology,
Executive Vice-Chair, Department of
Radiology and Biomedical Imaging, University
of California, San Francisco, San Francisco,
California, USA

JAVIER GALVAN, MD, MPH
Resident, Department of Imaging, Cedars-
Sinai Medical Center, Los Angeles, California,
USA

WENDE GIBBS, MD, MA
Director, Spine Imaging, Barrow Neurological
Institute, Associate Professor, Department of
Neuroradiology, St. Joseph's Hospital and
Medical Center, Phoenix, Arizona, USA

ALLISON GRAYEV, MD
Associate Professor, Department of Radiology,
University of Wisconsin-Madison School of
Medicine and Public Health, Madison,
Wisconsin, USA

JESSICA L. HOUK, MD
Assistant Professor, Department of Radiology,
Duke University Medical Center, Durham,
North Carolina, USA

JACK W. JENNINGS, MD, PhD
Professor, Department of Radiology,
Mallinckrodt Institute of Radiology, St Louis,
Missouri, USA

DAVID F. KALLMES, MD
Professor, Department of Radiology, Mayo
Clinic, Rochester, Minnesota, USA

SASAN KARIMI, MD
Attending Radiologist, Department of
Radiology, Memorial Sloan Kettering Cancer
Center, New York, New York, USA

HASSAN KOBEISSI, MD
Research Associate, Department of Radiology,
Mayo Clinic, Rochester, Minnesota, USA

PETER G. KRANZ, MD
Associate Professor, Department of Radiology,
Duke University Medical Center, Durham,
North Carolina, USA

VANCE T. LEHMAN, MD
Radiologist Department of Radiology, Mayo
Clinic, Rochester, Minnesota, USA

YENPO LIN, MD
Fellow, Radiology and Imaging, Hospital for
Special Surgery, Department of Medical
Imaging and Intervention, Chang Gung
Memorial Hospital, Taoyuan, Taiwan

ERIC LIS, MD
Associate Attending Radiologist, Department
of Radiology, Memorial Sloan Kettering Cancer
Center, New York, New York, USA

AJAY MADHAVAN, MD
Assistant Professor, Department of Radiology,
Mayo Clinic, Rochester, Minnesota, USA

SHARMILA MAJUMDAR, PhD
Margaret Hart Surbeck Distinguished
Professor in Advanced Imaging, Vice Chair for
Research, Executive Director, Center for
Intelligent Imaging, Director, Musculoskeletal
and Quantitative Imaging, Research Group,
Professor, Departments of Orthopedic
Surgery, and Bioengineering and Therapeutic
Sciences, University of California, San
Francisco, San Francisco, California, USA

TIMOTHY MAUS, MD
Professor Emeritus of Radiology, Department
of Radiology Mayo Clinic, Rochester,
Minnesota, USA

MARCEL MAYA, MD
Co-chair, Department of Imaging, Cedars-
Sinai Medical Center Los Angeles, California,
USA

ATAKAN ORSCELIK, MD
Research Fellow, Department of Radiology,
Mayo Clinic, Rochester, Minnesota, USA

KYUNG K. PECK, PhD
Attending Physicist, Department of Medical
Physics Memorial Sloan Kettering Cancer
Center, New York, New York, USA

JENIFER PITMAN, MD
Assistant Professor, Musculoskeletal Imaging,
Department of Radiology, Johns Hopkins
Hospital Baltimore, Maryland, USA

RAVI S. PRASAD, MD
Neuroradiologist, Department of Imaging
Cedars-Sinai Medical Center, Los Angeles,
California, USA

VARUN ROHATGI, BS
Research Assistant, Department of Radiology,
Weill Cornell Medicine, New York, New York,
USA

ATIN SAHA, MD, MS
Assistant Attending Radiologist, Department of
Radiology, Memorial Sloan Kettering Cancer
Center, New York, New York, USA

WOUTER SCHIEVINK, MD
Professor Department of Neurosurgery,
Cedars-Sinai Medical Center Los Angeles,
California, USA

YIGIT CAN SENOL, MD
Fellow Departments of Radiology and
Neurologic Surgery, Mayo Clinic, Rochester,
Minnesota, USA

VINIL SHAH, MD
Associate Professor of Radiology, Department
of Radiology and Biomedical Imaging, Chief,
Neuroradiology Division, University of
California, San Francisco, San Francisco,
California, USA

DARRYL SNEAG, MD
Director of MR Neurography and MRI
Research, Radiology and Imaging, Hospital for
Special Surgery, New York, New York, USA

JASON F. TALBOTT, MD, PhD
Assistant Professor, Department of Radiology
and Biomedical Imaging, Zuckerberg San
Francisco General Hospital and Trauma
Center, San Francisco, California, USA

EK TSOON TAN, PhD
Co-Director of MRI Lab, Radiology and
Imaging, Hospital for Special Surgery, New
York, New York, USA

CHRISTIN A. TIEGS-HEIDEN, MD
Fellow, Department of Radiology, Mayo Clinic,
Rochester, Minnesota, USA

ANDERANIK TOMASIAN, MD
Assistant Professor, Department of Radiology,
University of California, Irvine, Orange,
California, USA

VIKRAM S. WADWHA, MD
Cedars-Sinai Medical Center, Los Angeles,
California, USA

ALLEN Q. YE, MD, PhD
Assistant Professor, Department of Radiology
and Biomedical Imaging, Neuroradiology
Division, University of California, San
Francisco, Department of Radiology and
Biomedical Imaging, Zuckerberg San
Francisco General Hospital and Trauma
Center, San Francisco, California, USA

ONUR YILDIRIM, MD
Instructor Radiologist, Department of
Radiology, Memorial Sloan Kettering Cancer
Center, New York, New York, USA

Contents

The Anatomy, Technique, Safety, and Efficacy of Image-Guided Epidural Access   199

Timothy Maus

Epidural steroid injections have demonstrable efficacy and safety in treatment of radicular pain syndromes; transforaminal access has greater evidence of efficacy than interlaminar approaches. The interventionalist must understand epidural and foraminal anatomy and imaging to insure delivery of medication to the target, the ventral epidural space at the site of neural compression. This obligates pre-procedural planning. When performed with appropriate risk mitigation strategies, epidural injections by either access are safe. For transforaminal access, the use of dexamethasone as the injectate, and infraneural approaches, provides safety advantages.

Imaging of Discogenic and Vertebrogenic Pain   217

Frederik Abel, Franziska C.S. Altorfer, Varun Rohatgi, Wende Gibbs, and Joseph Levi Chazen

Chronic low back pain is a major source of pain and disability globally involving multifactorial causes. Historically, intervertebral disc degeneration and disruption have been associated as primary back pain triggers of the anterior column, termed "discogenic pain." Recently, the vertebral endplates have been identified as another possible pain trigger of the anterior column. This "endplate-driven" model, defined "vertebrogenic pain," is often interconnected with disc degeneration. Diagnosis of vertebrogenic and discogenic pain relies on imaging techniques that isolate pain generators and exclude comorbid conditions. Traditional methods, like radiographs and discography, are augmented by more sensitive methods, including SPECT, CT, and MRI. Morphologic MRI is pivotal in revealing indicators of vertebrogenic (eg, Modic endplate changes) and discogenic pain (eg, disc degeneration and annular fissures). More advanced methods, like ultra-short-echo time imaging, and quantitative MRI further amplify MRI's accuracy in the detection of painful endplate and disc pathology. This review explores the pathophysiology of vertebrogenic and discogenic pain as well as the impact of different imaging modalities in the diagnosis of low back pain. We hope this information can help identify patients who may benefit from personalized clinical treatment and image-guided therapies.

Magnetic Resonance Neurography of the Lumbosacral Plexus   229

Jenifer Pitman, Yenpo Lin, Ek Tsoon Tan, and Darryl Sneag

Pain and weakness in the low back, pelvis, and lower extremities are diagnostically challenging, and imaging can be an important step in the workup and management of these patients. Technical advances in magnetic resonance neurography (MRN) have significantly improved its utility for imaging the lumbosacral plexus (LSP). In this article, the authors review LSP anatomy and selected pathology examples. In addition, the authors will discuss technical considerations for MRN with specific points for the branch nerves off the plexus.

Video content accompanies this article at http://www.radiologic.theclinics.com

Spine pain is highly prevalent and costly, but evaluation with clinical features and anatomic imaging remain limited. Fat-suppressed MR imaging and molecular imaging (MI) may help identify inflammatory, lesional, and malignant causes. Numerous MI agents are available, each with advantages and disadvantages. Herein, FDG PET, prostate-specific membrane antigen (PSMA), bone radiotracers, and others are highlighted. No specific pain MI agents have been identified, but mechanisms of key agents are shown in video format, and the mechanism of PSMA as a theranostic agent is displayed. A multidisciplinary approach is needed to master this topic.

Localization of lesions in the spinal cord requires knowledge of the functional anatomy of gray and white matter tracts. Using decussation points for white matter tracts can help determine lesion level. Pathologies can affect gray and white matter tracts in distinct ways and pattern recognition can help narrow down the differential diagnosis.

Spinal cord pathologic condition often presents as a neurologic emergency where timely and accurate diagnosis is critical to expedite appropriate treatment and minimize severe morbidity and even mortality. MR imaging is the gold standard imaging technique for diagnosing patients with suspected spinal cord pathologic condition. This review will focus on the basic principles of diffusion imaging and how spinal anatomy presents technical challenges to its application. Both the promises and shortcomings of spinal diffusion imaging will then be explored in the context of several clinical spinal cord pathologies for which diffusion has been evaluated.

Significant advancements in cancer treatment have led to improved survival rates for patients, particularly in the context of spinal metastases. However, early detection and monitoring of treatment response remain crucial for optimizing patient outcomes. Although conventional imaging methods such as bone scan, PET, MR imaging, and computed tomography are commonly used for diagnosing and monitoring treatment, they present challenges in differential diagnoses and treatment response monitoring. This review article provides a comprehensive overview of the principles, applications, and practical uses of dynamic contrast-enhanced MR imaging and diffusion-weighted imaging in the assessment and monitoring of marrow-replacing disorders of the spine.

Recent advances in percutaneous minimally invasive thermal ablation and vertebral augmentation provide radiologists with important arsenal for treatment of selected patients with spinal metastases. These interventions have proven to be safe, effective, and durable in treatment of selected patients with vertebral metastases.

Attention to procedure techniques, including choice of ablation modality, vertebral augmentation technique, and thermal protection, is essential for improved patient outcomes. A detailed knowledge of such interventions and implementation of procedural safety measures will further heighten radiologists' role in the management of patients with spinal metastases.

Locating spinal cerebrospinal fluid (CSF) leaks can be a diagnostic dilemma for clinicians and radiologists, as well as frustrating for patients. Dynamic computed tomography myelography (dCTM) has emerged as a valuable tool in localizing spinal CSF leaks, aiding in accurate diagnosis, and guiding appropriate management. This article aims to provide insights into the technique, tips, tricks, and potential pitfalls associated with dCTM for spinal CSF leak localization. By understanding the nuances of this procedure, clinicians can optimize the diagnostic process and improve patient outcomes.

 Video content accompanies this article at http://www.radiologic.theclinics.com

Cerebrospinal fluid (CSF) leak can cause spontaneous intracranial hypotension (SIH) which can lead to neurologic symptoms, such as orthostatic headache. Over time, imaging techniques for detecting and localizing CSF leaks have improved. These techniques include computed tomography (CT) myelography, dynamic CT myelography, cone-beam CT, MRI, MR myelography, and digital subtraction myelography (DSM). DSM provides the highest sensitivity for identifying leak sites and has comparable radiation exposure to CT myelography. The introduction of the lateral decubitus DSM has proven invaluable in localizing leaks when other imaging tests have been inconclusive.

Spontaneous intracranial hypotension (SIH) is a treatable cause of orthostatic headaches secondary to pathologic loss of cerebrospinal fluid (CSF) from the subarachnoid space. SIH has several known pathologic causes including dural tears from disc osteophytes, leaks emanating from nerve root sleeve diverticula, and CSF-venous fistulas (CVFs). Depending on the type of leak, surgical repair or endovascular techniques may be options for definite treatment. However, epidural blood patching (EBP) remains first-line therapy for many patients due to its long track record, broad availability, and relatively lower risk profile. This review focuses on indications and techniques for the percutaneous treatment of SIH and provides an overview of post-procedural management of these patients.

Cerebrospinal fluid-venous fistula (CVF) is an important cause of spontaneous intracranial hypotension (SIH), a condition characterized by low cerebrospinal fluid (CSF)

volume and orthostatic headaches. The pathogenesis of CVF is thought to be direct connection of the spinal dura to one or more veins in the epidural space, allowing unregulated flow of CSF into the venous system. Herein, we provide a comprehensive review of the endovascular management of CVF in patients with SIH. We also focus on the various techniques and devices used in endovascular treatment, as well as the pathogenesis, diagnosis, and alternative treatment options of CVF.

Upasana Upadhyay Bharadwaj, Cynthia T. Chin, and Sharmila Majumdar

Artificial intelligence (AI), a transformative technology with unprecedented potential in medical imaging, can be applied to various spinal pathologies. AI-based approaches may improve imaging efficiency, diagnostic accuracy, and interpretation, which is essential for positive patient outcomes. This review explores AI algorithms, techniques, and applications in spine imaging, highlighting diagnostic impact and challenges with future directions for integrating AI into spine imaging workflow.

RADIOLOGIC CLINICS OF NORTH AMERICA

PROGRAM OBJECTIVE
The objective of the *Radiologic Clinics of North America* is to keep practicing radiologists and radiology residents up to date with current clinical practice in radiology by providing timely articles reviewing the state of the art in patient care.

TARGET AUDIENCE
Practicing radiologists, radiology residents, and other healthcare professionals who provide patient care utilizing radiologic findings.

LEARNING OBJECTIVES
Upon completion of this activity, participants will be able to:
1. Describe the principles of diffusion imaging and how spinal anatomy presents technical challenges to its application.
2. Discuss diagnostic dilemmas clinicians and radiologists encounter when locating spinal cerebrospinal fluid (CSF) leaks.
3. Recognize that significant advancements in cancer treatment have led to improved patient survival rates, particularly in spinal and vertebral metastases.

ACCREDITATION
The Elsevier Office of Continuing Medical Education (EOCME) is accredited by the Accreditation Council for Continuing Medical Education (ACCME) to provide continuing medical education for physicians.

The EOCME designates this journal-based CME activity for a maximum of 13 *AMA PRA Category 1 Credit*(s)™. Physicians should claim only the credit commensurate with the extent of their participation in the activity.

All other healthcare professionals requesting continuing education credit for this enduring material will be issued a certificate of participation.

DISCLOSURE OF CONFLICTS OF INTEREST
The EOCME assesses conflict of interest with its instructors, faculty, planners, and other individuals who are in a position to control the content of CME activities. All relevant conflicts of interest that are identified are thoroughly vetted by EOCME for fair balance, scientific objectivity, and patient care recommendations. EOCME is committed to providing its learners with CME activities that promote improvements or quality in healthcare and not a specific proprietary business or a commercial interest.

The planning committee, staff, authors, and editors listed below have identified no financial relationships or relationships to products or devices they or their spouse/life partner have with commercial interest related to the content of this CME activity:
Frederik Abel, MD; Franziska Altorfer, MD; Timothy J. Amrhein, MD; Upasana Upadhyay Bharadwaj, MD; Gokce B. Belge Bilgin, MD; Cem Bilgin, MD; Stephen M. Broski, MD; J. Levi Chazen, MD; Cynthia T. Chin, MD; Jeremy K. Cutsforth-Gregory, MD; William P. Dillon, MD; Javier Galvan, MD, MPH; Wende Gibbs, MD, MA; Allison Grayev, MD; Jessica L. Houk, MD; Jack W. Jennings, MD, PhD; Sasan Karimi, MD; Hassan Kobeissi; Peter G. Kranz, MD; Kothainayaki Kulanthaivelu, BCA, MBA; Vance T. Lehman, MD; Eric Lis, MD; Michelle Littlejohn; Ajay Madhavan, MD; Sharmila Majumdar, PhD; Timothy Maus, MD; Marcel Maya, MD; Atakan Orscelik, MD; Kyung K. Peck, PhD; Varun Rohatgi; Atin Saha, MD, MS; Wouter Schievink, MD; Yigit Can Senol, MD; Vinil Shah, MD; Jason F. Talbott, MD, PhD; Christin A. Tiegs-Heiden, MD; Anderanik Tomasian, MD; Allen Q. Ye, MD, PhD; Onur Yildirim, MD

The planning committee, staff, authors, and editors listed below have identified financial relationships or relationships to products or devices they or their spouse/life partner have with commercial interest related to the content of this CME activity:
Waleed Brinjikji, MD: Ownership: MIVI Neurovascular, Piraeus Medical, Sonoris Medical; Royalties Recipient: Balloon Guide Catheter Technology, Medtronic; Consultant: Asahi, Balt, Cerenovus, Imperative Care, Medtronic, Stryker, MicroVention, MIVI Neurovascular; Executive Role: Marblehead Medical LLC, MIVI Neurovascular, Piraeus Medical;

David F. Kallmes, MD: Ownershipn Interest: Conway Medical, Marblehead Medical, Piraeus Medical; Researcher: Balt, Insera Therapeutics, Medtronic, MicroVention; Advisor: Vesalio; Royalty Recipient: Medtronic

Yenpo Lin, MD: Research Support: GE HealthCare, Siemens

Jenifer Pitman, MD: Research Support: GE HealthCare, Siemens

Darryl Sneag, MD: Research Support: GE HealthCare, Siemens

Ek Tsoon Tan, PhD: Research Support: GE HealthCare, Siemens

UNAPPROVED/OFF-LABEL USE DISCLOSURE
The EOCME requires CME faculty to disclose to the participants:
1. When products or procedures being discussed are off-label, unlabelled, experimental, and/or investigational (not US Food and Drug Administration [FDA] approved); and
2. Any limitations on the information presented, such as data that are preliminary or that represent ongoing research, interim analyses, and/or unsupported opinions. Faculty may discuss information about pharmaceutical agents that is outside of

FDA-approved labelling. This information is intended solely for CME and is not intended to promote off-label use of these medications. If you have any questions, contact the medical affairs department of the manufacturer for the most recent prescribing information.

TO ENROLL
To enroll in the *Radiologic Clinics of North America* Continuing Medical Education program, call customer service at 1-800-654-2452 or sign up online at http://www.theclinics.com/home/cme. The CME program is available to subscribers for an additional annual fee of USD 340.00.

METHOD OF PARTICIPATION
In order to claim credit, participants must complete the following:
1. Complete enrolment as indicated above.
2. Read the activity.
3. Complete the CME Test and Evaluation. Participants must achieve a score of 70% on the test. All CME Tests and Evaluations must be completed online.

CME INQUIRIES/SPECIAL NEEDS
For all CME inquiries or special needs, please contact elsevierCME@elsevier.com.

Preface
Spine Imaging and Intervention

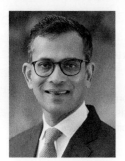

Vinil Shah, MD
Editor

I am honored to present this *Radiologic Clinics of North America* issue on Spine Imaging and Intervention. Disorders of the spine are common, and a leading cause of physician and emergency room visits worldwide. Imaging plays a crucial role in the evaluation and management of spinal disorders and for planning percutaneous intervention.

This issue of *Radiologic Clinics of North America* provides an up-to-date and comprehensive review of spinal and peripheral nerve imaging as well as minimally invasive image-guided spinal intervention. Each article has been written by a leading expert in the field, providing a unique and authoritative perspective on the topic covered. The text is richly illustrated with high-quality images, providing readers with a clear understanding of the relevant imaging findings and their clinical implications.

The articles cover practical and state-of-the-art applications of spinal diagnostic imaging relevant for the practicing radiologist. These topics include relevant spinal anatomy and techniques for safe and effective image-guided epidural access, an overview of the functional anatomy of the spinal cord, and technical and practical considerations for performing and interpreting MR Neurography, with a focus on the Lumbosacral Plexus. Advanced spinal imaging topics that are increasingly used in clinical practice are also covered, including diffusion-weighted imaging (DWI) of the spinal cord, and DWI and perfusion imaging of marrow replacing disorders of the spine. Up-to-date anatomic and molecular imaging of spinal pain generators, including discogenic and vertebrogenic pain, is also an important focus of this issue and will benefit both the practicing diagnostic radiologist and spine interventionalist.

This issue also covers state-of-the-art techniques for diagnosing, percutaneously treating, and managing patients with spinal cerebrospinal fluid (CSF) leaks, an increasingly important topic for the practicing radiologist to be aware of. These include techniques for effective and safe performance of dynamic CT Myelography, Digital Subtraction Myelography, and Endovascular Embolization of CSF Venous Fistulas. Increasingly, spine interventional radiologists have an important role to play in

Radiol Clin N Am 62 (2024) xv–xvi
https://doi.org/10.1016/j.rcl.2023.11.001
0033-8389/24/© 2023 Published by Elsevier Inc.

diagnosis and treatment of spinal tumors. To that end, this issue also addresses relevant considerations for percutaneous spinal tumor ablation. Finally, this issue also addresses practical applications of Artificial Intelligence in Spinal Imaging, a topic of increasing interest and relevance to the imaging community.

This issue is therefore intended for practicing radiologists, radiology trainees, and other health care professionals involved in the care of patients with spinal disorders. It provides essential information for the effective imaging evaluation and treatment of these patients and will be a valuable resource to diagnostic and spine interventional radiologists.

I extend my sincere gratitude to the authors, reviewers, and editorial staff, who have diligently contributed to developing this issue. I invite you to immerse yourself in the wealth of knowledge contained within these pages.

DISCLOSURE

No conflicts of interest. No relevant financial disclosures.

Vinil Shah, MD
Department of Radiology &
Biomedical Imaging
Neuroradiology
University of California at San Francisco
505 Parnassus Avenue #M-391
San Francisco, CA 94143, USA

E-mail address:
vinil.shah@ucsf.edu

The Anatomy, Technique, Safety, and Efficacy of Image-Guided Epidural Access

Timothy Maus, MD*

KEYWORDS

• Epidural steroid injection • Transforaminal • Interlaminar • Radicular pain

KEY POINTS

- The spine interventionalist must thoroughly understand spinal anatomy, and its representation on advanced imaging and planar fluoroscopy, for safe and efficacious epidural access.
- Transforaminal epidural steroid injections have demonstrable efficacy in treatment of radicular pain syndromes.
- Interlaminar epidural steroid injections have limited evidence of efficacy for radicular pain.
- Epidural steroid injections are not indicated for axial pain syndromes; there is minimal evidence for treatment of neurogenic intermittent claudication or cervical spondylotic myelopathy.
- Epidural access is safe when performed according to established practice guidelines.

INTRODUCTION

Radicular pain, a common clinical challenge, is the product of both neural compression and inflammatory response; there is face validity for the epidural administration of an anti-inflammatory agent.[1] This is particularly relevant for disc herniations whose natural history is resolution.[2] There is no mechanism, nor clinical evidence, whereby epidural administration of a corticosteroid may impact anterior or posterior column axial pain. There is scant evidence to support the use of epidural steroids for neurogenic intermittent claudication or cervical spondylotic myelopathy.[3,4] This discussion will address image-guided epidural access in the treatment of radicular pain. As thoracic radicular pain is uncommon, the discussion will be limited to the lumbar and cervical regions.

ANATOMY

The target epidural space, containing fat, venous structures, and traversing neural elements, is much smaller in the cervical than lumbar segments (Fig. 1). The distribution of epidural fat, where lipophilic medications are deposited and redistribute,

determines the access route. There is minimal or no dorsal epidural fat above C6–7.[5] The cervical ligamentum flavum, immediately dorsal to the epidural space, is frequently discontinuous in the midline, especially at C7–T1.[6] There is minimal cervical intraforaminal fat, and access to the neural foramen is challenged by surrounding vulnerable structures: the exiting nerve and contiguous plexus, vertebral artery, and carotid sheath.

The lumbar spine exhibits a prominent dorsal triangle of fat deep to the ligamentum flavum, maximal at L3–4. The lumbar dorsal epidural fat is discontinuous; recent investigations described fibrous tissue and veins separating the dorsal fat pads.[7] The midline lumbar dorsal fat thins considerably at L5 and S1 where the dura is often in contact with the ligamentum flavum. The lateral epidural compartment, containing the segmental nerve, vessels, and fat, is contiguous with the neural foramen. In the lumbar spine, there is no continuity of dorsolateral epidural fat with the foramen above L5; at the L5–S1 disc space, there is laterally situated fat inviting a parasagittal interlaminar access[7] (see Fig. 1). Fat fills the lower lumbar intervertebral foramen below the dorsal root ganglion–ventral root

Mayo Clinic, Rochester, MN, USA
* 588 Kaiola Street, Kihei, Hawaii 96753.
E-mail address: timpmaus@icloud.com

Radiol Clin N Am 62 (2024) 199–215
https://doi.org/10.1016/j.rcl.2023.09.006

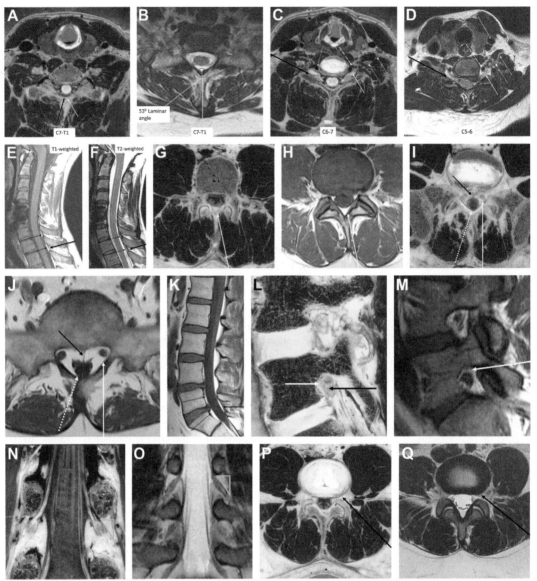

Fig. 1. Epidural anatomy/imaging. The cervical dorsal epidural space is 1 to 2 mm in depth as seen on the anatomic specimen (*black arrow, A*), just deep to the ligamentum flavum (*white arrow, A*). On fast spine echo (FSE) T2-weighted images, the ligamentum flavum is hypointense but may be dehiscent in the midline (*red circle, B*). The laminar angle is typically 50° to 55°; this identifies the angle of the contralateral oblique fluoroscopic view. The cervical foraminal and ventral epidural space is filled with venous channels (*dotted blue arrows, C*). Transforaminal access (*black arrows, C, D*) must avoid multiple vulnerable structures: vertebral artery (*dashed arrow*), plexus (*dotted arrows*, exiting nerve (*white arrow*), carotid artery (*red arrow*), and internal jugular vein (*blue arrow*). On sagittal imaging, dorsal epidural fat is seldom visible above C6–7 (*dotted arrows, E, F*). The ligamentum flavum is a hypointense band (*solid arrow, E, F*). The lumbar dorsal epidural space is more robust; fat is localized to a midline triangle L1–4 (*G, H*). Access via the ligamentum flavum (*arrows, G, H*) is paramedian. At L5, the thecal sac is contiguous with the ligamentum flavum in the midline (*dotted arrows, I, J*), but a lateral parasagittal approach is available (*solid arrows, I, J*). The midline sagittal T1-weighted image (*K*) illustrates the minimal dorsal epidural space in the midline at L5 (*black arrow*) and the more prominent ventral epidural space at L5 and S1 (*dotted arrow*). The ventral epidural space is divided by Hofmann ligaments (*black arrow, I, J*). The lumbar foramen contains the dorsal root ganglion (*black arrow, L*) and the ventral root (*white arrow, L*). These are inseparable on MR imaging. The supraneural transforaminal trajectory is identified in (*arrow, M*). In the coronal plane, the supraneural trajectory will place the needle superior and lateral to the exiting nerve (*green triangles, N, O*). An infraneural approach at the disc level interposes the needle between the exiting nerve and the superior articular process (*arrows, P, Q*). (Anatomic images A, C, G, I, P *modified from* the National Library of Medicine, Visible Human Project. Remainder of images modified from the forthcoming International Pain & Spine Intervention Society Technical Manual and Atlas, used with permission. Anatomic images B, D-F, H, J-O, Q Reproduced with permission from the International Pain and Spine Intervention Society (IPSIS).)

complex; there is also intraforaminal fat lateral to the exiting nerve as it moves caudally and anteriorly to leave the foramen. The ventral epidural space contains a robust venous plexus throughout the spine communicating with the centrally situated basivertebral vein. The ventral compartment is bisected longitudinally by Hofmann ligaments, which are variably fenestrated. Ventral epidural fat is minimal in the cervical and upper lumbar regions, becoming quite prominent at L4–S1.

GENERAL PROCEDURAL CONSIDERATIONS
Targeting: Diagnostic Procedures

If a symptom (pain, paresthesia) is mediated by a unique spinal nerve, anesthetizing that nerve should temporarily relieve the symptom; this is a selective nerve block. To maintain face validity, the block should occur with low-volume, high-concentration anesthetics to insure no other structures are anesthetized, confirmed by contrast media injection.[8] If anesthetic reaches the central epidural space or the extraforaminal plexus, specificity will be lost. This obligates a transforaminal (TF) approach, with needle placement more laterally and peripherally than for a therapeutic procedure, where central ventral epidural flow is necessary for efficacy.[9,10] Anesthetic volumes should be restricted to 0.2 to 0.3 cc of 2% to 4% lidocaine.[11] Segmental diagnostic information cannot be inferred from a therapeutic TF injection; these are distinct procedures. There is strong evidence that well-performed lumbar selective nerve blocks can improve identification of symptomatic segments, with moderate evidence of improved outcomes in decompression procedures.[12] There is less robust but moderate evidence for outcomes improvement in cervical decompressions.

Targeting: Therapeutic Procedures

The target for therapeutic epidural procedures in the radicular pain patient is the contact zone between the disc herniation (or fixed lesion, eg, synovial cyst, osteophyte) and neural tissue. Clinical effectiveness is associated with medication delivery to this contact zone, the dorsal root ganglion, and the preganglionic nerve in the ventral epidural space.[10,13] Purely peripheral flow to the ventral ramus will not be effective. The dorsal epidural space is insensate and only serves as a conduit to ventral flow in interlaminar access.

Guidance Modality

Interventional pain procedures have historically been performed with planar fluoroscopic guidance, as a widely available, cost/radiation-dose efficient

and learnable tool. Contrast media flow patterns can be observed in real time. Virtually all the high-quality evidence validating epidural procedures uses fluoroscopic guidance. Fluoroscopy is challenged, however, as the targets of injection (neural tissue) and potential vulnerable structures (vasculature, neural tissue, and thecal sac) are unseen and must be inferred by relationship to bony landmarks. Needle localization requires careful correlation of orthogonal planar views. The skill set of correlation of pre-procedural cross-sectional imaging with intraprocedural planar fluoroscopic observation must be mastered and is often underappreciated.

CT guidance has primarily been used within the radiologic community. Despite its inherent advantages of direct visualization of the target and vulnerable tissues, evidence supporting safety and efficacy of CT-guided epidural procedures is limited.[14] CT is more radiation intensive than fluoroscopy and has historically been ineffective in depicting contrast media flow in real time to detect vascularity (or other off-target flow). Recent studies with multislice pulsed CT fluoroscopy (CTF) have, however, demonstrated that epidural procedures can be performed with comparable radiation doses and similar vascular detection rates to conventional fluoroscopy.[15] Dose reduction techniques include limiting z-axis coverage of (or eliminating) planning scans and reducing tube current during needle placement before contrast injection.[16,17] Multislice acquisition during and immediately following contrast media injection (double-tap technique) can effectively detect vascular flow and document epidural flow.[15,18] CTF guidance has clinical efficacy equal to or greater than fluoroscopic guidance in limited studies.[19]

Ultrasound has the potential advantage of real-time guidance without ionizing radiation, allowing avoidance of contact with vascular and neural structures. It has been primarily used in the cervical spine where tissue depth is limited. Ultrasound is challenged by uncertainty of segment identification and accurate needle positioning.[20] It is blind within the confines of the bony foramen and central canal and cannot detect intraforaminal vascular uptake nor document epidural spread. It may have value as a hybrid guidance technique in combination with fluoroscopy.[20]

Enumeration

Variation in spinal enumeration is potentially confounding to segment correct epidural access. An altered number or distribution of thoracolumbar vertebrae is present in 11% to 20% of patients.[21] Transitional lumbosacral anatomy, present in 4% to 30% of patients, is strongly associated with an anomalous number of vertebrae. Fortunately, the cervical spine is homologous, and counting can occur from the cervicothoracic junction, where the first up-sloped transverse process identifies T1; this should be done routinely. It is the responsibility of the interventionalist to correctly correlate the lesion identified on cross-sectional imaging with the fluoroscopic access target. This obligates evaluation of pre-procedure imaging (PPI).

Therapeutic Injectate

Corticosteroids are the current class of anti-inflammatory agents used (off-label) for epidural injection. There have been numerous case reports of catastrophic neurologic complications, primarily cord infarcts, from TF epidural corticosteroid injections. Cervical cord infarcts have implicated direct vertebral artery injury or injection of particulate steroid formulations into the vertebral artery or reinforcing arteries traversing the neural foramen and communicating with the anterior spinal artery. In the low thoracic and lumbar region, inadvertent injection of particulate steroids into the great anterior radiculo-medullary artery is the likely proximate cause. The underlying pathophysiology of vascular insult to the cord was postulated to be embolization of steroid particles,[22,23] although the evidence was indirect. More recent, direct evidence suggests that particulate steroids deform red cell membranes resulting in red cell aggregation and vascular occlusion.[24] Multiple studies identify the non-particulate steroid dexamethasone (not credibly implicated in cord infarcts) as non-inferior or equivalent to particulate steroids in efficacy.[25-27] Practice guidelines suggest only dexamethasone be used in cervical transforaminal epidural steroid injections (TFESIs), and it should be the initial agent for lumbar TFESI.[28] There are no arterial communications between the dorsal epidural space and the neuroaxis; hence, particulate steroid may be used for interlaminar epidural steroid injections (ILESIs).

Although neurologic complications are rare, systemic side effects of corticosteroids are ubiquitous, to include hypothalamic–pituitary axis (HPA) suppression, immunosuppression, altered glucose metabolism, and diminished bone density (Benzon H.T., Maus T., Mina M., et al., A Multispecialty Multisociety Practice Guideline on the Safety of Steroid Injections Part I: Neuraxial Injections and Associated Topics). HPA suppression from epidural injections likely lasts 1 to 3 weeks; cumulative methylprednisolone (MP) equivalent doses of greater than 200 mg annually or greater than 300 mg more than 3 years significantly diminishes done density in postmenopausal women. The minimum effective steroid dose should be used; doses above 40 mg MP

equivalent (7.5–10 mg dexamethasone) are best avoided. Epidural corticosteroids should not be administered in a series for the same pain episode. Repeat injections are considered based on the response to a prior injection, either a substantial beneficial response that has since waned or an early repeat injection (2 weeks from initial injection) for a positive but incomplete response.[29] As steroid side effects are cumulative, ideally the interventionalist should quantify the patient's steroid consumption by all routes to identify high-risk patients. There is conflicting evidence regarding an increased infection risk post-lumbar decompression/fusion following epidural steroid injections; some investigators suggest delaying surgery by greater than 1 month after an injection.[30,31]

INTERLAMINAR ACCESS (INTERLAMINAR EPIDURAL STEROID INJECTION)

The dorsal epidural space may be accessed via an interlaminar approach with the intention of spread of therapeutic injectate to the lateral and ventral epidural compartments where nociception occurs. There is no therapeutic benefit to medication delivery to the dorsal epidural space itself; interlaminar access has no diagnostic role as injectate distribution will not be side or segment specific. A primary flaw in ILESI is that distribution to the ventral epidural compartment cannot be controlled nor guaranteed. Historically, ILESIs have been performed without image guidance using loss of resistance (LOR) technique. This relies on advancing a Touhy type needle with a side-facing bevel (which will not core tissue) in a midline or immediate paramedian location through the interspinous ligament to engage the dense ligamentum flavum. The needle is pressurized and advanced slowly through the ligamentum flavum until an LOR is felt, suggesting entry into the low pressure dorsal epidural space. Even in experienced hands, this technique fails to reach the epidural space in 25% of cases; injection may also be intradural or intravascular.[32] Even when image guidance is used in lumbar ILESI, injected contrast media reaches the target ventral epidural space in only 36% to 47% of procedures.[33,34]

Technique: Cervical Interlaminar Epidural Steroid Injection

ILESI may be performed with fluoroscopic or CTF guidance (Fig. 2). There is greater face validity for cervical (vs lumbar) ILESI in that the small volume of the cervical dorsal epidural space might promote flow to the desired ventral epidural compartment. This was suggested by earlier fluoroscopic studies. However, in a recent CT study using 5 cc of injectate, spread to the ventral epidural

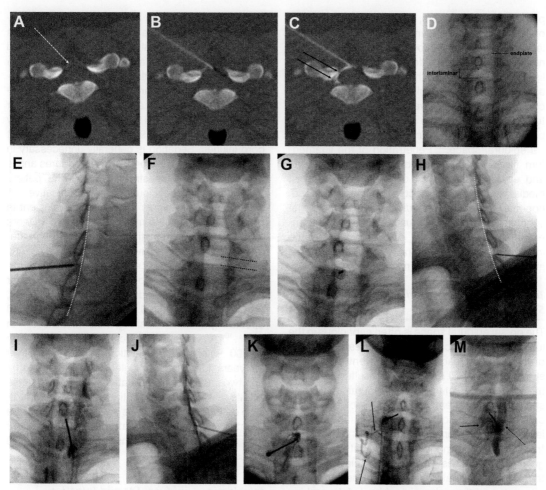

Fig. 2. CTF guidance for a C7-T1 ILESI (*A–C*). Note the relatively dense ligamentum flavum in (*A, dotted arrow*). A 22 G Touhy needle was used to access the dorsal epidural space (*B*). Note a vector of approach was constructed that did not intersect the cord. After loss of resistance, dilute contrast medium injection (0.2 cc) shows unilateral flow into the foramen (*C, arrows*). In (*D*), fluoroscopic guidance identifies the interlaminar space. A contralateral oblique (CLO) image (*E*) is parallel to the lamina (usually 50°–55°); the ventral interlaminar line (*dotted line, E*) connects the base of the lamina. The ligamentum flavum is at or minimally deep to this landmark. A cervical ILESI under fluoroscopic guidance identifies the interlaminar space (*F*) in slight ipsilateral obliquity; a Touhy needle is advance to the superior edge of the lamina (*G*), and the epidural space in entered in the CLO position (*H*) with loss of resistance. Contrast medium injection under live fluoro in AP and CLO planes (*I, J*) shows epidural flow dominant to the right. Note vacuolization—contrast medium flowing about fat globules—on the AP view, a positive marker of epidural distribution. The operator must recognize aberrant flow patterns. In (*K*), flow is extraspinal, in the multifidus muscle adjacent to the spinous process; this would be obvious on a CLO or lateral view. Extensive venous flow is seen in (*L*). A mixed pattern is apparent in (*M*); flow is partially epidural as marked by vacuolization (*solid arrow*), but partially intradural (central dural zone, *dotted arrow*). The procedure should be aborted. (*Reproduced with permission from* the International Pain and Spine Intervention Society (IPSIS).)

space occurred in only 65% of cases; there was longitudinal distribution in the ventral epidural space over only 1.6 ($\pm$ 1.6) segments.[18] Foraminal flow was favored by ipsilateral injection. Inspection of PPI to assure adequate dorsal epidural space is mandatory.[28] This is best done on T1-weighted sagittal images. Intervention should not be attempted at any level where there is significant

central canal compromise. Dorsal epidural fat is seldom identified above the C6–7 level; consensus practice guidelines suggest access at the C7–T1 level, but not above C6–7.[28] The practitioner must also be aware that the ligamentum flavum may be not be fused in the midline; this is unfortunately most prevalent at C7–T1, identified in 71% of subjects in a recent study.[6] This argues for paramedian, not midline, access, and assessment on PPI. Fluoroscopic image guidance is challenged by the inability to clearly visualize the spinolaminar line, which identifies the depth of the ligamentum flavum, on the lateral view. Contralateral oblique (CLO) imaging at approximately 50° can dramatically improve the practitioners ability to ascertain safe needle depth as it engages and penetrates the ligamentum flavum to enter the dorsal epidural space.[35] Penetration of the ligamentum flavum is identified by the LOR technique and epidural distribution confirmed by contrast media injection, with documentation of spread, hopefully to the ventral epidural space at the target segment, by imaging in multiple planes. Local anesthetics delivered to the epidural space by the interlaminar route serve no diagnostic purpose and should be avoided or minimized.

Technique: Lumbar Interlaminar Epidural Steroid Injection

The dorsal epidural space is often capacious in the lumbar region, which may require greater volumes of injectate to reach the target ventral epidural space (Fig. 3). PPI should be consulted to determine the location of the target epidural fat. Access should not be attempted at levels of significant central canal stenosis; consider a sub-adjacent level. At L1–L4, dorsal epidural fat is present in a triangle centered on the midline; far lateral parasagittal access raises concern for violation of the thecal sac. L5 anatomy is unique; here, there is often no midline dorsal epidural fat, making midline access fraught, whereas there is abundant lateral epidural fat, inviting a far lateral parasagittal access. This is a useful strategy for radicular pain due to L5 foraminal stenosis. The depth of needle penetration may be determined on a true lateral fluoroscopic view in the lumbar region, with the ligamentum flavum at and just deep to the spinolaminar line. If body habitus degrades the lateral view, a 45° CLO view provides depth information.[36] Epidural access is confirmed with LOR, documented in multiple planes with contrast media injection, and therapeutic injectate is delivered.

Interlaminar Epidural Steroid Injection: Safety

Epidural injections via an interlaminar approach are safe procedures. Adverse events may be categorized as major (neurologic deficit, intraspinal hemorrhage, infection) or minor (vasovagal reaction, dural puncture, acute systemic steroid effects, contrast reactions). Major adverse events have been limited to case reports. In an analysis of closed claims cases addressing cervical injuries, direct needle trauma to the cord (interlaminar injections)

was twice as common as cord infarcts (TF injections), emphasizing the need to carefully assess needle depth.[37] Epidural hematomas were reported in 8% of cord injury cases, as opposed to 53% caused by direct needle trauma. Epidural hematomas, although rare, are more commonly associated with interlaminar access. Deep sedation or general anesthesia was used in 67% of cord injury procedures but only 19% of procedures without cord injuries. Sedation is generally unnecessary in this and most interventional pain procedures and is a risk factor for catastrophic injury; the patient must always be conscious and communicative.[28]

Major adverse events are rare or nonexistent in prospective series. No major adverse events were recorded in a multi-institutional cohort of greater than 1500 patients receiving interlaminar injections performed in accordance with International Pain & Spine Intervention Society guidelines. Minor adverse events included dural punctures in 0.2%, vasovagal reactions in 0.5%, and systemic steroid effects (transient flushing, sleeplessness) in 2.6%.[38] A single-center review of greater than 18,000 interlaminar injections performed over 12 years identified a single epidural hematoma and two infectious complications as major adverse events.[39] A large retrospective evaluation of Medicare data revealed only nine serious spinal adverse events, all intraspinal hematomas, among greater than 832,000 interlaminar injections, a rate of 10.8 cases per million.[40]

Interlaminar Epidural Steroid Injection: Efficacy

Continuing the precedent of labor and delivery anesthesia, interlaminar epidural corticosteroid injections are performed without image guidance using the LOR technique despite the shortcomings noted above. A systematic review of nonimage-guided interlaminar injections (9 explanatory, 9 pragmatic, and 21 observational trials) found no evidence supporting benefit beyond 3 to 6 weeks in treatment of radicular pain. The evidence for short-term benefit was conflicting and low quality. The investigators concluded unguided interlaminar injections have no place in contemporary medical practice beyond rare settings where fluoroscopy is not available.[41] An explanatory trial of three unguided interlaminar injections versus placebo (saline interspinous ligament injection) in treatment of radicular pain (n = 228) found only transient benefit in pain and function at 3 weeks. There was no pain or function benefit from 6 to 52 weeks, no surgical sparing, and no benefit for three injections over a single injection.[42] Another explanatory trial treated radicular pain with one

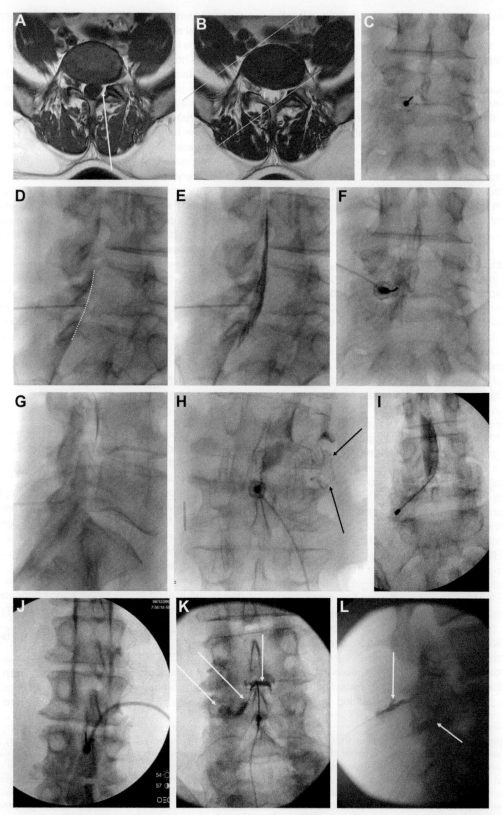

Fig. 3. Left L5 radicular pain, L5 foraminal narrowing. T1- and T2-weighted images at L5 (*A*, *B*) with the expected needle trajectory shown in (*A*). In (*B*), the gold lines indicate the x-ray beam trajectory for the contralateral

to three unguided ILESIs versus epidural saline ($n = 158$). There was improvement in mean leg pain scores in the epidural steroid group at 6 weeks, but not at 12 weeks, with no improvement in secondary outcomes; there was no improvement in categorical outcomes of global improvement at any time point.[43] The FDA Safe Use Initiative recommends that multi-planar image guidance be used for all epidural injections.[28]

Image-guided interlaminar injections provide documentation of epidural medication delivery, but the interventionalist cannot control injectate distribution in its laterality or its flow to the neural foramen and/or ventral epidural space where nociception occurs. Medication can be observed to reach the ventral epidural space in only about one-third to one-half of lumbar cases and in about two-thirds of cervical cases.[18,33,34] A systematic review ($n = 71$ trials) of lumbar interlaminar epidural injections found no explanatory trials; pragmatic trials were of low quality with evidence comparable to observational studies. There was no effectiveness for axial pain of any etiology. Evidence supported only short-term benefit for pain, but not function, in lumbar disc herniation patients.[44] A pragmatic trial of epidural steroid plus local anesthetic versus anesthetic alone ($n = 120$, radicular pain) showed improvement in both groups out to 12 months. There was no difference between the groups at 3 and 12 months; the 6-month data favored the steroid group. The study was confounded in that it allowed multiple injections, and the temporal relationship of the anesthetic injections and the assessments was not reported.[45] A small observational trial ($n = 21$, radicular pain) showed that less than one-third of patients achieved complete pain relief at 3 months, whereas 38% achieved 50% relief.[46]

Midline epidural injections, especially in the lumbar region, may leave much of the injectate in the dorsal fat pad. Lateral parasagittal injections are more likely to provide unilateral flow that reaches the neural foramen and/or ventral epidural space. Four controlled trials provide evidence that lateral parasagittal interlaminar injections are superior to placebo, superior to midline injections, and approach the efficacy of TF injections in treatment of unilateral radicular pain.[47–50] Parasagittal ILESIs have particular utility in the setting of foraminal stenosis, where TFESI may not achieve central and ventral epidural distribution.

Evidence for efficacy of cervical interlaminar injections is not robust. A systematic review of cervical interlaminar injections identified only three controlled trials and five observational studies. There was evidence of positive short-term benefit (<6 months) in the three controlled trials and longer term benefit in two trials; the observational studies were generally positive but with variability in study quality.[51] A pragmatic study of interlaminar delivery of steroids plus local anesthetic versus anesthetic alone ($n = 120$, nature of pain not defined) showed significant, similar benefit for both groups but was confounded by multiple injections and no reporting of the temporal relationship between injection and assessment.[52] A subsequent systematic review by the same investigator encompassed four self-authored pragmatic studies revealing similar results.[53] Finally, a review article concluded that cervical ILESIs are effective in short-term treatment of radicular pain, but the evidence base is lacking in true placebo-controlled trials.[54]

TRANSFORAMINAL ACCESS (TRANSFORAMINAL EPIDURAL STEROID INJECTION)

TF epidural injections are by definition image-guided, providing target specificity by delivering injectate directly to the neural foramen and subsequently to the lateral recess and the ventral epidural space. Intraforaminal needle placement implies proximity to vulnerable structures: the exiting nerve, vascular structures supplying the neuroaxis (vertebral and reinforcing arteries in the cervical spine, artery of Adamkiewicz in the lumbar spine), the lumbar disc, and the cervical/brachial plexus. This demands technique that is strategically chosen to deliver medication to the target space dependent on the anatomy of the index and adjacent foramina.

Technique: Cervical Transforaminal Epidural Steroid Injection

The cervical neural foramen is accessed from an anterolateral vector under fluoroscopic or CTF guidance in a supine patient; access is aided by

oblique view, parallel to the lamina. In (C), the Tuohy needle passes under the left L5 lamina. In the CLO view (D), the needle is at the expected level of the ligamentum flavum (ventral interlaminar line, dotted). After loss of resistance, contrast injection (E) shows epidural flow against the ligamentum flavum, which remains largely unilateral (F). On the lateral view (G) after delivery of steroid, only a small amount of contrast is seen in the ventral epidural space. The operator must be able to recognize aberrant, non-epidural flow such as venous uptake (H, *arrows*), intradural (central dural zone, *I*), intradural (boundary cell layer, *J*), or in the space of Okada (and interspinous ligament, facet joints, *arrows* in K, L). (*Reproduced with permission from* the International Pain and Spine Intervention Society (IPSIS).)

contralateral head rotation (**Fig. 4**). Although the path length for needle placement is short, the trajectory must avoid the carotid sheath, vertebral artery, exiting nerve, and its extension into the cervical or brachial plexus immediately posterior to the anterior scalene muscle. Evaluation of cross-sectional PPI is mandatory; in one series, the vertebral artery covered or nearly completely covered stenotic neural foramina in 65% of cases.[55] Nearly 40% of typical fluoroscopically constructed trajectories would have intersected the vertebral artery.[55] Some interventions are simply unwise. In addition to the vertebral artery, there may be reinforcing arteries traversing the foramen to the anterior spinal artery arising from deep and ascending cervical arteries; these will only be detected with contrast media injection before therapeutic injectate.[56] The foramen should be targeted at its inferior extent; the superior recess of the facet joint may lie in the posterior, superior foramen.

A small caliber needle (25–27 gauge) is directed parallel to the anterior surface of the superior articular process (SAP) in the inferior foramen. The anterior SAP often flattens toward the coronal plane, yielding a funnel-shaped foramen, especially at C6–7. Although this can be observed directly with CTF, at fluoroscopy this requires rotating into greater obliquity, beyond that of the lamina. Direct measurement of the SAP angle relative to true anteror-posterior (AP) on PPI forearms the fluoroscopic interventionalist and may prevent transgression of vulnerable structures.[57] The needle is advanced to a position half way across the articular pillar on an AP fluoroscopic view or axial CTF. Contrast media injection under real-time fluoroscopic observation or using the double-tap technique under CTF is necessary to exclude vascular uptake (arterial or venous) and document adequate central epidural distribution.[15] Documentary images in multiple planes should be included in the medical record. Test doses of local anesthetics are of uncertain value in the era of non-particulate steroid use.[58] Only dexamethasone should be used as a therapeutic injectate.[28]

Technique: Lumbar Transforaminal Epidural Steroid Injection

In the lumbar region, non-particulate steroids are recommended for initial injection; if the patient does not respond to an on-target injection or has a limited response, particulate steroids may be considered.[28] The lumbar neural foramen may be approached via supraneural, retroneural, or infraneural trajectories.

In the classic fluoroscopic supraneural approach (**Fig. 5**), a 10 to 15° ipsilateral oblique approach is used to place a 25 to 27 gauge needle under the margin of the pars interarticularis and subsequently along the inferior pedicle margin into the anterior foramen, with a lateral view endpoint just short of the junction of the pedicle and vertebra. The needle should not progress medial to the midpoint of the pedicle on a frontal view to minimize the risk of dural sleeve transgression. The needle thus lies above and lateral to the exiting nerve. Contrast injection typically reveals central epidural flow along the medial pedicle, progressing to the ventral epidural space if the lateral recess is patent. A 2.8 cc of injectate will reach the superior margin of the superjacent disc in 95% of cases.[59] This approach was derived to allow safe passage of the needle past the exiting nerve, but places it in proximity to a potential radiculomedullary artery, which transverses the foramen in its anterior-superior quadrant in 96% of subjects.[60]

A retroneural approach may be necessary when the exiting nerve is displaced superiorly or posteriorly into the path of a supraneural trajectory. Using a slight ipsilateral obliquity as above, the needle is placed into the mid or upper foramen but left in the posterior third of the foramen on a lateral view, posterior to the exiting nerve. This can be directly observed with CTF guidance. There are no data describing typical flow patterns, but this investigators' observation suggests a pattern similar to a supraneural approach if the needle is in close proximity to the nerve.

An infraneural trajectory can use more obliquity and bring the needle more medially, without the risk of violating the dural sleeve (see **Fig. 5**). Accessing the inferior foramen at the disc level reduces or eliminates the risk of encountering a radiculomedullary artery.[60,61] This trajectory is suggested if particulate steroids are used. Infraneural or retroneural approaches are necessary in intraforaminal extrusions, where the exiting nerve is displaced into a horizontal course.[62]

Using fluoroscopy, an obliquity determined by cross-sectional PPI is obtained, and the needle is advanced along the lateral margin of the SAP at the disc level; depth is assessed with periodic lateral imaging. The needle may approach, but not penetrate the disc. The trajectory can be directly visualized in the axial plane with CTF guidance. Contrast flow is often directly into the ventral epidural space, with less cephalad flow than a supraneural approach. At L4, 1 cc on contrast will cover the exiting L4 nerve 90% of the time and the L4 and L5 nerves 10%. At L5, the flow is more caudal, covering L5 alone 60%, L5 and S1 30%, and S1 alone 10%.[63]

The approach to the S1 dorsal foramen can be directly visualized in the axial plane with CTF, and

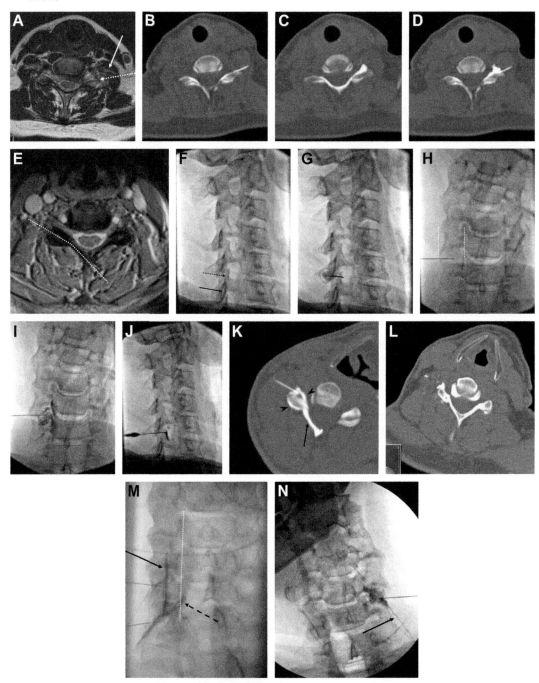

Fig. 4. A left C6–7 disc herniation (*A*) requires a nearly coronal plane trajectory (*dotted arrow*) to avoid the plexus (*solid arrow*). This is accomplished under CTF guidance (*B–D*) with central flow at the posterior aspect of the C7 nerve. In (*E*), mild right sided foraminal narrowing is causing radicular pain. Note that the SAP and laminar surfaces are not coincident (*dotted lines*). In (*F*), the fluoroscope is rotated to the measured angle of the SAP; note that the lamina (*solid arrow*) projects posterior to the SAP (*dotted arrow*). The SAP is the target landmark (*G*). The needle is advanced in the AP projection until it is approximately half way across the articular pillar (*dotted lines, H*). Subsequent contrast injection shows flow about the exiting nerve and into the central epidural space. The operator must recognize aberrant flow. In (*K*), off-target contrast media is seen in the facet joint capsule (*arrowheads*) with flow in the space of Okada to the midline (*arrow*). Venous uptake is demonstrated in (*L*), where there was transient opacification of multiple small veins as well as accumulation posterior to the exiting nerve. In (*M*), from the upper injection, there is vertical accumulation of contrast media (*arrow*), lateral to the uncinate line (*dotted line*): it therefore cannot be in the central epidural space. It should be in the interstitium of the venous plexus surrounding the vertebral artery. There is epidural flow from the lower injection (*dashed arrow*). Extraspinal venous flow is demonstrated in (*N*). (*Reproduced with permission from the International Pain and Spine Intervention Society (IPSIS).*)

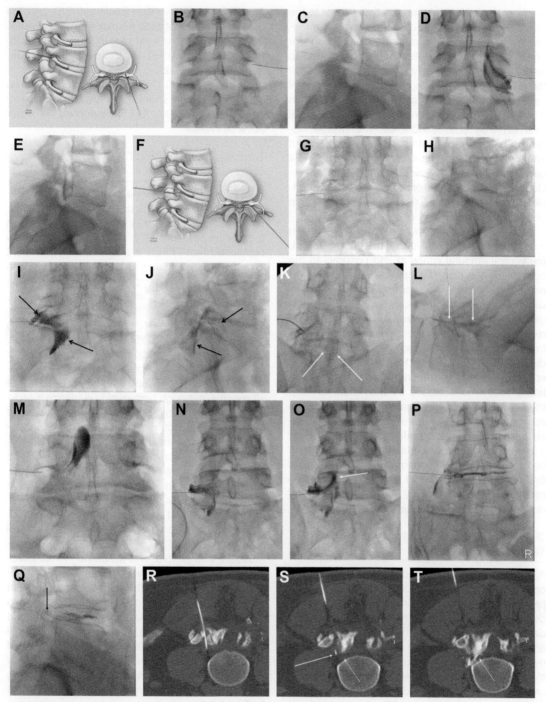

Fig. 5. The supraneural trajectory is depicted by the artist in (*A*). Only modest ipsilateral obliquity (10°–15°) is necessary, along with sufficient caudal to cranial angulation to pass under the pars interarticularis. (*B–E*) A supra-neural needle position and contrast flow pattern for a right L5 TFESI treating L5 radicular pain due to an L4–5 disc herniation. Note the needle does not pass the midpoint of the pedicle on the AP view (to avoid dural sleeve pene-tration) and is in close proximity to the undersurface of the pedicle. Contrast media flow is ventral, outlining the preganglionic nerve and dorsal root ganglion (DRG, *D, E*). An infraneural approach (*F*) is shown in (*G–J*). Note that a more oblique trajectory can be used without risk of dural transgression. At L5, an infraneural approach often provides coverage to the traversing S1 nerve as well as the L5 nerve (*arrows* in *I, J*).The operator must recog-nize aberrant flow, including intrathecal (*arrows, K, L*), intradural (central dural zone, *M*), and intra-articular (facet) distribution (*N*, resolved by needle advancement with epidural flow, *arrow* in *O*). An infraneural approach

the needle positioned immediately posterior to the nerve (**Fig. 6**). It is more challenging with fluoroscopy, where the beam is aligned to the S1 superior endplate and a slight ipsilateral obliquity added to visualize an arcuate line as the medial aspect of the S1 pedicle, continuing inferiorly as the lateral aspect of the S1 neural canal. The dorsal foramen is positioned immediately cephalad to the ventral foramen with craniocaudal tilt; the needle approaches the foramen at its inferolateral quadrant and is walked off bone to enter the foramen.[64] Final depth is then carefully assessed on the lateral view. Contrast media should predominantly flow cephalad; 3 cc of injectate will reach the superior margin of the L5–S1 disc in 92% of cases.[65]

The interventionalist must select the approach most likely to safely deliver contrast to the target, the ventral epidural space at and proximal to the contact zone between a compressive lesion and neural tissue. Evidence supports better outcomes with flow to the ventral epidural space and preganglionic nerve.[10,13] For example, when the lateral recess is patent, it is reasonable to expect flow from an infraneural approach (L4) at the level of a disc herniation (L4–L5) to reach the ventral epidural space and preganglionic nerve. If the lateral recess is occluded by disc material from the L4–5 herniation, a subjacent (L5) supraneural approach would be preferred. In foraminal stenosis cases, a superjacent infraneural approach, or a lateral parasagittal interlaminar approach may be preferred. The interventionalist should examine the relevant anatomy and enter the procedure room armed with a plan A, B, and C, to be used dependent on the flow patterns observed.

Transforaminal Epidural Steroid Injection: Safety

Although case reports of neurologic injury, primarily cord infarcts, created concern and even adverse practice recommendations in past decades, rational decision-making requires adverse event rates. Such data are now available, demonstrating that TFESIs are safe procedures. Safety has been enhanced by the evolving understanding of the risks of particulate steroids and practice guidelines addressing steroid use. A multi-institutional study of consecutive TFESI in all spine segments ($n = 14{,}956$) using International

Pain & Spine Intervention Society (IPSIS) practice guidelines demonstrated no major adverse events. Vasovagal reactions were seen in 1.3%, dural punctures in less than 0.1% and transient systemic steroid effects in 2.6%[38] A single-center study of greater than 24,000 TFESIs over 12 years identified no major adverse events.[39] A Medicare study of greater than 523,000 TFESIs identified no major adverse events.[40]

Transforaminal Epidural Steroid Injections: Efficacy

A 2020 systematic review addressing the effectiveness of lumbar TFESI examined 2 explanatory, 8 pragmatic, and 20 observational trials; it built on a prior review of 2013.[66,67] The investigators concluded that TFESIs are an effective treatment for radicular pain due to disc herniation, with strong evidentiary support. With greater than 50% reduction in pain as a categorical threshold, success rates were 63% (58%–68%) at 1 month, 74% (68%–80%) at 3 months, 64% (59%–69%) at 6 months, and 64% (57%–71%) at 12 months. There is evidence suggesting effectiveness for fixed lesions, with success rates of 48% (35%–61%) at 3 months and 59% (45%–73%) at 12 months, although high-quality evidence is lacking. A cohort study of imaging determinants of lumbar TFESI effectiveness demonstrated that patients with disc herniations also had better functional recovery (at 2 months) than those with fixed lesions.[68] However, patients with fixed lesions treated with dexamethasone had results equivalent to those with disc herniations.[68]

The most robust explanatory trial compared TF injection of steroid plus anesthetic to four control arms consisting of TF anesthetic, TF saline, intramuscular (IM) steroid, and IM saline.[69] This effectively controlled for the potential benefit of TF anesthetic alone or for the nonspecific delivery of steroid. Categorical outcomes of greater than 50% pain relief were superior for the TF steroid group 54% (36%–72%) when compared with all control groups 15% (8%–22%). Significant relief of pain was accompanied by functional recovery and significant reduction of consumption of other health care, including surgical sparing. A significant finding in this study was a bimodal outcome:

---

carries the risk of disc penetration (*P, Q*); cross-sectional imaging must be consulted in pre-procedure planning when herniation may bring the disc into the needle trajectory. CTF guidance offers the ability to negotiate obstacles insurmountable with fluoroscopy, such as the bone graft in (*R–T*). The 25 gauge needle passed through a gap in the graft to a final position adjacent to the DRG (needle tip at solid *arrow*; DRG at dotted *arrow* in *S*). In (*T*), contrast media flows about the DRG in the lateral recess. (Images 5A, F *Used with permission* of Mayo Foundation for Medical Education and Research, all rights reserved; Images 5 B-E, G-T *Reproduced with permission from* the International Pain and Spine Intervention Society (IPSIS).)

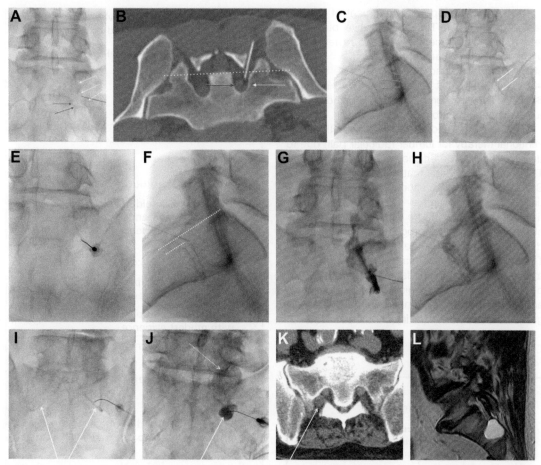

Fig. 6. Correlation of cross-sectional and projectional fluoroscopic anatomy (*A–C*). The lateral wall of the S1 foramen is the arcuate line of Aprill, white arrows in (*A, B*). The medial bony cortex is identifiable on the fluoroscopic (*A*) and CT (*B*) images (*red arrow*). The anterior cortical wall of the foramen is identified on the CT and lateral fluoroscopic view (*C*) by blue arrows. Note the posterior cortex of the S2 segment (*dotted line* in *B, C*). The needle needs to advance beyond this plane to approach the nerve. Slight ipsilateral obliquity (*D, arrows*) accentuates the arcuate line. A 25-gauge needle is advanced via a lateral to medial vector into the dorsal foramen (*E*) to reside just deep to the S2 cortex (*dotted lines, F*). Contrast media injection shows flow to the ventral aspect of the foramen, passing cephalad to the L5 level (*G, H*). Off-target venous flow is common in the highly vascular S1 foramen (*I*). One may also encounter synovial cysts (*arrow, J, K*) filling the L5 facet (*dotted arrow, J*) or meningeal (Tarlov) cysts (*L*). Pre-procedure planning using cross-sectional imaging is essential. (*Reproduced with permission from* the International Pain and Spine Intervention Society (IPSIS).)

success or no success. Group mean data concealed the clinical benefit, which was revealed with categorical outcomes of a predefined success threshold; subsequent methodological reviews suggest reporting categorical outcomes for pain.[70]

A pragmatic trial demonstrated 6-month success rates of 70% for greater than 50% pain relief and 65% for greater than 50% improvement in functional recovery. A study emphasizing the role of TFESI in holistic health care examined radicular pain patients who had failed non-interventional conservative care and were consented for surgery. Pain relief from TFESI then allowed participation

in a comprehensive mechanical diagnosis and treatment program; at 1-year follow-up 78% avoided surgery and 62% had minimal or no pain (visual analogue scale [VAS] <10/100) and essentially complete functional recovery.[71] A systematic review confirmed the surgical sparing effects of epidural injections.[72] A pragmatic trial compared TFESI versus microdiscectomy for disc herniation-related radicular pain. There was no difference in primary or secondary efficacy outcomes, but safety and cost-effectiveness favored TFESI, with a recommendation that TFESI is the initial procedural intervention in lumbar radicular pain.[73]

The evidence supporting treatment of cervical radicular pain with TFESI is positive but much less robust. Two recent systematic reviews note a paucity of explanatory studies.[74,75] Cohort studies demonstrated pooled response rates of 48% (34%–61%) at 1 month and 55% (45%–64%).[74] Better powered, high-quality studies with a true placebo control group are needed.

TFESI are safe and effective as an initial interventional therapy for lumbar radicular pain due to disc herniation. The efficacy evidence for lumbar TFESI greatly exceeds that of lumbar ILESI. TFESIs are also effective, although with less evidentiary support, for lumbar radicular pain due to fixed lesions. This is to be distinguished from the clinical syndrome of neurogenic intermittent claudication, where evidence is lacking. Cervical TFESI for radicular pain may be effective but with a lesser success rate and far less evidentiary support than in the lumbar region. When performed in accordance with evidence-based procedural guidelines, transforaminal injections are safe.

CLINICS CARE POINTS

Procedural considerations

- Diagnostic selective nerve blocks and therapeutic transforaminal injections are distinct procedures with different targeting.
- Although CT fluoroscopy guidance has unique advantages, virtually all the literature supporting interventional pain procedures use fluoroscopic guidance. US has a limited role.
- Spinal enumeration, as part of a systematic evaluation of pre-procedure imaging, is necessary for safe and effective procedures.
- Non-particulate steroid solutions (dexamethasone) are recommended for initial transforaminal access.
- Systemic side effects of corticosteroids are common and must be considered in a risk/benefit analysis.

Interlaminar epidural injections

- Interlaminar epidural steroid injections (ILESIs) are safe when performed in accordance with evidence-based procedural guidelines.
- Evidentiary support for ILESI efficacy is limited; thus, indications are constrained to:
  - Cervical radicular pain where a transforaminal approach is impeded by vulnerable structures
  - Lumbar radicular pain when a transforaminal approach is impeded by:
    - Foraminal stenosis, especially at L5
    - Bone graft
    - Instrumentation
    - Anatomic anomaly
  - A parasagittal approach is preferred when anatomy allows safe access.

Transforaminal epidural injections

- Transforaminal epidural steroid injections (TFESIs) are safe and effective when performed by evidence-based procedural guidelines.
- Indications for TFESI:
  - Lumbar radicular pain due to disc herniation, with strong evidentiary support
  - Lumbar radicular pain due to fixed lesions, with modest evidence
  - Cervical radicular pain, with modest evidence
- TFESIs require careful evaluation of pre-procedure imaging to optimize on-target delivery.
- TFESI should be used as one component of a holistic approach to the radicular pain patient.

DISCLOSURE

The author has nothing to disclose.

REFERENCES

1. Mulleman D, Mammou S, Griffoul I, et al. Pathophysiology of disk-related sciatica. I.–Evidence supporting a chemical component. Joint Bone Spine 2006; 73(2):151–8.
2. Bush K, Cowan N, Katz DE, et al. The natural history of sciatica associated with disc pathology. A prospective study with clinical and independent radiologic follow-up. Spine 1992;17(10):1205–12.
3. Friedly JL, Comstock BA, Turner JA, et al. A randomized trial of epidural glucocorticoid injections for spinal stenosis. N Engl J Med 2014;371(1): 11–21.
4. Manzur MK, Samuel AM, Vaishnav A, et al. Cervical Steroid Injections Are Not Effective for Prevention of Surgical Treatment of Degenerative Cervical Myelopathy. Global Spine 2021. https://doi.org/10. 1177/21925682211024573. 21925682211024573.

5. Hogan QH. Epidural anatomy examined by cryomicrotome section. Influence of age, vertebral level, and disease. Reg Anesth 1996;21(5):395–406.

6. Joshi J, Roytman M, Aiyer R, et al. Cervical spine ligamentum flavum gaps: MR characterisation and implications for interlaminar epidural injection therapy. Reg Anesth Pain Med 2022;47(8):459–63.

7. Boezaart AP, Prats-Galino A, Nin OC, et al. The Posterior Lumbar Epidural Space: Three-Dimensional Reconstruction of High-Resolution MRI: Real and Potential Epidural Spaces and Their Content In Vivo. Pain Med 2019;20(9):1687–96.

8. Bogduk N. Lumbar and sacral spinal nerve blocks. In: Bogduk N, editor. Practice Guidelines for spinal Diagnostic and treatment procedures. 2nd edition. San Fransisco, CA: International Spine Intervention Society; 2013. p. 443–56.

9. Wolff AP, Groen GJ, Wilder-Smith OH. Influence of needle position on lumbar segmental nerve root block selectivity. Reg Anesth Pain Med 2006;31(6):523–30.

10. Desai MJ, Shah B, Sayal PK. Epidural contrast flow patterns of transforaminal epidural steroid injections stratified by commonly used final needle-tip position. Pain Med 2011;12(6):864–70.

11. Makkar JK, Singh NP, Rastogi R. Volume of contrast and selectivity for lumbar transforaminal epidural steroid injection. Pain Physician 2015;18(1):101–5.

12. Cohen SP, Hurley RW. The ability of diagnostic spinal injections to predict surgical outcomes. Anesth Analg 2007;105(6):1756–75.

13. Jeong HS, Lee JW, Kim SH, et al. Effectiveness of transforaminal epidural steroid injection by using a preganglionic approach: a prospective randomized controlled study. Radiology 2007;245(2):584–90.

14. Bui J, Bogduk N. A systematic review of the effectiveness of CT-guided, lumbar transforaminal injection of steroids. Pain Med 2013;14(12):1860–5.

15. Kranz PG, Amrhein TJ, Gray L. Incidence of Inadvertent Intravascular Injection during CT Fluoroscopy-Guided Epidural Steroid Injections. AJNR Am J Neuroradiol 2015;36(5):1000–7.

16. Amrhein TJ, Schauberger JS, Kranz PG, et al. Reducing Patient Radiation Exposure From CT Fluoroscopy-Guided Lumbar Spine Pain Injections by Targeting the Planning CT. AJR Am J Roentgenol 2016;206(2):390–4.

17. Hoang JK, Yoshizumi TT, Toncheva G, et al. Radiation dose exposure for lumbar spine epidural steroid injections: a comparison of conventional fluoroscopy data and CT fluoroscopy techniques. AJR Am J Roentgenol 2011;197(4):778–82.

18. Amrhein TJ, Bozdogan E, Vekaria S, et al. Cross-sectional CT Assessment of the Extent of Injectate Spread at CT Fluoroscopy-guided Cervical Epidural Interlaminar Steroid Injections. Radiology 2019;292(3):723–9.

19. Lee JH, Lee S-H. Comparison of clinical effectiveness of cervical transforaminal steroid injection according to different radiological guidances (C-arm fluoroscopy vs. computed tomography fluoroscopy). Spine J 2011;11(5):416–23.

20. Ehsanian R, Kennedy DJ, Schneider B. Cervical ultrasound utilization in selective cervical nerve root injection for the treatment of cervical radicular pain: a review. Curr Phys Med Rehabil Rep 2019;7:386–96.

21. Thawait GK, Chhabra A, Carrino JA. Spine segmentation and enumeration and normal variants. Radiol Clin North Am 2012;50(4):587–98.

22. Benzon HT, Chew T-L, McCarthy RJ, et al. Comparison of the particle sizes of different steroids and the effect of dilution: a review of the relative neurotoxicities of the steroids. Anesthesiology 2007;106(2):331–8.

23. Okubadejo GO, Talcott MR, Schmidt RE, et al. Perils of intravascular methylprednisolone injection into the vertebral artery. An animal study. J Bone Joint Surg Am 2008;90(9):1932–8.

24. Laemmel E, Segal N, Mirshahi M, et al. Deleterious Effects of Intra-arterial Administration of Particulate Steroids on Microvascular Perfusion in a Mouse Model. Radiology 2016;279(3):731–40.

25. Kennedy DJ, Plastaras C, Casey E, et al. Comparative effectiveness of lumbar transforaminal epidural steroid injections with particulate versus nonparticulate corticosteroids for lumbar radicular pain due to intervertebral disc herniation: a prospective, randomized, double-blind trial. Pain Med 2014;15(4):548–55.

26. El-Yahchouchi C, Geske JR, Carter RE, et al. The noninferiority of the nonparticulate steroid dexamethasone vs the particulate steroids betamethasone and triamcinolone in lumbar transforaminal epidural steroid injections. Pain Med 2013;14(11):1650–7.

27. Mehta P, Syrop I, Singh JR, et al. Systematic review of the efficacy of particulate versus nonparticulate corticosteroids in epidural injections. PM&R 2017;9(5):502–12.

28. Rathmell JP, Benzon HT, Dreyfuss P, et al. Safeguards to prevent neurologic complications after epidural steroid injections: consensus opinions from a multidisciplinary working group and national organizations. Anesthesiology 2015;122(5):974–84.

29. Murthy NS, Geske JR, Shelerud RA, et al. The effectiveness of repeat lumbar transforaminal epidural steroid injections. Pain Med 2014;15(10):1686–94.

30. Lee Y, Issa TZ, Kanhere AP, et al. Preoperative epidural steroid injections do not increase the risk of postoperative infection in patients undergoing lumbar decompression or fusion: a systematic review and meta-analysis. Eur Spine J 2022;31(12):3251–61.

31. Kazarian GS, Steinhaus ME, Kim HJ. The Impact of Corticosteroid Injection Timing on Infection Rates Following Spine Surgery: A Systematic Review and Meta-Analysis. Global Spine J 2022;12(7):1524–34.

32. White AH, Derby R, Wynne G. Epidural injections for the diagnosis and treatment of low-back pain. Spine 1980;5(1):78–86.

33. Botwin KP, Natalicchio J, Hanna A. Fluoroscopic guided lumbar interlaminar epidural injections: a prospective evaluation of epidurography contrast patterns and anatomical review of the epidural space. Pain Physician 2004;7(1):77–80.

34. Weil L, Frauwirth NH, Amirdelfan K, et al. Fluoroscopic analysis of lumbar epidural contrast spread after lumbar interlaminar injection. Arch Phys Med Rehabil 2008;89(3):413–6.

35. Gill JS, Aner M, Jyotsna N, et al. Contralateral Oblique View is Superior to Lateral View for Interlaminar Cervical and Cervicothoracic Epidural Access. Pain Med 2015;16(1):68–80.

36. Gill JS, Nagda JV, Aner MM, et al. Contralateral Oblique View Is Superior to the Lateral View for Lumbar Epidural Access. Pain Med 2015;17(5):839–50.

37. Rathmell JP, Michna E, Fitzgibbon DR, et al. Injury and Liability Associated with Cervical Procedures for Chronic Pain. Anesthesiology 2011;114(4):918–26.

38. El-Yahchouchi CA, Plastaras CT, Maus TP, et al. Adverse Event Rates Associated with Transforaminal and Interlaminar Epidural Steroid Injections: A Multi-Institutional Study. Pain Med 2016;17(2):239–49.

39. Lee JW, Lee E, Lee GY, et al. Epidural steroid injection-related events requiring hospitalisation or emergency room visits among 52,935 procedures performed at a single centre. Eur Radiol 2018;28(1):418–27.

40. Eworuke E, Crisafi L, Liao J, et al. Risk of serious spinal adverse events associated with epidural corticosteroid injections in the Medicare population. Reg Anesth Pain Med 2021;46(3):203–9.

41. Vorobeychik Y, Sharma A, Smith CC, et al. The Effectiveness and Risks of Non-Image-Guided Lumbar Interlaminar Epidural Steroid Injections: A Systematic Review with Comprehensive Analysis of the Published Data. Pain Med 2016;17(12):2185–202.

42. Arden NK, Price C, Reading I, et al. A multicentre randomized controlled trial of epidural corticosteroid injections for sciatica: the WEST study. Rheumatology (Oxford) 2005;44(11):1399–406.

43. Carette S, Leclaire R, Marcoux S, et al. Epidural corticosteroid injections for sciatica due to herniated nucleus pulposus. N Engl J Med 1997;336(23):1634–40.

44. Sharma AK, Vorobeychik Y, Wasserman R, et al. The Effectiveness and Risks of Fluoroscopically Guided Lumbar Interlaminar Epidural Steroid Injections: A Systematic Review with Comprehensive Analysis of the Published Data. Pain Med 2017;18(2):239–51.

45. Manchikanti L, Singh V, Cash KA, et al. The Role of Fluoroscopic Interlaminar Epidural Injections in Managing Chronic Pain of Lumbar Disc Herniation or Radiculitis: A Randomized, Double-Blind Trial. Pain Pract 2013;13(7):547–58.

46. Furman MB, Kothari G, Parikh T, et al. Efficacy of fluoroscopically guided, contrast-enhanced lumbosacral interlaminar epidural steroid injections: a pilot study. Pain Med 2010;11(9):1328–34.

47. Ghai B, Bansal D, Kay JP, et al. Transforaminal versus parasagittal interlaminar epidural steroid injection in low back pain with radicular pain: a randomized, double-blind, active-control trial. Pain Physician 2014;17(4):277–90.

48. Ghai B, Kumar K, Bansal D, et al. Effectiveness of Parasagittal Interlaminar Epidural Local Anesthetic with or without Steroid in Chronic Lumbosacral Pain: A Randomized, Double-Blind Clinical Trial. Pain Physician 2015;18(3):237–48.

49. Ghai B, Vadaje KS, Wig J, et al. Lateral parasagittal versus midline interlaminar lumbar epidural steroid injection for management of low back pain with lumbosacral radicular pain: a double-blind, randomized study. Anesth Analg 2013;117(1):219–27.

50. Hashemi SM, Aryani MR, Momenzadeh S, et al. Comparison of Transforaminal and Parasagittal Epidural Steroid Injections in Patients With Radicular Low Back Pain. Anesthesiol Pain Med 2015;5(5):e26652.

51. Benyamin R, Singh V, Parr AT, et al. Systematic review of the effectiveness of cervical epidurals in the management of chronic neck pain. Database of Abstracts of Reviews of effects (DARE): Quality-assessed Reviews [Internet]. Pain Physician 2009;12(1):137–57.

52. Manchikanti L, Cash KA, Pampati V, et al. A randomized, double-blind, active control trial of fluoroscopic cervical interlaminar epidural injections in chronic pain of cervical disc herniation: results of a 2-year follow-up. Pain Physician 2013;16(5):465–78.

53. Manchikanti L, Nampiaparampil DE, Candido KD, et al. Do cervical epidural injections provide long-term relief in neck and upper extremity pain? A systematic review. Pain Physician 2015;18(1):39.

54. House LM, Barrette K, Mattie R, et al. Cervical Epidural Steroid Injection: Techniques and Evidence. Phys Med Rehabil Clin 2018;29(1):1–17.

55. Fitzgerald RT, Bartynski WS, Collins HR. Vertebral artery position in the setting of cervical degenerative disease: implications for selective cervical transforaminal epidural injections. Interv Neuroradiol 2013;19(4):425–31.

56. Huntoon MA. Anatomy of the cervical intervertebral foramina: vulnerable arteries and ischemic neurologic

injuries after transforaminal epidural injections. Pain 2005;117(1–2):104–11.

57. Levi D, Horn S, Murphy J, et al. Modification of the Cervical Transforaminal Epidural Steroid Injection Technique Based Upon the Anatomic Angle of the Superior Articular Process on MRI. Pain Med 2020; 21(10):2090–9.

58. Smuck M, Maxwell MD, Kennedy D, et al. Utility of the anesthetic test dose to avoid catastrophic injury during cervical transforaminal epidural injections. Spine J 2010;10(10):857–64.

59. Furman MB, Mehta AR, Kim RE, et al. Injectate volumes needed to reach specific landmarks in lumbar transforaminal epidural injections. Pm r 2010;2(7): 625–35.

60. Gregg L, Sorte D, Gailloud P. Intraforaminal location of thoracolumbar radicular arteries providing an anterior radiculomedullary artery using flat panel catheter angiotomography. Am J Neuroradiol 2017; 38(5):1054–60.

61. Murthy NS, Maus TP, Behrns CL. Intraforaminal location of the great anterior radiculomedullary artery (artery of Adamkiewicz): a retrospective review. Pain Med 2010;11(12):1756–64.

62. Kim HJ, Park JH, Shin KM, et al. The efficacy of transforaminal epidural steroid injection by the conventional technique in far-lateral herniation of lumbar disc. Pain Physician 2012;15(5):415–20.

63. Kim C, Choi HE, Kang S. Contrast spreading patterns in retrodiscal transforaminal epidural steroid injection. Ann Rehabil Med 2012;36(4):474–9.

64. Tiegs-Heiden C, Talsma J, Willard F, et al. The S1 dorsal foramen: Nuances of anatomy. Interventional Pain Medicine 2023;2(1):100172.

65. Furman MB, Butler SP, Kim RE, et al. Injectate volumes needed to reach specific landmarks in S1 transforaminal epidural injections. Pain Med 2012; 13(10):1265–74.

66. MacVicar J, King W, Landers MH, et al. The effectiveness of lumbar transforaminal injection of steroids: a comprehensive review with systematic analysis of the published data. Pain Med 2013; 14(1):14–28.

67. Smith CC, McCormick ZL, Mattie R, et al. The Effectiveness of Lumbar Transforaminal Injection of Steroid for the Treatment of Radicular Pain: A Comprehensive Review of the Published Data. Pain Med 2020;21(3):472–87.

68. Maus TP, El-Yahchouchi CA, Geske JR, et al. Imaging Determinants of Clinical Effectiveness of Lumbar Transforaminal Epidural Steroid Injections. Pain Med 2016;17(12):2176–84.

69. Ghahreman A, Ferch R, Bogduk N. The efficacy of transforaminal injection of steroids for the treatment of lumbar radicular pain. Pain Med. 2010;11(8): 1149–68.

70. Deyo RA, Dworkin SF, Amtmann D. Report of the NIH Task Force on Research Standards for Chronic Low Back Pain 1976, 39. (Phila) PA: Spine; 2014. p. 1128–43.

71. van Helvoirt H, Apeldoorn AT, Ostelo RW, et al. Transforaminal epidural steroid injections followed by mechanical diagnosis and therapy to prevent surgery for lumbar disc herniation. Pain Med 2014; 15(7):1100–8.

72. Bhatti AB, Kim S. Role of Epidural Injections to Prevent Surgical Intervention in Patients with Chronic Sciatica: A Systematic Review and Meta-Analysis. Cureus 2016;8(8):e723.

73. Wilby MJ, Best A, Wood E, et al. Surgical microdiscectomy versus transforaminal epidural steroid injection in patients with sciatica secondary to herniated lumbar disc (NERVES): a phase 3, multicentre, open-label, randomised controlled trial and economic evaluation. Lancet Rheumatology 2021; 3(5):e347–56.

74. Conger A, Cushman DM, Speckman RA, et al. The Effectiveness of Fluoroscopically Guided Cervical Transforaminal Epidural Steroid Injection for the Treatment of Radicular Pain; a Systematic Review and Meta-analysis. Pain Med 2020;21(1):41–54.

75. Borton ZM, Oakley BJ, Clamp JA, et al. Cervical transforaminal epidural steroid injections for radicular pain : a systematic review. Bone Joint J 2022; 104-b(5):567–74.

Imaging of Discogenic and Vertebrogenic Pain

Frederik Abel, MD[a], Franziska C.S. Altorfer, MD[b,c], Varun Rohatgi, BS[d],
Wende Gibbs, MD, MA[e], Joseph Levi Chazen, MD[a,*]

KEYWORDS

• Vertebrogenic pain • Discogenic pain • MRI • CT • Discography • UTE • Quantitative MRI

KEY POINTS

- Discogenic and vertebrogenic pain are 2 major entities causing chronic lower back pain, involving painful intervertebral disc degeneration and vertebral endplate deterioration.
- Conventional imaging faces challenges in identifying specific findings indicative of both pain forms, with MRI offering the highest diagnostic value.
- Advanced techniques like single photon emission computed tomography (SPECT)/CT, ultra-short echo time, and quantitative MRI aim to enhance precision and accuracy in detecting early discogenic and vertebrogenic changes.

INTRODUCTION

Lower back pain (LBP) is a burdensome medical condition that affects a substantial portion of the global population, with a life-time prevalence reported to be 60% to 80%.[1] Remaining a primary contributor to disability, global LBP patient count is projected to rise from 619 to 843 million by 2050, mainly attributed to global population growth and aging.[2]

Two major sources of chronic, axial LBP are discogenic and vertebrogenic pain. Discogenic pain is associated with abnormal intervertebral disc (IVD) degeneration, while vertebrogenic pain, a more recently described entity, relates to deterioration of vertebral endplates.[3,4]

In diagnosing LBP, imaging is becoming more crucial to pinpoint the potential cause of chronic LBP, although many imaging findings lack specificity.

Various imaging modalities are available to aid in diagnosis and management of LBP. Radiographs,

CT, and mainly MRI are common in clinical practice. Advanced techniques (eg, SPECT/CT or quantitative MRI) can be appropriate depending on the patient history, clinical suspicion, or in research settings. Provocative discography is considered the gold standard for discogenic pain, but due to its invasiveness and potential acceleration of IVD degeneration, it is generally not a first-line study and only applied to selected patients. Basivertebral nerve blocks, while theoretically useful for vertebrogenic pain, are similarly invasive and not ideal for an early detection method.[4]

This review aims to 1) cover the current understanding of the pathophysiology of discogenic and vertebrogenic pain, 2) explore the value of diagnostic imaging modalities in discriminating both entities, and 3) briefly outline treatment trends for these pain sources.

PATHOPHYSIOLOGY

Vertebrogenic pain results from structural alterations of the highly innervated endplates of a

[a] Department of Radiology and Imaging, Hospital for Special Surgery, 535 East 70th Street, NY 10021, USA;
[b] Department of Spine Surgery, Hospital for Special Surgery, 535 East 70th Street, NY 10021, USA;
[c] Department of Orthopedic Surgery, Balgrist University Hospital, University of Zurich, Forchstrasse 340, Zurich 8008, Switzerland; [d] Department of Radiology, Weill Cornell Medicine, 525 East 68th Street, NY 10065, USA;
[e] Barrow Neurological Institute, St. Joseph's Hospital and Medical Center, 350 West Thomas Road, Phoenix, AZ 85013, USA
* Corresponding author.
E-mail address: chazenjl@hss.edu

Radiol Clin N Am 62 (2024) 217–228
https://doi.org/10.1016/j.rcl.2023.10.003
0033-8389/24/© 2023 Elsevier Inc. All rights reserved.

segment leading to chronic LBP. Discogenic pain involves IVD degeneration, including structural defects resulting in biomechanical instability and inflammation. These changes closely intersect with the peripheral and central nervous systems to cause nerve sensitization and ingrowth.[3] To comprehend the pathophysiology of vertebrogenic and discogenic pain, a thorough understanding of the histologic and biomechanical properties as well as the innervation of the IVD is essential.

The IVD comprises a central nucleus pulposus (NP) surrounded by the annular fibrosus (AF), bordered by cartilage endplates (CEP) of the adjacent segments. The CEP are thin layers of hyaline cartilage weakly binding the disc to the vertebrae. The NP primarily consists of 70% to 90% water, proteoglycans, and Type II collagen fibers, maintaining its high-water content via proteoglycans and distributing the hydraulic pressure.[5] The AF exhibits a laminar structure with crisscross layers, including the inner (primarily type II collagen) and outer AF (primarily type I collagen). Biomechanically, the central NP resists axial compression upright, while the AF withstands circumferential loads and allows limited rotation and bending.[6] Together, these components contribute to spinal stability and flexibility. Nerves only exist in the outer third of the AF.[7] The CEP are densely innervated by the basivertebral nerves (BVN), a branch of the sinuvertebral nerve entering the vertebral body via the posterior foramen. In degenerative disc disease, CEP develop fissures and tears leading to depletion of proteoglycan in the cartilage, microfractures, and bony sclerosis of the vertebra resulting in the release of inflammatory mediators.[8] These changes manifest as abnormal signals on MRI as Modic changes (MC)[9] and are strongly linked to chronic LBP.[10] Vertebrogenic pain arises from damaged, chronically inflamed CEP. In this state, the BVN carries painful sensations due to higher nociceptor density tracing back to the BVN compared to normal endplates.[11]

The pathophysiology for discogenic pain follows a different pattern. Compromised vertebral endplates impact the disc, leading to acidic conditions and degeneration.[12] Consequently, the NP undergoes dehydration with disc height loss and eventual fibrosis.

Biomechanically, NP dehydration reduces elasticity, diminishing its ability to withstand axial forces. This hinders effective force absorption and distribution. The resulting NP displacement leads to inner layer-focused outward lamella bowing, affecting primarily the inner layers. Stress may lead to AF tears, gradual loss of disc height, biomechanical shifts, and increased facet joint stress. Inflammation and degeneration unlock proinflammatory cytokines, promoting vascular growth and sensory fiber ingrowth. The nervous ingrowth into the previously aneural degenerative disc precipitated by inflammatory insults induces nociception, and contributes to discogenic pain.[13]

Clinically differentiating between discogenic and vertebrogenic pain can be challenging and often remains inconclusive. Both are associated with degenerative changes of the IVD. Imaging can assist in detecting endplate changes linked to vertebrogenic pain and advanced IVD degeneration in cases of discogenic pain.

RADIOGRAPHS

Radiographs are often the initial diagnostic modality to evaluate the lumbar spine in patients presenting with LBP. Radiographs provide a comprehensive overview of the spinal anatomy and alignment, and can identify major pathology causing LBP, including compression fractures and alignment and curvature abnormalities including spondylolisthesis or scoliosis.

The utility of radiographs in diagnosing both vertebrogenic and discogenic pain is limited to evaluating degenerative osseous changes. Radiographs can identify IVD degeneration through disc space height loss, vacuum phenomenon, calcified discs, and bone spurs. These stigmata can be associated with discogenic pain, although not all degenerated discs are painful.[3] However, since IVD is common in older individuals, these are nonspecific imaging findings, and inadequate for distinguishing symptomatic from pain-free patients. Radiographs also fall short in visualizing disc herniations and annular fissures, potentially linked to painful discs.

Endplate-driven vertebrogenic pain can appear as sclerotic endplate changes (**Fig. 1**) and/or endplate defects, often accompanied by manifestations of IVD degeneration. Given the high resolution of radiographs for osseous structures, endplate changes are often evident at lower lumbar spine levels, revealing painful motion segments. However, for most of these findings, CT or MRI has higher sensitivity. Particularly MC have been associated with vertebrogenic pain and are best assessed on MRI.[14]

DISCOGRAPHY

Historically, provocation discography has been frequently used to assess discogenic pain, yet ongoing challenges arise from methodological heterogeneity in the literature and accuracy debates.[15] Provocation discography entails fluoroscopic-guided disc puncture using a spinal needle,

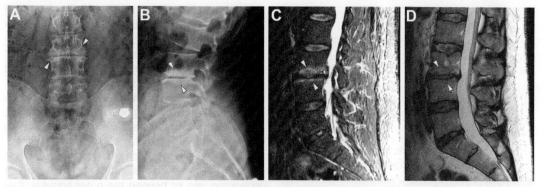

Fig. 1. Radiographs and MR images in a 44-year-old male experiencing axial low back pain for 6 months. Coronal (*A*) and sagittal (*B*) plain radiographs of the lumbar spine demonstrate endplate sclerosis and marked reduced disc height (*arrows*) at L3/4 with corresponding endplate edema signal (*arrows*) on the sagittal short-tau inversion recovery (*C*) and T2-weighted (*D*) MR images, reflecting Modic changes Type 1.

followed by contrast media injection to pressurize the disc. Pressurization may provoke pain, and post-interventional CT can reveal disc morphology, radial fissures, or contrast extravasation into the ventral epidural space (**Fig. 2**). Such findings in the presence of a concordant pain response can facilitate the diagnosis of a painful disc.[16] Discography is not routinely performed in many orthopedic centers, as considerable drawbacks lie in its invasiveness, and potentially higher risk of accelerated disc degeneration, disc herniations, and discitis-osteomyelitis.[17,18] Moreover, there is controversy surrounding its ability to elicit a concordant painful response in asymptomatic patients, although 1 meta-analysis suggests a low false-positive rate of approximately 6% per disc.[19]

For standardization of provocation discography, it is recommended to adhere to the Spine Intervention Society (SIS)/ (International Association for the Study of Pain (IASP) technical guidelines (**Box 1**). These guidelines lower false positives compared to earlier, high-pressure techniques.[20] Notably, pain likelihood rises significantly in patients with endplate damage.[19] Hence, discography's efficacy in distinguishing pain originating from the disc AF versus the vertebral endplate remains unclear, as pressurization might trigger nociception from both the annulus (sinuvertebral nerve) and endplate (basivertebral nerve).[21]

CT AND CT-MYELOGRAPHY

CT is a valuable imaging modality in the diagnosis and management of LBP, facilitated by its three-dimensional (3D) multiplanar reformation (MPR)

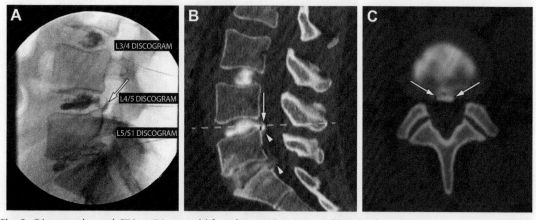

Fig. 2. Discography and CT in a 54-year-old female experiencing axial low back pain for 3 years. Discography (*A*) demonstrates needles within the L3/4–L5/S1 discs with injected contrast extending into the posterior annulus at L4/5 (*arrow*). Sagittal post-discography CT (*B*) shows moderate disc degeneration with associated disc protrusions (*arrowheads*) and an annular fissure at L4/5 (*arrow*), which is seen to better advantage on the corresponding axial section (*C*) at L4/5 (*dashed line, b*).

capabilities, excellent bone visualization, and ultra-high spatial resolution (approaching territories of 0.2 mm isotropic) that is driven by advances in photon-counting CT.[22] These attributes permit thorough spinal anatomy analysis and detection of many disorders such as spinal stenosis, spondylolisthesis, fractures, and bone tumors.

In patients with suspected discogenic pain, post-discography CT offers more detailed imaging of damaged IVD than discograms (two-dimensional fluoroscopy). Common findings include fissured/ruptured discs and contrast agent extending into or beyond the outer annulus, that have been shown to be positive in 94% and 97% of concordant painful discs at discography, respectively (see **Fig. 2**).[23]

CT also facilitates detection of degenerative endplate defects owing to its superior spatial resolution and osseous detail. Endplate defects are closely linked to MC,[24] which are primary indicators (particularly MC Type 1) for vertebrogenic pain, reflecting subchondral inflammation and bone marrow alterations. MC are often associated with endplate sclerosis and can help identify a painful vertebrogenic motion segment on CT. Endplate sclerosis can exist in all MC types (1–3) and is not a characteristic feature of MC Type 3 (**Fig. 3**).[25]

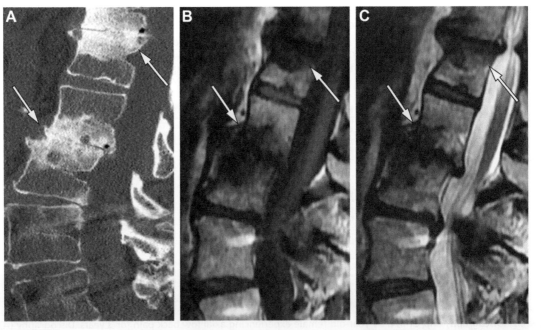

Fig. 3. CT and MR images in a 65-year-old male with chronic low back pain for 2 years. Sagittal CT (*A*) demonstrates sclerotic endplate changes (*arrows*) at L1/2 and L3/4 with collapsed discs. Corresponding T1-weighted (*B*) and T2-weighted (*C*) MR images show hypointense endplate changes, indicative of sclerosis (Modic changes Type 3).

Nonetheless, CT is less effective for soft tissue discrimination (including spinal cord and nerve roots) and IVD imaging compared to MRI. CT-Myelography, combining CT with contrast injection into the subarachnoid space, enhances soft tissue details and enables assessment of spinal cord, nerve roots, and disc contours. It is valuable for diagnosing disc herniations and ruling out nerve root(let) or spinal cord compression causing radicular pain.[26] CT-Myelography is sometimes obtained to evaluate the thecal sac in instances of severe susceptibility from implants/instrumentation, but MRI in most cases remains the primary imaging modality for discogenic and vertebrogenic pain evaluation.

SPECT/CT

Single photon emission computed tomography (SPECT/CT), a hybrid technique merging bone scintigraphy with radiotracer uptake (often Tc-99m methylene diphosphonate) and anatomic accuracy of CT, has shown promise in detecting metabolically active vertebral endplates. Increased tracer uptake in bone scintigraphy strongly correlates with MC Type 1,[27] showing high agreement between MCs and metabolic activity on bone SPECT/CT imaging (**Fig. 4**).[28] In particular, MC Type 1, along with severe disc degeneration, may predict positivity on SPECT/CT scans,[29] and increased tracer uptake occurs

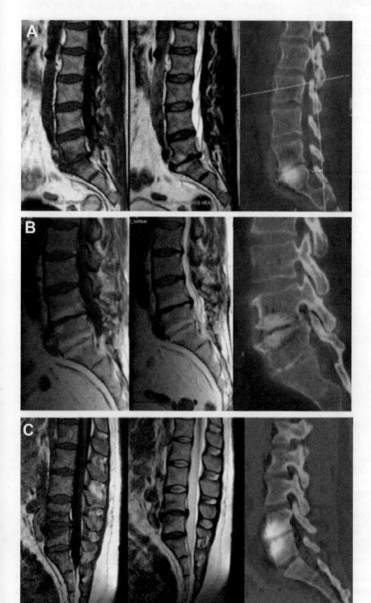

Fig. 4. Correlation between Modic changes on MRI and osteoblastic activity on hybrid single photon emission computed tomography (SPECT/CT) imaging. Modic change type I (*A*), type II (*B*), and type III (*C*). (*Adapted from* Reference 28 with permission.)

more frequently in patients with LBP compared to those without.[30] Thus, SPECT/CT holds potential in the diagnostic workup of patients with LBP to unmask painful endplate changes and/or severely degenerated discs or facet joints with greater specificity than conventional methods like qualitative MRI. Since SPECT/CT detects increased metabolic activity in both severe IVD degeneration and MC, it might prove clinically useful in managing vertebrogenic and discogenic pain, though its discriminative role requires further clarification.

QUALITATIVE MRI

MRI provides both osseous and excellent soft tissue detail without using ionizing radiation, positioning it as the favored imaging modality for working up LBP. Three-dimensional (3-D) sequences enable MPR capabilities, bolstered by spatial resolution improvements via deep learning reconstruction.[31] T2-weighted signal changes can assess IVD and endplate degeneration, and more recently, ultra-short echo time (UTE) sequences are emerging to characterize discogenic and/or vertebrogenic pain sources.

T2-weighted Changes

Multifactorial changes leading to discogenic pain can yield nonspecific late IVD degeneration findings. IVD degeneration reduces signal on T2-weighted sequences, blurred AF-NP boundary, irregular cartilage layers, and sparse horizontal trabeculae. High-intensity zones (HIZ) and Pfirrmann scores[32] are widely accepted to assess

disc degeneration in clinical practice and research settings.

HIZ describe T2 prolongation in the posterior AF, separated from the signal of the NP and are often best visible on sagittal slices (**Fig. 5**). HIZ may represent annular fissures and are strongly associated with painful discs during discography.[33] While HIZ pose a risk factor for discogenic LBP, they are also frequently found (prevalence: ~25%) in asymptomatic patients with degenerative disc disease.[34]

The Pfirrmann score (**Table 1**) grades disc degeneration severity from I to V (none to severe) on routine T2-weighted sequences based on signal characteristics, height, and distinction between NP and AF (**Fig. 6**). Although higher Pfirrmann grades reportedly correlate with discogenic pain,[35] they have a similar specificity challenge as HIZ in that they are often seen in asymptomatic patients.

Modic Changes

Advanced disc degeneration and herniations are associated with vertebral bone marrow changes, termed "Modic changes (MC)," visible adjacent to discs on MRI and are specific to painful responses during provocation discography.[36] Therefore, MC traditionally were established as possible discogenic pain triggers. However, recent findings of nerve ingrowth into damaged endplates, sensitizing endplate nociceptors through chemical and mechanical stimuli, support their role as vertebrogenic pain triggers.[4]

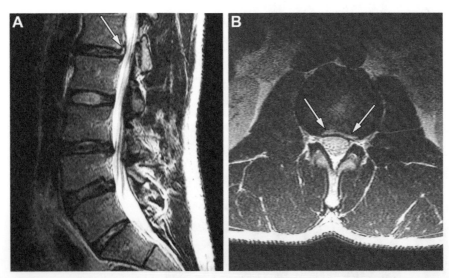

Fig. 5. MR images in a 35-year-old male experiencing low back pain for 3 months. Sagittal (*A*) and axial (*B*) T2-weighted MR images demonstrate a degenerated disc with prominent crescentic fissure (*arrows*) in the posterior outer annulus at L1–2.

Table 1
Pfirrmann grading system for lumbar disc degeneration

Grade	Structure	Distinction of Nucleus and Annulus	Signal Intensity	Disc Height
I	Homogeneous, bright white	Clear	Hyperintense, isointense to cerebrospinal fluid	Normal
II	Inhomogeneous with or without horizontal bands	Clear	Hyperintense, isointense to cerebrospinal fluid	Normal
III	Inhomogeneous, gray	Unclear	Intermediate	Normal to slightly decreased
IV	Inhomogeneous, gray to black	Lost	Intermediate to hypointense	Normal to moderately decreased
V	Inhomogeneous, black	Lost	Hypointense	Collapsed disc space

Three distinct types of MC are classified based on signal characteristics in T1-weighted and T2-weighted sequences (see **Fig. 4**). MC Type 1 are hypointense on T1-weighted and hyperintense on T2-weighted sequences, histologically representing vascularized granulation tissue and endplate edema as a sign of inflammation. MC Type 2 are hyperintense on both T1-weighted and T2-weighted sequences, signifying fatty bone marrow replacement. MC Type 3 are hypointense on both T1-weighted and T2-weighted sequences, indicative of stable sclerotic changes. MC prevalence is higher in LBP patients (43% vs 6% in asymptomatic patients),[37] with MC Type 1 more often being associated with LBP compared to MC Type 2/3.[38] On MRI, MC are more common at lower lumbar levels (L4–S1), typically symmetric, and frequently pronounced at the anterior third of endplates. MC Type 1 and Type 2 can transition over time, eventually forming MC Type 3. The exact contribution of MC, whether discogenic or vertebrogenic pain, remains a dynamic research area, given evidence of proinflammatory crosstalk between bone marrow and adjacent disc in MC-associated back pain[39]

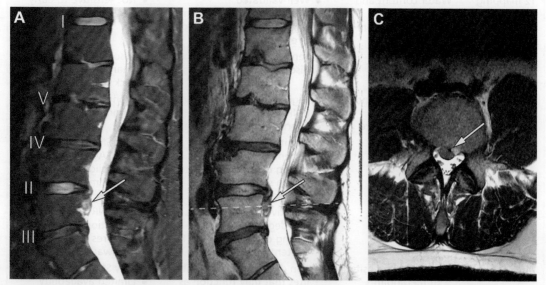

Fig. 6. MR images in a 56-year-old female presenting with acute on chronic low back pain. Sagittal short-tau inversion recovery (*A*) and T2-weighted (*B*) MR images demonstrate different grades of disc degeneration (Pfirrmann I-V). Additionally, a caudally oriented disc extrusion is apparent (*arrow*) originating from the L4/5, seen to better advantage on the axial T2-weighted section (*C*).

Ultra-short Echo Sequences

Ultra-short echo (UTE) sequences drastically reduce the effective echo time, permitting visualization of highly organized structures with very short T2 and T2* values (eg, cortical bone, cartilage) with rapid decay of transverse magnetization. Lately, the UTE disc sign (hyper- or hypointense changes within the disc) emerged as a novel biomarker linked to IVD degeneration, disc bulges/extrusions, MC, spondylolisthesis, and reduced T1ρ (rho) values within the disc. The UTE disc sign correlates with chronic LBP and disability,[40] suggesting its potential in assessing painful discs. Its morphologic counterpart might reflect disc calcifications.[41] Therefore, the UTE disc sign may serve as a sensitive biomarker for early degeneration often unnoticed on conventional T2-weighted sequences. However, additional validation is needed to determine its correlation with discogenic pain. The enhanced bone detail afforded by UTE sequences might also aid in detecting CEP damage responsible for vertebrogenic pain.[42] Similar to the UTE disc sign, the value of UTE for assessment of vertebrogenic pain needs further confirmatory studies.

QUANTITATIVE MRI

Quantitative MRI (qMRI) techniques capture biochemical information and are sensitive to pathologic microstructural changes earlier than qualitative MRI. Particularly well-studied for cartilage, qMRI has been mainly applied to assess the painful disc. Various qMRI techniques have been proposed for evaluation of IVD degeneration, aiming to establish imaging biomarkers more specific to clinical symptoms to aid in diagnosis, treatment, and prognostication (Table 2).

T2 and T1ρ (rho) mapping are among the most established and well-validated techniques, derived from quantifying T2 and T1 relaxation times. In IVD degeneration, water content and proteoglycan content decreases, resulting in decrease of both T2 values and T1ρ,[43] respectively. Particularly T1ρ might excel in early changes detection due to its correlation with early proteoglycan loss preceding water loss. T1ρ holds promise in predicting discogenic pain, correlating with painful discs during discography[44] and popular clinical outcome measures like SF-36 or Oswestry Disability Index in chronic LBP patients.[45]

Another experimental method to assess painful IVD degeneration is glycosaminoglycan chemical

Table 2
Summary of popular quantitative MRI imaging techniques for painful disc evaluation

Technique	Evaluated Structure	Advantages	Disadvantages
T2 mapping	Water content and extracellular matrix structure	• Well-validated • Available on most systems and across different field strengths	• Not sensitive to early disc degeneration
T1ρ	PG/GAG content	• Sensitive to early stages of disc degeneration	• Susceptible to quantification errors • Lack of standardization
T2* mapping	Water content and extracellular matrix structure	• High signal to noise ratio (SNR) • Short scan times	• Prone to field inhomogeneities
GagCEST	PG/GAG content	• Sensitive to early degeneration • Strong discrimination accuracy in severity of disc degeneration	• Low SNR at 3T for low GAG content • Less validated than T1p/T2 mapping
Sodium MRI	PG/GAG content, pH changes	• Sensitive to early stages of disc degeneration • Strong correlation with PG content	• Low SNR and spatial resolution • Requires specialized hardware
MRS	Chemical composition of metabolites	• Can detect several metabolites that may function as biomarkers	• Low SNR • Limited availability

GAG, glycosaminoglycan, GagCEST, GAG chemical exchange saturation transfer, MRS, magnetic resonance spectroscopy, PG, proteoglycan.

exchange saturation transfer (gagCEST). GagC-EST exploits the exchange of protons between bulk water protons and the hydroxyl and amine groups of glycosaminoglycans (GAGs), enabling an indirect measurement of GAG content and its loss within IVD. GagCEST shows a moderate negative correlation with IVD degeneration severity and has been linked to LBP in patients[46]

Sodium MRI is emerging for estimation of PG content in degenerated discs, utilizing the attraction of cationic sodium to negatively charged GAG. Sodium MRI correlates with a modified Pfirrmann score (Fig. 7), and its value may be increased be combination with T2 mapping[47] to assess both water content and PG content. Although promising, sodium MRI's impact in detecting painful discs has yet to be evaluated.

UTE imaging affords evaluation of rapidly decaying T2* species and has been evaluated in discs and their adjacent CEP. A study revealed that compositional deficits of the cartilage endplate, reflected by low T2* values, were associated with T1ρ changes of the NP and severity of disc degeneration in chronic LBP patients.[48] Similar to other qMRI biomarkers, UTE-T2* significantly inversely correlates with Pfirrmann grades[49] and is feasible for whole IVD characterization including the CEP,[50] highlighting its potential for quantitatively assessing both discogenic and vertebrogenic painful motion segments.

Until now, these findings are constrained by heterogeneous and small cohorts, discrepancies in protocols and hardware setups, and the absence of direct histopathological correlates. Despite these limitations, non-invasive techniques remain valuable and have potential in identifying discogenic and painful by characterization of discs and CEP, respectively.

TREATMENT

Non-surgical interventions to target vertebrogenic or discogenic pain triggers most commonly include epidural injections or radiofrequency ablation. Epidural injections, including steroids and anesthetics, are widely applied clinically to address radicular pain, but are also used for LBP with questionable efficacy.

For vertebrogenic pain, a focused and enduring approach is achieved by intraosseous basivertebral nerve radiofrequency ablation (BVN RFA), which has recently demonstrated improvements in pain and functionality in patients with chronic vertebrogenic LBP and MC Type 1 or 2[4]. Typically, BVN RFA utilizes a transpedicular access and bipolar RFA to ablate the BVN at painful motion segments in the lower lumbar spine (Fig. 8). The reported benefits, including pain reduction and improvements in Oswestry Disability Index scores, lasting up to 5 years and longer,[51] make BVN RFA an attractive treatment choice for selected patient cohorts.

For non-surgical treatment of discogenic pain, thermal (intradiscal) techniques in painful discs

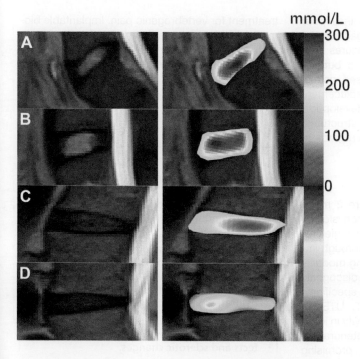

Fig. 7. Sagittal T2-weighted fast spin echo MR images of the lumbar spine, representing different Pfirrmann grades with corresponding 3-T quantitative sodium concentration images. Pfirrmann grade I (A), II (B), III (C), and IV (D) demonstrate decrease in the tissue sodium concentration with increasing disc degeneration, which is pronounced from grade III (C) to IV (D).

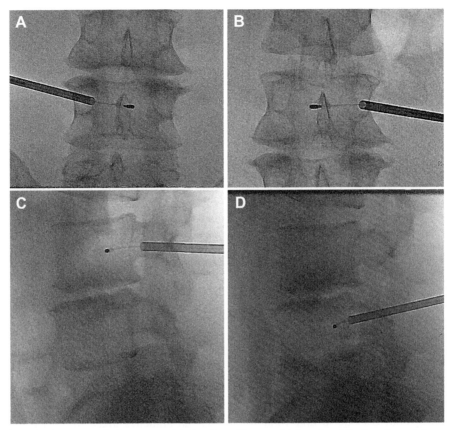

Fig. 8. Basivertebral nerve radiofrequency ablation in a 51-year-old female with chronic vertebrogenic lower back pain for 12 months. Anterior-posterior (A,B) and lateral (C,D) fluoroscopy show the radiofrequency tip through a transpedicular approach on the right side (A, C) at L4 and on the left side (B,D) at L5.

have been largely abandoned due to their poor outcomes. Currently, promising approaches aim to implant biomaterials for annulus closures and/or NP replacements to repair the disc but are controversial due to potential increased risk of re-herniation. Many AF repair and NP replacement devices and biomaterials have been developed,[3] including whole IVD tissue-engineered structures, that are currently being evaluated with regards to their efficacy in IVD repair.[52]

SUMMARY

Discogenic and vertebrogenic pain are 2 major pain triggers in the multifactorial pathophysiology of chronic LBP. Distinguishing these etiologies remains challenging, both clinically and through imaging. While MRI is the primary imaging modality for detecting painful vertebrogenic or discogenic segments, findings often lack specificity. Advanced techniques like SPECT/CT, UTE, or quantitative MRI could enhance sensitivity in identifying painful endplate and disc deterioration. Basivertebral nerve ablation is a promising

treatment for vertebrogenic pain. Implantable biomaterials are a promising emerging treatment to address painful intervertebral discs, although further studies are needed to assess safety and efficacy.

CLINICS CARE POINTS

- Radiographs can reveal disc degeneration through disc space height loss, vacuum phenomenon, calcified discs, and bone spurs. These findings often lack specificity.

- Computed tomography (CT) provides detailed visualization of disc degeneration stigmata, with post-discography CT enhancing accuracy in detecting painful discogenic segments such as the presence of high-grade radial fissures.

- CT can identify vertebrogenic painful endplate alterations by detecting endplate defects and sclerotic changes.

- Key findings for painful disc degeneration on MRI include signal loss on T2-weighted sequences, blurred boundaries, irregular cartilage layers, and high-intensity zones in the posterior annulus.
- Modic Type 1 changes on MRI exhibit the strongest correlation with chronic low back pain and particularly vertebrogenic pain.

DISCLOSURE

The authors have no conflicts to disclose.

REFERENCES

1. Ohtori S, Inoue G, Miyagi M, et al. Pathomechanisms of discogenic low back pain in humans and animal models. Spine J 2015;15(6):1347–55.
2. Collaborators G 2021 LBP., Ferreira ML, Luca K de, et al. Global, regional, and national burden of low back pain, 1990–2020, its attributable risk factors, and projections to 2050: a systematic analysis of the Global Burden of Disease Study 2021. Lancet Rheumatol 2023;5(6):e316–29.
3. Fujii K, Yamazaki M, Kang JD, et al. Discogenic Back Pain: Literature Review of Definition, Diagnosis, and Treatment. JBMR Plus 2019;3(5):e10180.
4. Conger A, Smuck M, Truumees E, et al. Vertebrogenic Pain: A Paradigm Shift in Diagnosis and Treatment of Axial Low Back Pain. Pain Med: Off J Am Acad Pain Med 2022;23(Suppl 2):S63–71.
5. Newell N, Little J, Christou A, et al. Biomechanics of the human intervertebral disc: A review of testing techniques and results. J Mech Behav Biomed Mater 2017;69:420–34.
6. Molladavoodi S, McMorran J, Gregory D. Mechanobiology of annulus fibrosus and nucleus pulposus cells in intervertebral discs. Cell Tissue Res 2020; 379(3):429–44.
7. Groh AMR, Fournier DE, Battié MC, et al. Innervation of the Human Intervertebral Disc: A Scoping Review. Pain Med 2021;22(6):1281–304.
8. Steffens D, Hancock MJ, Maher CG, et al. MRI predicting future LBP. Eur J Pain 2014;18(6):755–65.
9. Dudli S, Fields AJ, Samartzis D, et al. Pathobiology of Modic changes. Eur Spine J 2016;25(11): 3723–34.
10. Teraguchi M, Hashizume H, Oka H, et al. Detailed Subphenotyping of Lumbar Modic Changes and Their Association with Low Back Pain in a Large Population-Based Study: The Wakayama Spine Study. Pain Ther 2022;11(1):57–71.
11. Bailey JF, Liebenberg E, Degmetich S, et al. Innervation patterns of PGP 9.5-positive nerve fibers within the human lumbar vertebra. J Anat 2011;218(3): 263–70.
12. Bibby SRS, Urban JPG. Effect of nutrient deprivation on the viability of intervertebral disc cells. Eur Spine J 2004;13(8):695–701.
13. Freemont AJ, Watkins A, Maitre CL, et al. Nerve growth factor expression and innervation of the painful intervertebral disc. J Pathol 2002;197(3):286–92.
14. Brinjikji W, Diehn FE, Jarvik JG, et al. MRI Findings of Disc Degeneration are More Prevalent in Adults with Low Back Pain than in Asymptomatic Controls: A Systematic Review and Meta-Analysis. Am J Neuroradiol 2015;36(12):2394–9.
15. Manchikanti L, Soin A, Benyamin RM, et al. An Update of the Systematic Appraisal of the Accuracy and Utility of Discography in Chronic Spinal Pain. Pain Physician 2018;21(2):91–110.
16. Derby R, Kim B-J, Lee S-H, et al. Comparison of discographic findings in asymptomatic subject discs and the negative discs of chronic LBP patients: Can discography distinguish asymptomatic discs among morphologically abnormal discs? Spine J 2005;5(4):389–94.
17. Carragee EJ, Don AS, Hurwitz EL, et al. ISSLS Prize Winner: Does Discography Cause Accelerated Progression of Degeneration Changes in the Lumbar Disc. Spine 2009;34(21):2338–45.
18. Fraser R, Osti O, Vernon-Roberts B. Discitis after discography. J Bone Jt Surg Br 1987;69-B(1):26–35.
19. Wolfer LR, Derby R, Lee J-E, et al. Systematic review of lumbar provocation discography in asymptomatic subjects with a meta-analysis of false-positive rates. Pain Physician 2008;11(4):513–38.
20. Carragee EJ, Lincoln T, Parmar VS, et al. A Gold Standard Evaluation of the "Discogenic Pain" Diagnosis as Determined by Provocative Discography. Spine 2006;31(18):2115–23.
21. Bartynski WS, Agarwal V, Kahn AS, et al. Motion Characteristics of the 'Functional Spinal Unit' During Lumbar Disc Injection (Discography) including Comparison between Normal and Degenerative Levels. Pain Med 2021;22(8):pnab121.
22. Kijowski R, Fritz J. Emerging Technology in Musculoskeletal MRI and CT. Radiology 2023;306(1):6–19.
23. Lim C-H, Jee W-H, Son BC, et al. Discogenic lumbar pain: association with MR imaging and CT discography. Eur J Radiol 2005;54(3):431–7.
24. Määttä JH, Rade M, Freidin MB, et al. Strong association between vertebral endplate defect and Modic change in the general population. Sci Rep 2018;8(1):16630.
25. Kuisma M, Karppinen J, Haapea M, et al. Modic changes in vertebral endplates: a comparison of MR imaging and multislice CT. Skeletal Radiol 2009;38(2):141–7.
26. Huang Z, Zhao P, Zhang C, et al. Value of imaging examinations in diagnosing lumbar disc herniation: A systematic review and meta-analysis. Front Surg 2023;9:1020766.

27. Järvinen J, Niinimäki J, Karppinen J, et al. Does bone scintigraphy show Modic changes associated with increased bone turnover? Eur J Radiol Open 2020;7:100222.

28. Russo VM, Dhawan RT, Dharmarajah N, et al. Hybrid Bone Single Photon Emission Computed Tomography Imaging in Evaluation of Chronic Low Back Pain: Correlation with Modic Changes and Degenerative Disc Disease. World Neurosurg 2017;104: 816–23.

29. Varga M, Kantorová L, Langaufová A, et al. Role of Single-Photon Emission Computed Tomography Imaging in the Diagnosis and Treatment of Chronic Neck or Back Pain Caused by Spinal Degeneration: A Systematic Review. World Neurosurg 2023;173: 65–78.

30. Kelft EV de, Verleye G, Kelft A-SV de, et al. Validation of topographic hybrid single-photon emission computerized tomography with computerized tomography scan in patients with and without nonspecific chronic low back pain. A prospective comparative study. Spine J 2017;17(10):1457–63.

31. Chazen JL, Tan ET, Fiore J, et al. Rapid lumbar MRI protocol using 3D imaging and deep learning reconstruction. Skeletal Radiol 2023;1–8. https://doi.org/10.1007/s00256-022-04268-2.

32. Pfirrmann CWA, Metzdorf A, Zanetti M, et al. Magnetic Resonance Classification of Lumbar Intervertebral Disc Degeneration. Spine 2001;26(17):1873–8.

33. Schellhas KP, Pollei SR, Gundry CR, et al. Lumbar Disc High-intensity Zone. Spine 1996;21(1):79–86.

34. Carragee EJ, Paragioudakis SJ, Khurana S. Lumbar High-Intensity Zone and Discography in Subjects Without Low Back Problems. Spine 2000;25(23): 2987–92.

35. Borthakur A. Sensitivity of T1ρ MRI and Pfirrmann Grade to Discogenic Pain. Glob Spine J 2012;2(1_suppl). https://doi.org/10.1055/s-0032-1319979. s-0032-1319979-s-0032-1319979.

36. Thompson KJ, Dagher AP, Eckel TS, et al. Modic Changes on MR Images as Studied with Provocative Diskography: Clinical Relevance—A Retrospective Study of 2457 Disks. Radiology 2009;250(3):849–55.

37. Jensen TS, Karppinen J, Sorensen JS, et al. Vertebral endplate signal changes (Modic change): a systematic literature review of prevalence and association with non-specific low back pain. Eur Spine J 2008;17(11):1407.

38. Järvinen J, Karppinen J, Niinimäki J, et al. Association between changes in lumbar Modic changes and low back symptoms over a two-year period. BMC Muscoskel Disord 2015;16(1):98.

39. Dudli S, Sing DC, Hu SS, et al. ISSLS PRIZE IN BASIC SCIENCE 2017: Intervertebral disc/bone marrow cross-talk with Modic changes. Eur Spine J 2017;26(5):1362–73.

40. Pang H, Bow C, Cheung JPY, et al. The UTE Disc Sign on MRI. SPINE 2018;43(7):503–11.

41. Zehra U, Bow C, Cheung JPY, et al. The association of lumbar intervertebral disc calcification on plain radiographs with the UTE Disc Sign on MRI. Eur Spine J 2018;27(5):1049–57.

42. Ji Z, Li Y, Dou W, et al. Ultra-short echo time MR imaging in assessing cartilage endplate damage and relationship between its lesion and disc degeneration for chronic low back pain patients. BMC Med Imag 2023;23(1):60.

43. Wang Y-XJ, Zhao F, Griffith JF, et al. T1rho and T2 relaxation times for lumbar disc degeneration: an in vivo comparative study at 3.0-Tesla MRI. Eur Radiol 2013;23(1):228–34.

44. Borthakur A, Maurer PM, Fenty M, et al. T1ρ Magnetic Resonance Imaging and Discography Pressure as Novel Biomarkers for Disc Degeneration and Low Back Pain. Spine 2011;36(25):2190–6.

45. Blumenkrantz G, Zuo J, Li X, et al. In vivo 3.0-tesla magnetic resonance T1ρ and T2 relaxation mapping in subjects with intervertebral disc degeneration and clinical symptoms. Magn Reson Med 2010;63(5): 1193–200.

46. Wada T, Togao O, Tokunaga C, et al. Glycosaminoglycan chemical exchange saturation transfer in human lumbar intervertebral discs: Effect of saturation pulse and relationship with low back pain. J Magn Reson Imag 2017;45(3):863–71.

47. Moon CH, Jacobs L, Kim J-H, et al. Part 2. Spine 2012;37(18):E1113–9.

48. Bonnheim NB, Wang L, Lazar AA, et al. The contributions of cartilage endplate composition and vertebral bone marrow fat to intervertebral disc degeneration in patients with chronic low back pain. Eur Spine J 2022;31(7):1866–72.

49. Wu L-L, Liu L-H, Rao S-X, et al. Ultrashort time-to-echo T2* and T2* relaxometry for evaluation of lumbar disc degeneration: a comparative study. BMC Muscoskel Disord 2022;23(1):524.

50. Wei Z, Lombardi AF, Lee RR, et al. Comprehensive assessment of in vivo lumbar spine intervertebral discs using a 3D adiabatic T 1ρ prepared ultrashort echo time (UTE-Adiab-T 1ρ) pulse sequence. Quant Imag Med Surg 2021. https://doi.org/10.21037/qims-21-308.

51. Fischgrund JS, Rhyne A, Macadaeg K, et al. Long-term outcomes following intraosseous basivertebral nerve ablation for the treatment of chronic low back pain: 5-year treatment arm results from a prospective randomized double-blind sham-controlled multi-center study. Eur Spine J 2020;29(8):1925–34.

52. Sloan SR, Lintz M, Hussain I, et al. Biologic Annulus Fibrosus Repair: A Review of Preclinical In Vivo Investigations. Tissue Eng Part B 2018;24(3):179–90.

Magnetic Resonance Neurography of the Lumbosacral Plexus

Jenifer Pitman, MD[a],*, Yenpo Lin, MD[b,c], Ek Tsoon Tan, PhD[b],
Darryl Sneag, MD[b]

KEYWORDS

• Magnetic resonance neurography • Lumbosacral plexus • MRI techniques • Peripheral nerves

KEY POINTS

• Protocols for magnetic resonance neurography in the lumbosacral plexus should be customized to optimize imaging of the nerve in question, with the radiologist preferably remaining involved throughout the examination.

• A combination of 2-dimensional high-resolution anatomic (proton density–weighted) and T2-weighted fast spin-echo sequences and 3-dimensional high-resolution isotropic sequences allow for optimal nerve visualization and assessment.

• Gadolinium contrast can highlight nerve pathology in the setting of tumor, entrapment, and inflammatory neuropathies.

• Dixon or dual-echo steady-state free precession type fat suppression is preferred for higher signal-to-noise ratio, although short-tau inversion recovery may be useful when more homogeneous fat suppression is not achievable.

• When imaging around metal, 3T often remains preferable to maintain the highest resolution possible, but the use of 1.5 T may be necessary if the nerve in question is in close proximity to hardware.

INTRODUCTION

Low back, pelvic, and lower extremity pain and weakness are ubiquitous issues that present a diagnostic challenge for referring clinicians and radiologists. The complex anatomy of the lumbosacral plexus (LSP) and overlapping clinical presentations often make it difficult to pinpoint the precise site of pathology. Electrodiagnostic testing of the LSP is difficult due to a relative paucity of reliable sites for nerve conduction velocity studies and deep-seated muscles difficult to access by needle electromyography.[1]

Magnetic resonance neurography (MRN) is still evolving as a technique to evaluate the LSP, but technical advances over the past decade have significantly improved its diagnostic utility.[2] This article will first review normal LSP anatomy. Specific technical considerations for MRN, particularly as they relate to branch nerves off the plexus, will then be discussed. Lastly, the authors will review a select range of pathologies affecting the LSP, focusing on those most likely to necessitate adjustments to standard protocols to optimize diagnostic yield.

ANATOMY

Lower motor neurons originate from the anterior horns of the spinal cord and then exit as ventral nerve roots to combine with the dorsal nerve roots and form spinal nerves.[3] Spinal nerves then divide

[a] Musculoskeletal Imaging, Department of Radiology, Johns Hopkins Hospital, 601 N Caroline Street, 3rd Floor, Baltimore, MD, USA; [b] Radiology Department, Hospital For Special Surgery, 535 East 70th Street, 3rd Floor, New York, NY, USA; [c] Department of Medical Imaging and Intervention, Chang Gung Memorial Hospital, Taoyuan, Taiwan
* Corresponding author.
E-mail address: jenifer.pitman@gmail.com

Radiol Clin N Am 62 (2024) 229–245
https://doi.org/10.1016/j.rcl.2023.09.008

into dorsal and ventral rami. Dorsal rami supply the paraspinal musculature and ventral rami provide sensory and motor innervation to the pelvis and lower extremities. The LSP comprises separate lumbar and sacral plexi, with some fibers of the lumbar plexus providing contributions to the sacral plexus via the lumbosacral (LS) trunk.[3] The lumbar plexus is formed from the ventral rami of the L1 to L4 nerves, with a small contribution from the T12 nerve root or subcostal nerve (**Fig. 1**). The LS trunk, comprising L4 and L5 ventral rami contributions, joins with the S1 to S3 nerve roots along the anterior aspect of the piriformis muscle to form the sacral plexus.

Within the lumbar plexus, the iliohypogastric (L1, with variable contribution from T12), ilioinguinal (L1, with variable contribution from T12), and genitofemoral (L1–L2) nerves branch directly from the ventral rami. The remaining ventral rami divide into anterior (L2–L5) and posterior (L2–L4) divisions. The posterior divisions give rise to the lateral femoral cutaneous (L2–L3, **Fig. 2**), and femoral (L2–L4, see **Fig. 2**) nerves, which exit lateral to the psoas muscle along with the nerves arising from the ventral rami.[3] The anterior divisions give

rise to the obturator nerve (L2–L4, see **Fig. 2**) and the lumbar plexus' contribution to the lumbosacral trunk (L4–L5), which exit medial to the psoas muscle.[3] (**Table 1**)

Branches of the sacral plexus include the sciatic nerve, inferior and superior gluteal nerves, and the pudendal nerve.[3] The anterior divisions of the L4 to S2 ventral rami form the tibial component of the sciatic nerve, while the posterior divisions of the L4 to S2 ventral rami, inclusive of the LS trunk, form the common peroneal component of the sciatic nerve (see **Fig. 2**). The superior (L4–S1) and inferior gluteal (S1–S2) nerves arise from the posterior divisions of their respective ventral rami prior to formation of the sciatic nerve. The anterior divisions of S2 to S4 also give rise to the pudendal nerve, and the posterior femoral nerve is formed from anterior divisions of S2 to S4 and a contribution from the posterior division of S1.[3] (see **Table 1**)

The coccygeal plexus consists of a network of nerves arising from the ventral rami of the S4 to C1 nerve roots, as well as the dorsal rami of the sacral sympathetic trunk, which converge in the region of the iliococcygeus muscle. This plexus

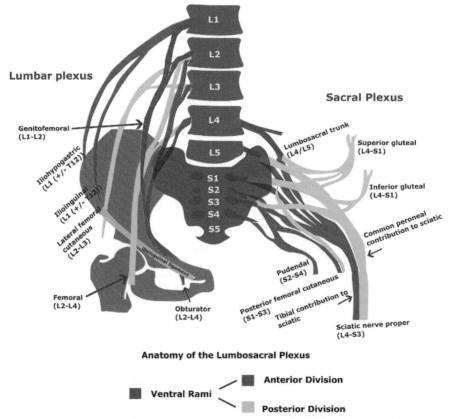

Anatomy of the Lumbosacral Plexus

Fig. 1. Diagram of the lumbosacral plexus and main branch root origins. Image components are not drawn to scale.

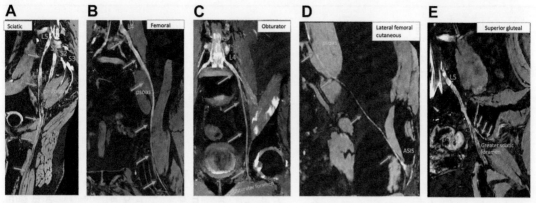

Fig. 2. 3-dimensional double-echo steady-state (DESS)-curved multiplanar reconstruction images show normal appearance of selected nerves of the lumbosacral plexus.

supplies the vertebrae and coccygeal muscles as well as the sacrospinous, sacrotuberous, and coccygeal ligaments, and the periosteum. Ano-coccygeal nerves, which supply the subcutaneous tissues around the coccyx, are also part of the coccygeal plexus[4] but are not typically visible on MRN (see **Table 1**).

TECHNICAL CONSIDERATIONS
General Protocol Considerations and Pulse Sequences

Technological progress, namely higher field strength, multichannel receiver coils, and accelerated imaging techniques, has contributed to improvement in MRN.[2,5] Imaging at 3.0 T is favored given almost double the signal-to-noise ratio (SNR) compared to 1.5 T, which enables higher spatial resolution for a given acquisition time.[6,7] For LSP evaluation, the authors recommend a spine posterior array coil and an anterior (16–30 channel) surface array flexible coil wrapped around the lumbar-pelvic region.

MRN protocols used at the authors' institution typically include 2-dimensional (2-D) high-resolution axial intermediate-weighted (~0.2–0.5 mm in-plane) and fat-suppressed fluid-sensitive (~0.4–0.8 mm in-plane) sequences obtained with slice thicknesses of 3 to 4.5 mm (**Tables 2** and **3**). A 3-dimensional (3-D) sequence such as short tau inversion recovery-fast spin echo (STIR-FSE) or steady-state free precession (SSFP) sequence such as dual-echo SSFP (DESS) may be added. Although the primary purpose of the MRN examination is not to evaluate the lumbar spine itself (ie, canal/foramina), it is important to assess this region (particularly if a dedicated lumbar spine MRI is not concurrently performed), as spine-related abnormalities are more common than primary nerve pathology.[8] Incorporating a

single, isotropic T2-weighted 3-D FSE sequence of the spine with deep learning reconstruction can thus be considered.[9]

Prior clinical notes and results of electrodiagnostic testing, if performed, should be reviewed in advance to cater the MRN protocol to the clinical question(s). Close communication between the examining clinician and radiologist is crucial in accurately identifying the target of investigation, as patient-reported symptoms alone can be non-localizing. A radiologist experienced in MRN is recommended to oversee the examination in real time. The technologist's interactions with the patient are also critical for ensuring a successful study; these include recording the patient's most symptomatic site (and as indicated, placing a skin marker over the site of pain or surgical scar), coaching the patient to remain still during image acquisition, and breathing regularly. In the authors' experience, it is helpful to empty the urinary bladder to reduce flow-related motion artifact, particularly with SSFP sequences (**Fig. 3**).

2-dimensional versus 3-dimensional imaging
2-D T2-weighted sequences typically enable higher in-plane spatial resolution (~0.4–0.8 mm), although at the expense of lower through-plane spatial resolution. 3-D MRN enables higher through-plane isotropic resolution (~0.9–1.2 mm), which in turn accommodates multiplanar reformations to better depict the curvilinear trajectories, and pathologic changes, of nerves.[10,11] To optimize 3-D MRN using STIR-FSE, the flip angle train can be adjusted to balance between relaxation-induced signal loss and blurring effects.[12] Utilizing acceleration techniques like parallel imaging or compressed sensing can be helpful to mitigate the long scan time inherent to 3-D imaging.[13]

3-D diffusion-weighted time-reversed fast imaging with SSFP (PSIF) and DESS are T2-weighted

Table 1
Innervation, root origins, anatomic course, and common mechanisms of injury of the lumbosacral plexus

| | | Lumbosacral Plexus Nerve Innervation | | | |
| | | Innervation | | | |
Nerve	Root Origins	Muscular	Sensory Distribution	Course	Common mechanism/Site of injury
Iliohypogastric	L1, ± T12	Lower fibers transverse abdominis, internal oblique	Blue-lateral gluteal region and skin superior to the pubis	• Courses anteroinferiorly along anterior border quadratus lumborum • Penetrates posterior fascia of transversus abdominis superior to posterior iliac crest. • Courses parallel and above iliac crest between transversus abdominis and internal oblique • Separates into abdominal and genital terminal branches	Iatrogenic-abdominal surgeries
Ilioinguinal	L1, ± T12	Lower fibers transverse abdominis, internal oblique	Green-pubic symphysis, superior and medial aspect femoral triangle, root of penis and anterior scrotum/mons pubis and labia majora Yellow-femoral branch-thigh adjacent to inguinal ligament and surrounding femoral triangle	• Parallel and inferior to iliohypogastric • Pierces lower border internal oblique • Passes anterior to spermatic cord into superficial inguinal ring • Traverses psoas muscle from posterior to anterior at L3-L4 • Runs along anterior psoas deep to peritoneum/transversalis fascia • Bifurcates into genital and femoral branches • Genital branch pierces transversalis and spermatic fascia, then passes through internal inguinal ring along dorsal aspect of spermatic cord (round ligament in females)	Latrogenic-abdominal surgeries Iatrogenic-abdominal surgeries, iliac bone graft harvest

Nerve	Roots	Motor	Sensory	Course	Etiology
Genitofemoral	L1–L2	Cremaster	Pink-genital branch-spermatic cord and scrotum/labia majora	• Femoral branch courses with external iliac artery beneath inguinal ligament, entering femoral sheath lateral and superficial to femoral artery.	
Lateral femoral cutaneous	L2–L3	None	Purple-anterior and lateral thigh	• Travels anteroinferiorly across superficial aspect of iliacus muscle toward anterior superior iliac spine • Pierces, passes deep to, or courses laterally around inguinal ligament • Runs in fat plane between sartorius and tensor fascia lata • Divides into anterior and posterior branches	Obesity, tight belts Iatrogenic-iliac bone graft harvest, psoas muscle traction, compression against ASIS in spine surgery
Femoral	L2–L4	Quadriceps, pectineus, sartorius, psoas, iliacus	Purple-upper and anterior thigh, hip and knee joints	• Descends between psoas and iliacus muscles, deep to inguinal ligament into femoral triangle (most lateral structure) • Divides into anterior and posterior divisions ~4 cm distal to inguinal ligament. • Posterior divisions continue into lower leg as saphenous nerve.	Intrapelvic-iatrogenic-pelvic/hip/gynecologic surgery (ie, hysterectomy) Mass/collection/hematoma along iliopsoas Extrapelvic-distal to inguinal ligament
Obturator	L2–L4	Adductor magnus, adductor brevis, adductor longus, obturator externus, pectineus, gracilis	Green-medial and distal thigh	• Courses along iliopectineal line, descending through psoas muscle fibers into pelvis • Emerges from medial border of psoas near the pelvic brim • Courses along lateral pelvic sidewall, posterior to common iliac artery, then lateral to internal iliac artery distal ureter, then anterior to obturator vessels • Passes through obturator canal into medial thigh	Iatrogenic prolonged lithotomy position, traction during THA, pelvic surgery Entrapment-within obturator canal or near pubic symphysis

(continued on next page)

Table 1
(continued)

Lumbosacral Plexus Nerve Innervation

Nerve	Root Origins	Innervation — Muscular	Sensory Distribution	Course	Common mechanism/ Site of injury
				• Near obturator, canal, branches into anterior and posterior divisions • Anterior division passes between pectineus branch abd adductor longus, then between adductor longus and brevis and terminates as cutaneous branch of obturator nerve • Posterior division passes between adductor brevis and magnus; Also send articular branches to the hip and knee.	
Sciatic	L4–S3	Biceps femoris, semitendinosus, semimembranosus, adductor magnus	Orange, green, and blue-gluteal region, posterior thigh, perineum, hip joint, popliteal fossa, lower leg except medial portion	• Exits pelvis through greater sciatic foramen, most commonly inferior to piriformis • Pudendal nerve and vessels course with the nerve through greater sciatic notch • Nerve courses through posterior compartment of the thigh deep to long head biceps femoris	Iatrogenic-posterior approach THA Compression-by hematoma/ paralabral cyst
Nerve to quadratus femoris	L4–S1	Quadratus femoris, inferior gemellus	None	• Exits pelvis through greater sciatic foramen, below piriformis and anterior to sciatic nerve	Intrapelvic masses

Nerve	Roots	Motor	Sensory	Course	Pathology
Nerve to obturator internus	L5–S2	Obturator internus, superior gemellus (± inferior gemellus)	None	• Exits pelvis through greater sciatic foramen, below piriformis, between posterior cutaneous nerve of the thigh and pudendal nerve • Courses lateral to ischial spine, re-enters pelvis through lesser sciatic foramen	Intrapelvic masses
Nerve to piriformis	S2±,S1,L5	Piriformis	None	• Remains intrapelvic, supplies piriformis by piercing anterior surface	Intrapelvic masses
Pudendal	S2–S4	Urinary bladder and rectal sphincters	External genitalia	• Courses through greater sciatic foramen superiorly, above piriformis • Passes along posterior aspect of ischial spine superficial to coccygeus muscle within pudendal canal • Re-enters pelvis via lesser sciatic foramen • Gives off inferior rectal nerve followed by perineal nerve and dorsal nerve of the penis/clitoris	Entrapment–Within Alcock's canal, often in cyclists
Superior gluteal	L4–S1	Gluteus medius, gluteus minimus, tensor fascia lata	None	• Exits pelvis through greater sciatic foramen superiorly, above piriformis • Courses between gluteus medius and minimus muscles • Divides into superior and inferior branches	Iatrogenic–iliosacral screw placement Posttraumatic productive changes in sacrum/greater sciatic notch
Inferior gluteal	L4–S1	Gluteus maximus	None	• Exits pelvis through greater sciatic foramen, below piriformis and medial to sciatic nerve	Iatrogenic–lateral or anterolateral approach THA Posttraumatic productive changes in sacrum/greater sciatic notch

(continued on next page)

Table 1
(continued)

Nerve	Root Origins	Innervation		Course	Common mechanism/ Site of injury
		Muscular	**Sensory Distribution**		
Posterior femoral cutaneous	S1–S3	None	Skin of posterior thigh, buttock, posterior scrotum/labia	• Exits pelvis through greater sciatic foramen, below piriformis • Descends superficial to long head biceps femurs, deep to fascia lata, giving three branches • Cutaneous branch courses midline along posterior thigh, deep to fascia lata, superficial to hamstrings • Gluteal branch = inferior cluneal nerve Perineal branch, courses medially between gracilis and fascia lata	Referred pain—from within pelvis Compression—often in cyclists

Lumbosacral Plexus Nerve Innervation

Table 2
Recommended protocol parameters for lumbosacral plexus magnetic resonance neurography at 3.0 T

Parameters	2-D IW-FSE	2-D T2-w-FSE	Oblique 2-D T2-w-FSE	3-D DESS	3-D STIR-FSE
			Sequence Types		
Imaging plane(s)	axial; axial oblique	axial, coronal or sagittal	oblique sagittal	coronal or oblique	coronal
TR/TE/TI (ms)	3500–6000/30/-	3500–6000/80/-	8660/80/-	14.7/5.1–9.7/-	3300/80/250
FOV (cm)	29–32	28–30	20	30–32	30–32
Matrix size (FE × PE)	512 × 320	320 × 192	320 × 192	356 × 356	288 × 288
Slice thickness/ gap (mm)	4.5/0.0	4.5/0.0 (axial) 3.0/0.0 (coronal)	2.5/0.0	0.9/0.0	1.2/0.0
Echo train length	10	15	17	-	130
Bandwidth (Hz/pixel)	195	391 (axial) 521 (coronal)	521	234	347
Fat suppression technique	-	Dixon	Dixon	Water-excitation	STIR
Parallel imaging factor (PE × SE)	1.75	1–1.5	1–1.5	2 × 1–1.5	1.5 × 1
Scan time (min)	3–5	4–6	6–8	5–6	5–6

Abbreviations: DESS, dual-echo steady-state; FE, frequency encoding; FOV, field of view; FSE, fast/turbo spin echo; IW, intermediate-weighted; PE, phase encoding; SE, slice encoding; STIR, short-tau inversion recovery; TI, inversion time; TR/TE, repetition time/echo time.

and utilize diffusion gradients to dephase vascular signal and provide predominantly T2 contrast which depicts nerve pathology well.[14] They are commonly acquired with water excitation for fat suppression and diffusion-sensitizing gradients for vascular suppression.[15,16] Multi-echo in steady-state acquisition (MENSA), a type of DESS sequence, simultaneously acquires 2 SSFP echoes, in which the first echo, from free induction decay, has higher signal but less T2-weighting, and the second echo has lower signal but higher T2-weighting and less vascular contamination. The 2 images can either be combined to generate a single image[17] or

evaluated individually. In the authors' experience, the second echo, alone, is most relevant for MRN due to its greater T2-weighting and vascular suppression. Field inhomogeneity may be a concern in cases of suboptimal shimming and larger craniocaudal coverage (>15 cm). Additionally, the diffusion gradients in PSIF and DESS and spoiler gradients in FSE are sensitive to bulk motion, which can cause signal loss.[18] In the authors' experience, the SSFP technique is preferable to STIR-FSE for 3-D imaging in the authors' practice as higher spatial resolution (~0.9 mm) may be attained than with STIR-FSE (~1.1–1.2 mm) for the same scan time,

Table 3
Common 2-dimensional and 3-dimensional imaging options on major vendors

	GE	Siemens	Philips
2-D T2-weighted fat-suppressed		FLEX	Dixon	mDixon
3-D nerve selective sequence	3-D isotropic fast/turbo spin echo and STIR	CUBE-STIR	SPACE -STIR	VISTA-STIR and SHINKEI
	Steady-state	SSFP	PSIF	PSIF
	DESS	MENSA	DESS	DESS

Abbreviations: DESS, dual-echo steady-state; MENSA, multi-echo in steady-state acquisition; PSIF, time-reversed fast imaging with steady-state free precession; SHINKEI, nerve-sheath signal increased with inked rest-tissue rare imaging; SPACE, sampling perfection with application optimized contrasts using different flip angle evolution; SSFP, steady-state free precession; STIR, short-tau inversion recovery; VISTA, volume isotropic turbo spin echo acquisition.

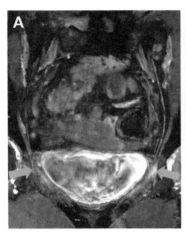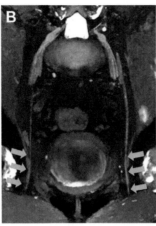

Fig. 3. The effect of bladder voiding on 3-dimensional double-echo steady-state (DESS) images in 2 different patients. Coronal maximal intensity projection (MIP) image (A) in a 57-year-old woman depicts the obturator nerve segments within the obturator canal obscured amidst significant phase ghost artifact from motion of the filled bladder (arrows). Coronal MIP image (B) in a postvoided 77-year-old male shows improved conspicuity of the bilateral obturator nerves (arrows).

and images are sharper due to lower interecho spacing with SSFP sequences. However, STIR-FSE may provide increased T2-weighting and superior fat suppression, especially in the presence of metallic implants.[19]

A type of 3-D STIR-FSE, SHINKEI (nerve-SHeath signal increased with INKed rest-tissue RARE Imaging) uses spectral adiabatic inversion recovery for fat suppression and improved motion-sensitized driven-equilibrium (iMSDE) for vascular suppression.[20] iMSDE improves SNR by utilizing an extra refocusing pulse and 2 extra gradients in addition to the motion sensitization gradients used in traditional MSDE. While SHINKEI may have superior conspicuity of LSP small branches and increased nerve SNRs compared to 3-D STIR-FSE, banding artifacts may occur.[20]

Fat suppression

Nerve abnormalities demonstrate T2 hyperintensity on MRN and this is thought to be related to impeded axoplasmic flow, increased endoneurial fluid, and/or perineurial edema.[21] Fat suppression improves nerve contrast-to-background ratio as peripheral nerves course along fat planes and both fat and nerves are T2 hyperintense on FSE imaging.[22] Typically robust suppression techniques in the LSP include nonspectrally selective STIR and chemical shift imaging (Dixon).[23] STIR offers uniform fat suppression, but at lower SNR.[24] The Dixon fat-water separation technique is favored for its higher SNR.[23] A "2-point" Dixon acquires images at 2 different echo times in which the precession of fat relative to water is at opposite phases.[25] By providing "water" and "fat" images, additional evaluation can be made with regard to active or chronic muscle denervation by edema or fatty infiltration, respectively. Fat-water swapping artifacts can sometimes occur; thus, retaining "fat" images for comparison is important.[26–28]

Bowel and respiratory motion

Bowel motion is a challenge in LSP MRN. Several strategies can be employed although they are not routinely done in practice. First, patients can be advised to fast (typically for 4 hours) prior to the examination to minimize bowel content. Conducting imaging in the prone position, as commonly used in magnetic resonance enterography, could aid in compressing bowel loops, thereby mitigating peristalsis and minimizing motion from the anterior abdominal wall.[27] In addition, the use of antispasmodic agents such as glucagon or hyoscine butylbromide prior to the scan can reduce bowel motility. Finally, swapping phase-encoding and frequency-encoding directions may mitigate motion through a specific region, at the expense of lengthened scan time.

Respiratory motion can degrade image quality through motion and ghosting artifacts, especially when evaluating the lower thoracic (T12) and upper lumbar nerve roots (L1–L2) near the diaphragm. The use of intermittent breath-holding in LSP is considered impractical due to the lengthy scan time of T2-weighted sequences.[28] Prospective respiratory gating is frequently employed in brachial plexus MRN but its use in the LSP MRN has not been thoroughly evaluated.[28] Occasionally, radial k-spaced sampling imaging techniques, such as PROPELLER (Periodically Rotated Overlapping ParallEL Lines with Enhanced Reconstruction) or BLADE, are used to mitigate motion artifact but due to their oversampling scheme, these typically involve longer acquisition times.[29]

Use of gadolinium contrast

Conditions which result in breakdown of the blood-nerve barrier will result in the enhancement of peripheral nerves. Examples include diffuse processes such as diabetic and inflammatory neuropathies and traumatic nerve injury involving the perineurium and endoneurial vessels, which are the main components of the blood-nerve barrier.[30] At the authors' institution, postcontrast imaging is often employed when an inflammatory neuropathy is considered, a mass requires further characterization, or for delineation of postoperative granulation tissue that may entrap nerves.[31] (**Fig. 4**)

The use of intravenous contrast agents can also aid in vascular suppression, especially for evaluation of small nerve branches as accompanying hyperintense vascular structures can impede visualization.[32] By using gadolinium, both T1 and T2 signals of blood are shortened, which allows for suppression of vascular signal after applying an inversion pulse. This technique has proven to be useful in MRN of both the brachial plexus and LSP.[33–35]

Imaging around metal

Susceptibility effect from indwelling metallic hardware can degrade image quality and hinder interpretation, but several mitigating techniques, previously summarized by Sneag and colleagues, are often successful.[33] As mentioned earlier, LSP MRN performed at 3.0 is still preferable for higher SNR and better spatial resolution, unless the susceptibility effect specifically obscures the targeted

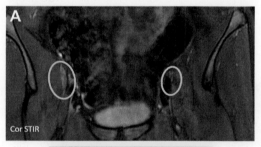
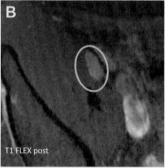

Fig. 4. Femoral nerve perineurioma in a 15-year-old girl with right thigh atrophy for 1 year prior to imaging. Large–field of view coronal short-tau inversion recovery (STIR) (*A*) and oblique axial T2 Dixon fat sat postcontrast images (*B*) demonstrate focal enlargement and homogeneous enhancement of the femoral nerve within the pelvis. In (*A*) the contralateral femoral nerve is also shown for comparison.

nerve at 3.0 T, in which case it may be necessary to (re)image the patient at 1.5 T. Particularly when metal is present, it is critically important for real-time monitoring by a radiologist to ensure a diagnostic examination (**Fig. 5**).

Other considerations

The application of diffusion tensor imaging (DTI) in the LSP has also been evaluated with proposed acquisition parameters including a b-value of 600 to 800 and 15 to 20 directions at 3.0 T.[34–36] However, the small size of many peripheral nerves (<5 mm) compared to the typical spatial resolution achievable with DTI ($\sim$1.5 mm in-plane, 2–4 mm through-plane) poses a challenge. Additionally, image distortion and accompanying blood vessels compromise contrast resolution and hinder accurate DTI tractography.[34,35,37] Currently, quantitative DTI measurements such as apparent diffusion coefficient, fractional anisotropy, and derivative visualization with diffusion tractography have focused on assessing the nerve roots and the larger sciatic nerve in research settings.[34,38,39]

Deep learning (DL) can improve MRN by denoising, minimizing artifacts, and reconstructing under-sampled data in sequences acquired with acceleration techniques.[40,41] Application in LSP MRN can improve 2-D images by increasing the conspicuity of the outer epineurium and fascicular architecture, two important features to evaluate when determining presence and severity of peripheral nerve injury.[42] Recently, DL reconstruction has been used in 3-D MRN of the LSP to improve visibility of nerve branches, resulting in higher diagnostic confidence.[43] (**Fig. 6**)

Specific Protocols for Common Lumbosacral Plexus MRI Examinations and Selected Examples of Pathology

Lumbosacral plexus and sciatic nerve

The authors' standard protocol for imaging the LSP and sciatic nerve begins with a large–field of view (FOV) (28–30 cm) bilateral axial 2-D proton density (PD)–weighted sequence, followed by bilateral axial and coronal Dixon fat-suppression techniques, with the coronal sequences plotted from the level of the lumbar neural foramina extending posteriorly to include the sciatic nerves. A unilateral, smaller FOV (18–20 cm), oblique-sagittal, T2-weighted Dixon fat-suppressed sequence is then acquired to more clearly delineate fascicular detail. This latter sequence is plotted off the coronal, orthogonally to the side of the lower LS plexus/sciatic nerve of interest. PD-weighted sequences are preferred to T1 as the former provides equivalent to higher spatial resolution in addition to improved contrast

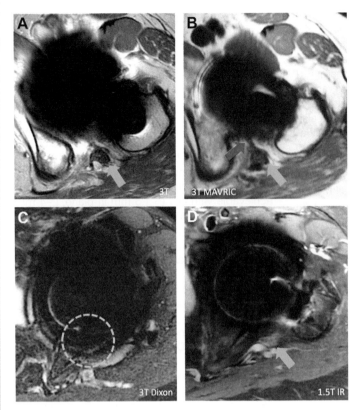

Fig. 5. Comparison of different magnetic resonance techniques in a 74-year-old woman presenting with left drop foot after left total hip arthroplasty 1 year earlier. Axial 3.0-T intermediate-weighted image (A) shows preserved fascicular architecture of the left sciatic nerve with tented morphology (blue arrow). Axial 3.0-T intermediate-weighted multi-acquisition variable-resonance image combination (MAVRIC) (B) allows for improved evaluation of structures surrounding the arthroplasty, with linear low signal intensity scar/granulation tissue (red arrow), tethering the sciatic nerve (blue arrow) to the posterior pseudocapsule and resultant anterior deviation of the nerve from its expected course. Axial 3.0-T Dixon water image (C) shows the nerve was obscured by artifact (circle). Axial 1.5-T inversion recovery image (D) allows visualization of the hyperintense and mildly swollen sciatic nerve (blue arrow).

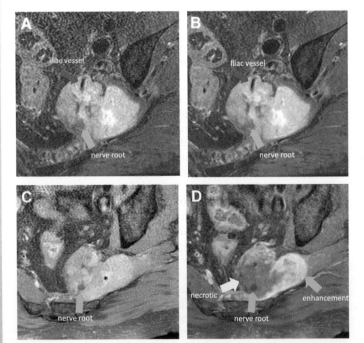

Fig. 6. Deep learning reconstruction and contrast enhancement techniques in a 61-year-old male with an intramuscular solid mass within the left piriformis. Axial T2-weighted Dixon water image processed with deep learning reconstruction (DLRecon) (B) demonstrates superior image quality and denoising as compared to the same images processed with the standard reconstruction method (A). Encasement of the left internal iliac vessels (red arrows) and left S3 nerve root (blue arrows) are also demonstrated. Avid-enhancing and necrotic components are more conspicuous on the postcontrast axial T1 fat-suppressed image (D) as compared to the precontrast image (C). Intrinsic T1 hyperintensity within the mass (asterisk, C) may reflect hemorrhage.

resolution, given longer echo times that contribute to a degree of T2-weighting.

The sciatic nerve may be injured following various types of traumatic injury, including hamstring tear. In the acute setting, hemorrhage and edema may extend around the sciatic nerve within the thigh. With time, scarring may lead to mass effect upon the nerve and/or tethering (**Fig. 7**). The sciatic nerve is also susceptible to iatrogenic injury during intrapelvic operations and posterior approach hip arthroplasty (**Fig. 8**). The tibial and common peroneal nerve contributions are frequently topographically visible as separate bundles, with the common peroneal component positioned anterolateral relative to the tibial component. As such, injury to the nerve may be localized to either of these components, more commonly the common peroneal, in which case the patient may present with a foot drop.

Processes involving the LSP more diffusely include inflammatory hypertrophic neuropathies such as Charcot-Marie-Tooth and chronic inflammatory demyelinating polyneuropathy, and post-radiation changes (**Fig. 9**).

Femoral and obturator nerves

Imaging protocols follow those for the LSP and sciatic nerve; however, coronal coverage instead extends from the neural foramina anteriorly to include these nerves. A 3-D gradient-echo–based fat-suppressed technique, such as DESS, is frequently added at the radiologist's discretion to evaluate for subtle abnormalities of either nerve. The femoral nerve may be injured following direct anterior and anterolateral approaches for total hip arthroplasty, which may place excessive retraction on the femoral nerve or result in postoperative perineural scarring.

The obturator nerve may be compressed during surgery secondary to prolonged time spent in the lithotomy position, or in pelvic trauma related to impingement by displaced fracture fragments in the acute setting, or later by heterotopic bone formation. It is also susceptible to excessive retraction in medial approach hip surgeries such as the modified Stoppa technique.[44]

Lateral femoral cutaneous nerve

The lateral femoral cutaneous nerve (LFCN) arises from the posterior divisions of the L2 and L3 nerve roots, surfaces along the psoas major, and travels anterior to the iliacus muscle before exiting the pelvis medial to the anterior superior iliac spine (ASIS). The coronal coverage of the LFCN typically extends from the upper margin of the third lumbar vertebra (L3) to the lesser trochanter of the femur. Although there are anatomic variations of the course of the LFCN, this nerve is frequently vulnerable to injuries and compression where it pierces the inguinal ligament and courses anterior to the ASIS.[45,46] Thus, it is crucial to include the anterior skin and subcutaneous tissues in the imaging field in the evaluation of meralgia paresthetica, ie, mononeuropathy of the LFCN (**Fig. 10**). The recommended LFCN protocol is similar to the sciatic nerve except that oblique-sagittal scans are plotted orthogonal to the LFCN rather than the sciatic nerve. The oblique-sagittal scan employs a unilateral, smaller FOV, T2-weighted Dixon fat-suppressed sequence, focusing on the symptomatic side(s) and extending from the upper margin of L3 inferior to the level of the lesser trochanter. This nerve may also become injured during surgery or be compressed more proximally by a disc herniation. Another potential cause of injury is during iliac bone graft harvest, particularly

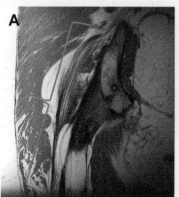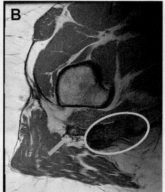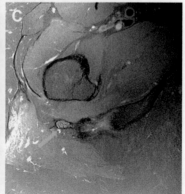

Fig. 7. 45-year-old woman with scar tethering of the sciatic nerve after hamstring repair 1 year prior. Coronal (*A*) and axial proton density–weighted (*B*), and axial T2 fat-saturated (FS) (*C*) sequences show dense circumferential perineural scar (*blue arrows*) surrounding the right sciatic nerve (*bracket, A*). Postsurgical changes related to the hamstring repair are also seen (*orange circle, B*). The fascicular architecture and signal intensity of the nerve are maintained.

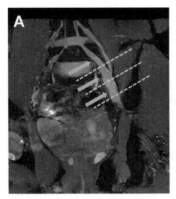
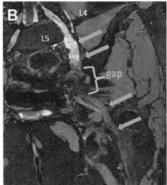
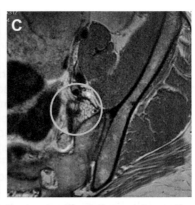

Fig. 8. 38-year-old woman with left foot drop after excision of a rectal tailgut cyst, with sciatic nerve transection. Straight coronal multi-echo in steady-state acquisition (MENSA) maximal intensity projection (MIP) (*A*), coronal curved multiplanar reconstruction (MPR) reformatted MENSA (*B*), and axial proton density–weighted images (*C*) demonstrate enlargement and signal hyperintensity of the proximal left sciatic nerve (*blue arrows*). In (*B*) the distal nerve is visible (*green arrows*), as is the gap. In (*A*), the plane of acquisition of oblique axial sequence perpendicular to the nerve's course (*orange grid lines*) is also seen.

when the nerve passes more laterally along the ilium.

Pudendal nerve

The course of the pudendal nerves (S2–S4) can be appreciated in the axial plane as they insinuate between the sacrospinous and sacrotuberous ligaments near the ischial spine before entering pudendal (Alcock's) canal, where nerve entrapments often occur. We typically employ axial and coronal nonfat-suppressed PD-weighted and T2-weighted Dixon sequences from the superior margin L5 vertebra, inferiorly to include the external genitalia. Additional nonfat-suppressed PD-weighted and T2-weighted Dixon sequences in an oblique axial plane are plotted off the

pubococcygeal line in the sagittal plane, connecting the inferior border of the symphysis pubis to the coccygeal joint. A unilateral, smaller FOV, oblique-sagittal scan is also plotted bilaterally to evaluate the extraforaminal sacral nerve root contributions to the pudendal nerve.

Imaging of the pudendal nerve is most commonly indicated at the authors' institution in the setting of chronic pelvic floor/perineal pain. In the absence of prior trauma or surgery, frequently no abnormal findings are detected as the nerve and its branches are difficult to visualize. However, postsurgical or posttraumatic scarring can occasionally be identified, and the nerve may be visible when abnormally enlarged and hyperintense (**Fig. 11**).

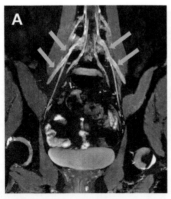
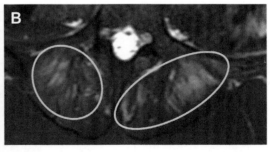

Fig. 9. Radiation plexitis: Magnetic resonance neurography (MRN) of the lumbosacral plexus (LSP) in a 45-year-old woman with bilateral lower extremity weakness and numbness after pelvic radiation for breast cancer metastases. Oblique coronal 3-dimensional multi-echo in steady-state acquisition (MENSA) (*A*) image demonstrates thickening and increased T2 signal within the L4 spinal nerves and dorsal root ganglion bilaterally, extending into the femoral nerves. T2 hyperintensity within the left greater than right dorsal paraspinal musculature is seen in axial short-tau inversion recover (STIR) image (*B*) reflecting radiation myositis.

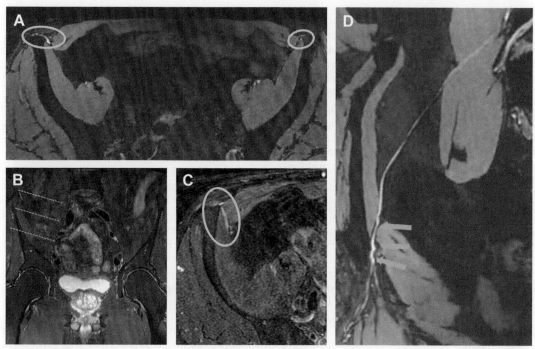

Fig. 10. A 78-year-old man with chronic burning along the right anterolateral thigh. (A) reformatted oblique axial multi-echo in steady-state acquisition (MENSA) from oblique coronal acquisition, (C) oblique sagittal T2 Dixon, and (D) MENSA curved multiplanar reconstruction (MPR) images demonstrate thickening and hyperintensity of the right lateral femoral cutaneous nerve along a short segment after the nerve passes into the thigh over the anterior superior iliac spine, and proximally within the intrapelvic portion. In (A), comparison to the contralateral, unaffected side is shown. (B) straight coronal T2 Dixon demonstrates plane of acquisition of oblique sagittal sequence (C) perpendicular to the nerve's course (orange grid lines).

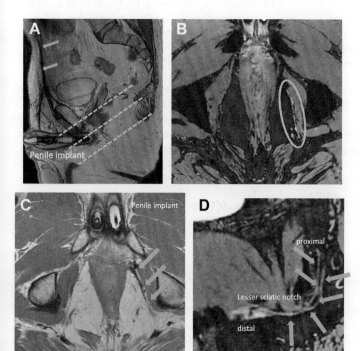

Fig. 11. A 58-year-old man with urinary bladder and penile pain after neuroma resection 1 year prior to imaging. Sagittal proton density (PD) (A) demonstrates dense scar along suprapenile tissues (blue arrows), as well as the plane of acquisition of oblique axial sequences perpendicular to the nerve's course (orange grid lines). Oblique axial PD (C) sequence demonstrates dense scar along the pudendal (Alcock's) canal (blue arrows) Thickening and signal hyperintensity of the pudendal nerve is demonstrated on oblique axial multi-echo in steady-state acquisition (MENSA) and curved multiplanar reconstruction (MPR) reformats (B, D) as the nerve re-enters the pelvis through the lesser sciatic notch. In (D), a vessel coursing with the nerve is also seen (green arrows).

SUMMARY

MRN is a useful tool in the workup of patients with sensorimotor disturbances of the pelvis and lower extremities. Technological improvements have increased image quality of MRN in recent years, particularly advances in gradient performance, coil technology, and sequence design to increase spatial and contrast resolution. Knowledge of the regional anatomy and familiarity with available techniques as well as the range of pathologies is important to maximize the diagnostic yield of LSP examinations.

CLINICS CARE POINTS

- Spine-related pathology is a more common cause of lower extremity nerve symptoms than primary nerve pathology in the LSP.
- Image quality may be improved by having patients empty their bladder prior to the examination.
- Due to its close proximity, the sciatic nerve is susceptible to injury/entrapment after hamstring tears as scar forms.
- The femoral and sciatic nerves may be injured iatrogenically during anterior and posterior approach hip arthroplasty, respectively.

DISCLOSURE

Hospital for Special Surgery maintains institutional research agreements with GE Healthcare and Siemens.

REFERENCES

1. Laughlin RS, Dyck PJB. Electrodiagnostic testing in lumbosacral plexopathies. Phys Med Rehabil Clin N Am 2013;24(1):93–105.
2. Sneag DB, Queler S. Technological Advancements in Magnetic Resonance Neurography. Curr Neurol Neurosci Rep 2019;19(10):75.
3. Liyew WA. Clinical Presentations of Lumbar Disc Degeneration and Lumbosacral Nerve Lesions. Int J Rheumatol 2020;2020:1–13.
4. Mostafa E, Varacallo M. Anatomy, Back, Coccygeal Vertebrae. In: StatPearls. Treasure Island FL: StatPearls Publishing; 2023.
5. Chhabra A, Flammang A, Padua A, et al. Magnetic Resonance Neurography Technical Considerations. Neuroimaging Clin N Am 2014;24(1):67–78.
6. Tagliafico A, Succio G, Emanuele Neumaier C, et al. MR imaging of the brachial plexus: comparison between 1.5-T and 3-T MR imaging: preliminary experience. Skeletal Radiol 2011;40(6):717–24.
7. Soher BJ, Dale BM, Merkle EM. A Review of MR Physics: 3T versus 1.5T. Magn Reson Imaging Clin N Am 2007;15(3):277–90.
8. Chazen JL, Cornman-Homonoff J, Zhao Y, et al. MR Neurography of the Lumbosacral Plexus for Lower Extremity Radiculopathy: Frequency of Findings, Characteristics of Abnormal Intraneural Signal, and Correlation with Electromyography. American Journal of Neuroradiology 2018;39(11):2154–60.
9. Sun S, Tan ET, Mintz DN, et al. Evaluation of deep learning reconstructed high-resolution 3D lumbar spine MRI. Eur Radiol 2022;32(9):6167–77.
10. Chhabra A, Rozen S, Scott K. Three-Dimensional MR Neurography of the Lumbosacral Plexus. Semin Musculoskelet Radiol 2015;19(02):149–59.
11. Sims GC, Boothe E, Joodi R, et al. 3D MR Neurography of the Lumbosacral Plexus: Obtaining Optimal Images for Selective Longitudinal Nerve Depiction. American Journal of Neuroradiology 2016;37(11):2158–62.
12. Cervantes B, Bauer JS, Zibold F, et al. Imaging of the lumbar plexus: Optimized refocusing flip angle train design for 3D TSE. J Magn Reson Imag 2016;43(4):789–99.
13. Aoike T, Fujima N, Yoneyama M, et al. Development of three-dimensional MR neurography using an optimized combination of compressed sensing and parallel imaging. Magn Reson Imaging 2022;87:32–7.
14. Chhabra A, Subhawong TK, Bizzell C, et al. 3T MR neurography using three-dimensional diffusion-weighted PSIF: technical issues and advantages. Skeletal Radiol 2011;40(10):1355–60.
15. Qin Y, Zhang J, Li P, et al. 3D Double-Echo Steady-State with Water Excitation MR Imaging of the Intraparotid Facial Nerve at 1.5T: A Pilot Study. American Journal of Neuroradiology 2011;32(7):1167–72.
16. Zhang Z, Meng Q, Chen Y, et al. 3-T imaging of the cranial nerves using three-dimensional reversed FISP with diffusion-weighted MR sequence. J Magn Reson Imag 2008;27(3):454–8.
17. Chavhan GB, Babyn PS, Jankharia BG, et al. Steady-State MR Imaging Sequences: Physics, Classification, and Clinical Applications1. Radiographics 2008;28(4):1147–60.
18. Gras V, Farrher E, Grinberg F, et al. Diffusion-weighted DESS protocol optimization for simultaneous mapping of the mean diffusivity, proton density and relaxation times at 3 Tesla. Magn Reson Med 2017;78(1):130–41.
19. Hu S, Li Y, Hou B, et al. Multi-echo in steady-state acquisition improves MRI image quality and lumbosacral radiculopathy diagnosis efficacy compared with T2 fast spin-echo sequence. Neuroradiology 2023;65(5):969–77.

20. Kasper JM, Wadhwa V, Scott KM, et al. SHINKEI—a novel 3D isotropic MR neurography technique: technical advantages over 3DIRTSE-based imaging. Eur Radiol 2015;25(6):1672–7.

21. Filler AG, Kliot M, Howe FA, et al. Application of magnetic resonance neurography in the evaluation of patients with peripheral nerve pathology. J Neurosurg 1996;85(2):299–309.

22. Delfaut EM, Beltran J, Johnson G, et al. Fat Suppression in MR Imaging: Techniques and Pitfalls. Radiographics 1999;19(2):373–82.

23. Grande F, Santini F, Herzka DA, et al. Fat-Suppression Techniques for 3-T MR Imaging of the Musculoskeletal System. Radiographics 2014;34(1):217–33.

24. Wang X, Greer JS, Dimitrov IE, et al. Frequency Offset Corrected Inversion Pulse for B0 and B1 Insensitive Fat Suppression at 3T: Application to MR Neurography of Brachial Plexus. J Magn Reson Imag 2018;48(4):1104–11.

25. Dixon WT. Simple proton spectroscopic imaging. Radiology 1984;153(1):189–94.

26. Hardy PA, Hinks RS, Tkach JA. Separation of fat and water in fast spin-echo MR imaging with the three-point dixon technique. J Magn Reson Imag 1995; 5(2):181–5.

27. Chatterji M, Fidler JL, Taylor SA, et al. State of the Art MR Enterography Technique. Top Magn Reson Imag 2021;30(1):3–11.

28. Sneag DB, Mendapara P, Zhu JC, et al. Prospective respiratory triggering improves high-resolution brachial plexus MRI quality. J Magn Reson Imag 2019;49(6):1723–9.

29. Pipe JG. Motion correction with PROPELLER MRI: Application to head motion and free-breathing cardiac imaging. Magn Reson Med 1999;42(5):963–9.

30. Neufeld EA, Shen PY, Nidecker AE, et al. MR Imaging of the Lumbosacral Plexus: A Review of Techniques and Pathologies. J Neuroimaging 2015; 25(5):691–703.

31. Endo Y, Miller TT, Sneag DB. Imaging of the Peripheral Nerves of the Lower Extremity. Radiol Clin North Am 2023;61(2):381–92.

32. Delaney H, Bencardino J, Rosenberg ZS. Magnetic Resonance Neurography of the Pelvis and Lumbosacral Plexus. Neuroimaging Clin N Am 2014; 24(1):127–50.

33. Sneag DB, Zochowski KC, Tan ET. MR Neurography of Peripheral Nerve Injury in the Presence of Orthopedic Hardware: Technical Considerations. Radiology 2021;300(2):246–59.

34. Foti G, Lombardo F, Fighera A, et al. Role of diffusion tensor imaging of sciatic nerve in symptomatic patients with inconclusive lumbar MRI. Eur J Radiol 2020;131:109249.

35. Chalian M, Chhabra A. Top-10 Tips for Getting Started with Magnetic Resonance Neurography. Semin Musculoskelet Radiol 2019;23(04):347–60.

36. Lemos N, Melo HJF, Sermer C, et al. Lumbosacral plexus MR tractography: A novel diagnostic tool for extraspinal sciatica and pudendal neuralgia? Magn Reson Imaging 2021;83:107–13.

37. Jeon T, Fung MM, Koch KM, et al. Peripheral nerve diffusion tensor imaging: Overview, pitfalls, and future directions. J Magn Reson Imag 2018;47(5): 1171–89.

38. Chhabra A, Kanchustambham P, Mogharrabi B, et al. MR Neurography of Lumbosacral Plexus: Incremental Value Over XR, CT, and MRI of L Spine With Improved Outcomes in Patients With Radiculopathy and Failed Back Surgery Syndrome. J Magn Reson Imag 2023;57(1):139–50.

39. Sakai T, Aoki Y, Watanabe A, et al. Functional Assessment of Lumbar Nerve Roots Using Coronal-plane Single-shot Turbo Spin-echo Diffusion Tensor Imaging. Magn Reson Med Sci 2020;19(2): 159–65.

40. Zhang K, Zuo W, Chen Y, et al. Beyond a Gaussian Denoiser: Residual Learning of Deep CNN for Image Denoising. IEEE Trans Image Process 2017;26(7): 3142–55.

41. Hammernik K, Klatzer T, Kobler E, et al. Learning a variational network for reconstruction of accelerated MRI data. Magn Reson Med 2018;79(6):3055–71.

42. Zochowski KC, Tan ET, Argentieri EC, et al. Improvement of peripheral nerve visualization using a deep learning-based MR reconstruction algorithm. Magn Reson Imaging 2022;85:186–92.

43. Ensle F, Kaniewska M, Tiessen A, et al. Diagnostic performance of deep learning–based reconstruction algorithm in 3D MR neurography. Skeletal Radiol 2023. https://doi.org/10.1007/s00256-023-04362-z.

44. Kim JW, Shon HC, Park JH. Injury of the obturator nerve in the modified Stoppa approach for acetabular fractures. Orthop Traumatol Surg Res 2017; 103(5):639–44.

45. de Ridder VA, de Lange S, Popta JV. Anatomical Variations of the Lateral Femoral Cutaneous Nerve and the Consequences for Surgery. J Orthop Trauma 1999;13(3):207–11.

46. Ivins GK. Meralgia Paresthetica, The Elusive Diagnosis. Ann Surg 2000;232(2):281–6.

Beyond Anatomy
Fat-Suppressed MR and Molecular Imaging of Spinal Pain Generators

Vance T. Lehman, MD*, Christin A. Tiegs-Heiden, MD,
Stephen M. Broski, MD

KEYWORDS

- Molecular imaging • Facet joint • Back pain • Spine pain • Spondyloarthropathy • Sacroiliac joint
- Intervertebral disc • Neck pain

KEY POINTS

- Many spinal pain generators cannot be reliably identified with either clinical examination or anatomic imaging.
- Nonanatomic imaging findings may facilitate identification of spine pain generators in some settings, but the radiologist needs to be aware of the limitations of a given technique and the current literature.
- Contrast enhancement and T2 hyperintensity on fat-suppressed MR imaging are useful for characterizing certain spinal pain generators, particularly in the setting of an underlying spondyloarthropathy.
- Numerous molecular imaging agents can help identify inflammatory or oncologic causes of spinal pain.
- Molecular imaging agents that target pain-specific molecular pathways would be useful but remain in the early stages of evaluation.

 Video content accompanies this article at .http://www.radiologic.theclinics.com

INTRODUCTION

Spine pain (neck and low back) is the leading cause of disability worldwide.[1] A few entities are thought to account for most chronic cases. Specifically, neck pain is facetogenic in 26% to 70% of cases, whereas low back pain (LBP) is attributed to the intervertebral disc, facet joint, or sacroiliac joint (SIJ) in more than 90% of cases.[1,2] Other causes of pain such as compression fractures, inflammatory arthropathies, and metastases also contribute to disabling spine pain. Procedures directed toward spinal pain generators are common. For example, several hundred thousand percutaneous facet joint interventions and SIJ injections are performed in the Medicare population each year.[3,4]

Identifying specific pain generators is useful for directing targeted therapy and averting unnecessary interventions or diagnostic procedures. However, the spine is a challenging area to assess clinically and radiologically for numerous reasons. Although anatomic imaging findings can identify certain pathologic lesions and MR imaging findings have been correlated to discogenic pain,[5] radiologic findings are not considered highly useful for the diagnosis of specific degenerative axial pain generators. For example, a recent international multispecialty working group reported that imaging is not useful for directing cervical facet joint intervention.[1] Age-related changes overlap with degenerative changes on anatomic examinations and are frequently asymptomatic.

Department of Radiology, Mayo Clinic, 200 1st Street SouthWest, Rochester, MN 55905, USA
* Corresponding author.
E-mail address: lehman.vance@mayo.edu

Radiol Clin N Am 62 (2024) 247–261
https://doi.org/10.1016/j.rcl.2023.09.005

Beyond anatomic imaging, molecular imaging (MI) may be useful for the diagnosis and management of spinal pain. In 2005, a large multidisciplinary summit of physicians and scientists defined MI as follows: "MI techniques directly or indirectly monitor or record the spatiotemporal distribution of molecular or cellular processes for biochemical, biologic, diagnostic, or therapeutic applications."[6] Nonanatomic findings on fat-suppressed (FS) MR imaging such as increased T2 signal (edema) or contrast enhancement (both grouped here as "signal change") are also commonly encountered in clinical assessment for potential pain generators.

The clinical implementation of MI for inflammatory or pain-related indications has been outpaced by oncologic indications. Further, theranostic evaluation and treatment of metastatic disease has emerged in recent years and seems poised for exponential growth. The spine is a frequent location of painful metastases managed with theranostics; thus, it is useful for spine radiologists to understand basic theranostic principles. This review briefly describes the main challenges of clinical and imaging diagnosis of spinal pain, introduces the essential concepts of MI for oncologic and inflammatory evaluation, and discusses the use of anatomic and FS MR imaging sequences.

Challenges of Spinal Pain Assessment

The diagnostic challenges related to spinal pain are numerous: overlapping pain patterns of multiple juxtaposed potential pain generators, limitations of physical examination maneuvers, variable nerve routes and dermatomes, incompletely understood pathomechanisms, lack of pathoanatomic gold standard tests, poorly understood pharmacokinetics of local anesthetic nerve blocks, overlapping appearance of degenerative findings and age-related changes, and a high incidence of asymptomatic findings (**Fig. 1**).[5] Criterion standard tests are cumbersome, invasive, and subjective. These include provocation discography for discogenic pain, comparative medial branch blocks (cMBBs) for facet joints, and intra-articular anesthetic injection for sacroiliac (SI) joints.[7]

Subclassification of some common pain generators has emerged in the literature. Some clinicians now differentiate pain arising from the lumbar intervertebral disc (discogenic) from the endplates (vertebrogenic) and pain arising from the articular SIJ from the overlying posterior ligaments.[8–10] Further, joints throughout the spine have variable biomechanics, including a large degree of rotational freedom at the C1–2 joint, relatively fixed positions of the thoracic joints, and highly fixed interlocking SI joints. In our experience, joints with higher mobility

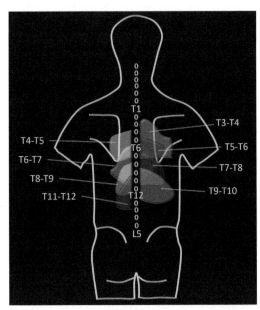

Fig. 1. Composite pain diagrams have been produced for the cervical, thoracic, and lumbar spine facet joints and other potential pain generators such as the costotransverse joints. An example of the thoracic facet joint pain patterns *adapted from* Dreyfuss and colleagues[8] is shown. This demonstrates marked overlap of pain among adjacent facet joints, highlighting the challenge of pinpointing a single target facet joint clinically.

are more likely to develop surrounding edema in the absence of an inflammatory (spondylo)arthropathy.

Brief History of Molecular Imaging

Modern MI builds on experiences and a knowledge base acquired over the past century, which has accelerated substantially in recent years. Early radiotracer and fluorescein use in the first half of the twentieth century was followed by development of single-photon emission computerized tomography (SPECT) and PET technologies in the second half. At the turn of this century, it was said we were on the dawn of an MI revolution with the convergence of several scientific advances.[11]

Nearly a quarter century later, countless new MI probes have been reported, and we have seen marked advances in theranostic treatments. Still, techniques that use newly discovered probe-target pairs are less common in clinical use than repurposing and optimization of known targets and probe categories. For example, the most commonly used radiotracers discussed below target pathways that have long been elucidated. Moreover, flourine-18 fluorodeoxyglucose (^{18}F-FDG) remains the most commonly used radiotracer for PET scans. Numerous features must coalesce to bring new probes into clinical practice, including proven clinical utility, availability, favorable radiobiopharmakokinetics, safety, and high target-to-background signal.

Methods of MI of pain can target either inflammation or an underlying painful lesion such as neoplasm. Although numerous radiotracers can target inflammation (Fig. 2), most have not found use in routine clinical practice. Many of these are adapted from other indications, primarily oncologic applications. Central and peripheral nociception molecular pathways are being explored on multiple fronts, including imaging correlates and early testing in human subjects.[12] However, most direct pain pathway imaging endeavors remain in the preclinical realm with limited clinical translation.[13,14]

Theranostics has been ushered in by MI, placing the diagnosis and treatment planning, execution, and response assessment under the same umbrella. Theranostic imaging probes generally consist of a radionuclide, a linker (chelator), and a target. A diagnostic radionuclide for these probes can be swapped with a therapeutic tracer. The diagnostic probe can confirm sufficient target binding, and then a therapeutic radionuclide can precisely deliver targeted radiation (Video 1). Currently, most therapeutic agents are beta-emitters (^{177}Lu, ^{90}Y), but alpha-emitter (^{211}At, ^{225}Ac) use is emerging due to high linear energy transfer (>a factor 500 greater) and short tissue penetration (<100 μm vs several millimeters).[15] Numerous clinical trials are currently underway and may herald a new theranostic era.

Other modalities also have potential MI applications for pain evaluation in the future. For example, spectral imaging with photon-counting computed tomography (CT) could potentially image the biodistribution of targeted nanoparticle cages containing specific elements like gold and optical imaging of inflammatory cells.[16,17]

Nonanatomic MR Imaging

Although numerous nonanatomic MR imaging techniques are relevant, this discussion will focus on FS sequences, as these have been incorporated into most MR imaging pain protocols. T2 or gadolinium-enhanced T1 FS MR can demonstrate edema and enhancement in the setting of a variety of axial pain generators. Multiple MR imaging findings associated with discogenic pain have been extensively correlated to outcomes of provocation discography.[18] These include type 1 and type 2 Modic endplate changes, which are highly

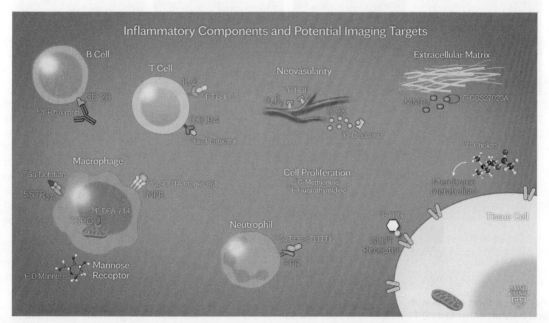

Fig. 2. Numerous components of the inflammatory cascade are amenable to targeting with PET radiotracers, including inflammatory cell receptors, glucose receptors, receptors associated with neovascularity, and other inflammatory mediators. Despite the high number of possibilities (including many beyond the examples shown here), few are used routinely in clinical practice. Barriers to implementation can include factors related to availability, kinetics, biodistribution, target specificity, and target-to-background ratios. (*Adapted from* Wu C et al. PET imaging of inflammation biomarkers Theranostics 2013; 3 (7): 448–466 & Kircher M et al. Infection and inflammation imaging: beyond FDG. PET Clin 2020: 215–229.)

associated with positive provocation discography in patients with axial LBP (vertebrogenic). Recent evidence suggests that these Modic changes can be used to help select patients for basivertebral nerve ablation.[10]

Beyond the intervertebral disc, evidence demonstrating a correlation of MR imaging findings to axial pain generators is far less robust. Retrospective findings demonstrate that high-grade peri-facet signal change (involving >50% of the perimeter of the joint with or without extension to adjacent structures) correlates to the side of unilateral axial LBP,[19] but comparison to the results of cMBBs or radiofrequency ablation is lacking. Peri-facet signal change is more common in the setting of anterolisthesis, scoliosis, and compression fractures, although the diagnostic significance is not well established (Figs. 3 and 4).[20,21] Available evidence and clinical experience suggest that the significance varies by anatomic site and pathology. In the cervical spine,

evidence is largely derived from patients with an underlying inflammatory arthropathy such as rheumatoid arthritis (RA).[22]

Typical MR imaging findings of spondyloarthropathies, infection, and degenerative change differ in pattern, though many of the same structures can be involved such as facet joints, costovertebral joints, and intervertebral disc. Spondyloarthropathies can demonstrate numerous characteristic features such as multilevel involvement of posterior element ligaments, vertebral body corner signal change, enthesitis, and marked inflammatory change surrounding the SI joints (Figs. 5 and 6).[23] MR imaging also helps select patients for anti-tumor necrosis factor (TNF)-alpha treatment and treatment response assessment (Fig. 7).[23]

In some cases, differentiating between infectious, degenerative, and inflammatory conditions of the spine can be challenging (Fig. 8). In our experience, infectious facetitis is more likely to

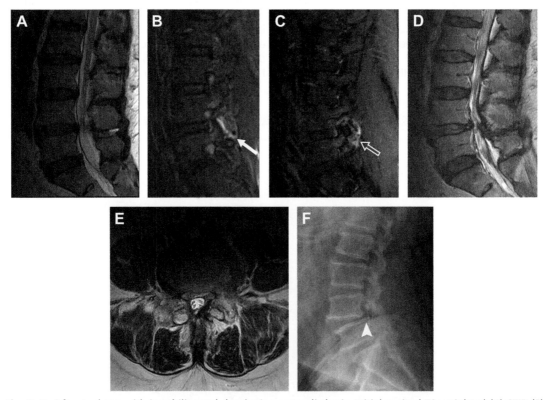

Fig. 3. Peri-facet edema with instability and developing anterolisthesis. Initial sagittal T2-weighted (A) STIR (B) and contrast-enhanced (C) T1-weighted images in a 53-year-old male demonstrate no significant anterolisthesis. There is marked bilateral peri-facet edema and enhancement (open *arrow*) at L4–L5 with facet joint effusions (*arrow*) (right side not shown). No plain films were obtained at this time. A follow-up MR imaging 3 years later demonstrates slight anterolisthesis at L4–L5. (D) The joint effusions had resolved, the peri-facet enhancement had decreased, and the facet joints appeared fused. (E) Standing lateral plain film at this time (F) demonstrates grade 1 anterolisthesis (*arrowhead*) which was more marked than the recumbent MR imaging, consistent with positional instability. Both effusion and peri-facet signal change can be seen at levels with instability and in our experience can predate development of anterolisthesis, though this concept is not well characterized in the literature.

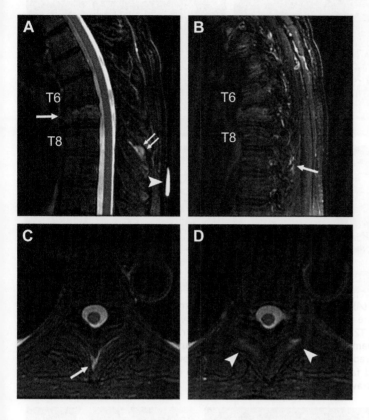

Fig. 4. Posterior element edema associated with a compression fracture. An 82-year-old woman with osteoporosis and recent fall presented with severe mid-thoracic pain. Midline fat-suppressed sagittal T2-weighted MR imaging demonstrates a T7 compression fracture with edema (*arrow*), interspinous region edema at T7–T8 (double *arrows*), and a skin marker placed directly over the level of focal pain (*arrowhead*). (*A*) Off-midline sagittal fat-suppressed T2-weighted MR imaging shows T8–T9 peri-facet edema (*arrow*). (*B*) Axial fat-suppressed T2-weighted MR imaging examinations at the T7–T8 level (*C*) and the T8–T9 level (*D*) demonstrate edema in the T7–T8 interspinous region (*arrow*) and muscular edema adjacent to the bilateral T8–T9 facet joints (*arrowheads*). This figure demonstrates that posterior element edema can be associated with compression fractures near, but not always directly at the fracture level. Thoracic compression fractures have various patterns of pain, which can be directly at the site or referred pain. However, the utility of such edema as a biomarker of the specific location of posterior element pain in this setting has not been definitively investigated.

demonstrate increasing effusion and marked muscular enhancement and can be associated with paraspinal abscess. In the SIJ, edema and contrast enhancement in the adjacent musculature suggests infection (**Fig. 9**).[24] Correlation with clinical findings, further evaluation with nuclear medicine techniques, and/or aspiration may be required.

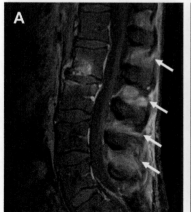
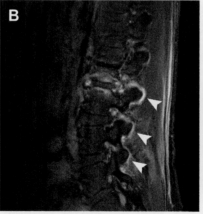
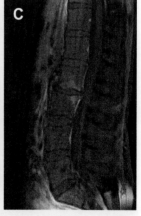

Fig. 5. Inflammatory spondyloarthropathy. A 48-year-old woman presented to the emergency department with abdominal and low back pain. CT abdomen and pelvis demonstrated colitis (not shown). Midline (*A*) and off-midline (*B*) sagittal fat-suppressed T1 MR imaging with gadolinium demonstrates extensive multilevel enhancement of the interspinous regions (*arrowheads*) and the overlying supraspinous ligament as well as diffuse peri-facet joint enhancement (*arrowheads*). The patient was diagnosed with spondyloarthropathy in the setting of inflammatory bowel disease. A 9-month follow-up MR imaging after medical treatment demonstrates complete resolution of the posterior element enhancement. (*C*) This pattern of profound, multilevel posterior element ligament enhancement is typical of some early spondyloarthropathies and would be atypical in other settings.

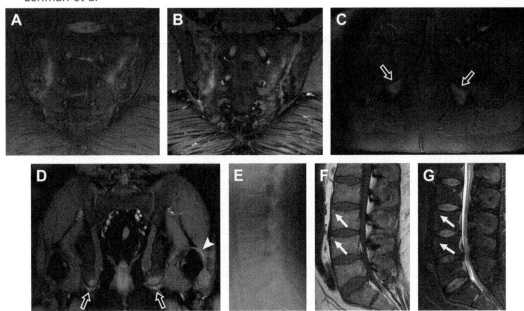

Fig. 6. Coronal oblique T2 fat-saturated (*A*) and IV contrast-enhanced (*B*) MR images in a 33-year-old patient with ankylosing spondylitis demonstrate bone marrow edema, osteitis, and synovitis around both sacroiliac joints, compatible with active sacroiliitis. Axial T2 fat-saturated (*C*) and coronal contrast-enhanced (*D*) images show inflammatory enthesitis involving the hamstrings origins (open *arrows*), gluteal insertions (*arrowhead*), and adductor origins (not shown). Lateral radiograph (*E*) was unremarkable; however, sagittal T1 (*F*) and T2 fat-saturated (*G*) MR images demonstrated fatty infiltration and bone marrow edema in the anterior corners of several vertebral body endplates. IV, intravenous.

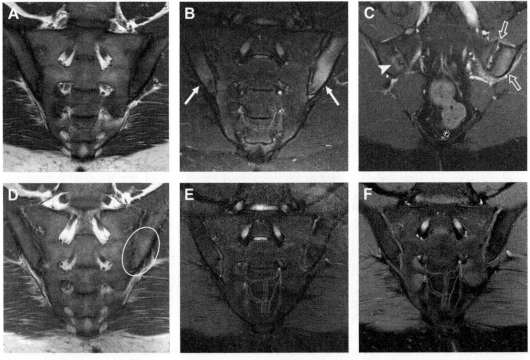

Fig. 7. Sacroiliitis with response to treatment. Coronal oblique T1 (*A*) T2 fat-saturated (*B*) and T1-weighted contrast-enhanced (*C*) MR images in an 18-year-old male patient with ankylosing spondylitis demonstrate erosive change (*arrowhead*), bone marrow edema (*arrows*), and enhancement (open *arrows*) about the sacroiliac joints, compatible with sacroiliitis. Repeat examination 2 years later (*D–F*) shows complete resolution of inflammation, with no residual bone marrow edema or enhancement. On coronal T1-weighted image (*D*) there is some new fatty bone marrow replacement around the left sacroiliac joint, compatible with chronic sequelae of sacroiliitis. The degree of enhancement would not be typical of osteoarthritis in this location.

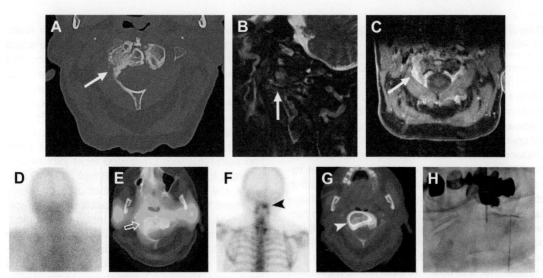

Fig. 8. Axial non-contrast CT (*A*) sagittal T2 fat-saturated MR imaging (*B*) and axial contrast-enhanced MR (*C*) images in a 71-year-old woman with advanced degenerative arthritis of the right C1–2 facet joint (*arrows*). There are osteophyte formation, periarticular bone marrow edema, and surrounding enhancement. Planar (*D*) and fused SPECT/CT (*E*) images from a 67Gallium citrate scan of the cervical spine demonstrates low-level uptake about the joint (*E, open arrow*). Planar (*F*) and fused SPECT/CT (*G*) images from a subsequent 99mMDP bone scan showed marked increased radiotracer uptake about the joint (*arrowhead*), indicative of osteoarthritis, rather than infection. The patient was subsequently treated with a fluoroscopically guided C1–2 facet joint injection (*H*). 99mMDP, technetium-99m-methyl diphosphonate.

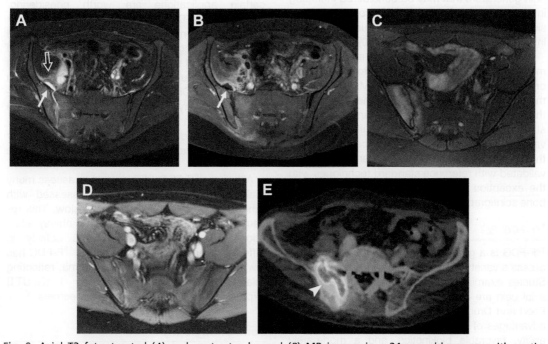

Fig. 9. Axial T2 fat-saturated (*A*) and contrast-enhanced (*B*) MR images in a 24-year-old woman with septic arthritis of the right sacroiliac joint demonstrate cortical irregularity, bone marrow edema-like signal around the joint, and a joint effusion which communicates with a peripherally enhancing abscess (*arrows*). There is marked soft tissue edema with enhancement about the joint, a hallmark of sacroiliac joint septic arthritis (open *arrow*). In comparison, axial T2 fat-saturated (*C*) and contrast-enhanced (*D*) MR images in a 16-year-old man with inflammatory sacroiliitis also demonstrate asymmetric bone marrow edema about the right sacroiliac joint; however, there is notable lack of periarticular soft tissue and enhancement in this case. (*E*) Companion axial 18F-FDG fused PET/CT image in an 80-year-old man with culture-proven septic arthritis of the right sacroiliac joint demonstrates intense FDG uptake within and surrounding the joint (*arrowhead*). This degree of 18F-FDG is not characteristic of bland sacroiliitis.

Overview of Molecular Imaging Assessment of Pain Generators

Numerous potential pain-specific pathway targets for MI have been described, but clinical implementation remains challenging.[25] For instance, there are challenges in identifying common chronic pain pathways, evaluating small structures, and potential agent toxicity[26] superimposed on the numerous challenges inherent to MI agent development such as optimization of target specificity, target-to-background activity, incorporation of amplification strategies, and biokinetics.[11] Conversely, advantages of MI can include whole-body imaging as patterns of referred pain from spinal and extraspinal pain generators can overlap, ability to determine semiquantitative standard uptake values with PET radiotracers, and ability to treat some metastatic lesions.

Spine assessment by MI typically benefits from hybrid imaging with CT or MR imaging for anatomic localization and lesion characterization. CT is more widely available and commonly used. In addition to lower radiation dose, MR imaging offers improved characterization of many potential pain generators that may be considered including intervertebral disc findings, neural compressive lesions, spinal canal stenosis, osseous lesions, and inflammatory signal change (**Fig. 10**).

This review focuses on the few MI agents that are most widely used and most relevant to inflammatory or oncologic spine pain, listed by MI agent rather than by pain generators. Many of these MI probes that primarily assess malignancy can also demonstrate activity in the setting of inflammation to varying degrees. For degenerative causes of pain, the agents listed below have not been meaningfully validated with reference standard techniques with the exception of technetium-99m (^{99m}Tc)-based bone scintigraphy.

^{18}F-FDG PET

^{18}F-FDG is a glucose analog and can be used to assess a variety of malignancies and inflammation. Studies examining its specific use for evaluating axial pain are emerging, but the indication is not Food and Drug Administration (FDA) cleared. The advantages of ^{18}F-FDG include widespread availability, favorable biokinetics, and a moderately long half-life (110 minutes). Numerous factors can increase ^{18}F-FDG activity including blood flow, cellular factors, and biochemical factors (see animation). Many of the mechanisms that increase ^{18}F-FDG activity are similar for both neoplastic and inflammatory conditions, although not identical (Video 2).[27,28]

^{18}F-FDG activity has been assessed in the setting of degenerative change and pain evaluation. In principle, ^{18}F-FDG activity could offer higher specificity for inflammation compared with bone scans (**Fig. 11**). Moderate to high activity associated with degenerative changes of the spine (either facet joint or intervertebral disc) has been reported in 22% of patients undergoing ^{18}F-FDG PET examinations for evaluation of malignancy.[29] One ^{18}F-FDG PET/MR imaging study reported that six of six (100%) patients with ^{18}F-FDG avid facet joints had pain relief with CT-guided facet joint blocks, whereas four of four (100%) without ^{18}F-FDG avid joints did not respond.[30] Another pilot study assessed 10 patients with suspected lumbar facet joint pain with ^{18}F-PET/MR imaging,[31] demonstrating that ^{18}F-FDG activity in principle has the potential to alter management by identifying differences in clinically and metabolically implicated facet joints. However, larger studies using cMBBs would be needed to confirm the utility.

Both of the previously mentioned facet joint studies suggest that ^{18}F-FDG activity may have high concordance to inflammatory change on more standard MR imaging examinations.[30,31] Thus, the utility of ^{18}F-FDG over standard MR imaging alone for facet joint assessment is unclear. Still, certain applications are worth considering. Possibly, ^{18}F-FDG PET may be more useful for early assessment of treatment response compared with MR imaging findings as suggested in RA and osteoarthritis of the appendicular skeleton, though more work would be needed for confirmation in the spine.[32,33] One study found that ^{18}F-FDG activity could identify areas of inflammation that were not apparent on MR imaging in the knee.[34] In addition, limited evidence indicates that ^{18}F-FDG PET/CT can alter management of chronic neuropathic pain.[35]

Although ^{18}F-FDG PET is used to assess many malignancies, some are better assessed with other radiotracers, as discussed below. This reflects, in part, different metabolic pathway alterations and mechanisms of FDG activity in different neoplasms.[36] For example, ^{18}F-FDG has low sensitivity for renal cell carcinoma, reflecting relatively low glucose transporter 1 (GLUT1) expression and sometimes central necrosis.[37]

Bone Scintigraphy

The two major categories of bone radiotracers are ^{99m}Tc-based agents and ^{18}F-NaF. Uptake of bone-specific radiotracers is due to a combination of factors, including increased blood flow, osteoblastic activity with bone formation, and bone remodeling, which may occur in both benign and malignant processes (Video 3). The precise mechanisms differ and ^{18}F-NaF has favorable biokinetic

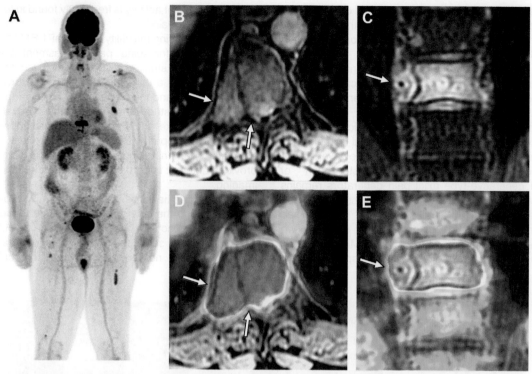

Fig. 10. A 61-year-old man with relapsed multiple myeloma and back pain undergoing restaging PET/MR imaging. ^{18}F-FDG PET MIP image (*A*) demonstrates multiple FDG-avid osseous lesions. Axial and coronal fat-saturated LAVA flex (*B*, *C*) and fused PET/MR imaging (*D*, *E*) images demonstrate an FDG-avid osseous lesion in the T8 vertebra, with extraosseous extension into the right neural foramen and epidural space (*arrows*). MIP, maximum intensity projection.

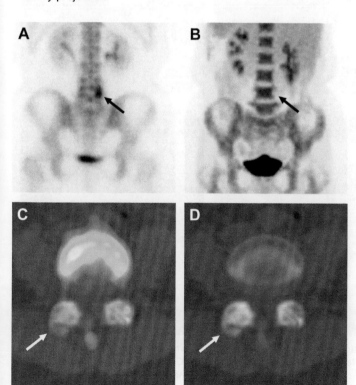

Fig. 11. Increased ^{99m}Tc MDP activity without increased ^{18}F-FDG activity. A 63-year-old woman with breast cancer and several imaging investigations within a 1-month period to evaluate for metastatic disease. A posterior planar bone scan image demonstrates markedly increased ^{99m}Tc activity in the right L4–L5 facet joint (*arrow*) (*A*). A posterior MIP image from an ^{18}F-FDG PET examination (*B*) and corresponding axial PET/CT (*C*) demonstrate no evidence of corresponding increased ^{18}FDG activity (*arrows*). An axial CT image (*D*) demonstrates hypertrophic change of the right L4–L5 facet joint (*arrow*). The cumulative findings suggest increased bone scan activity associated with bone metabolism and hypertrophy without substantially increased inflammation.

features, but the biodistribution and clinical significance are similar. ^{18}F-NaF has the previously mentioned advantages of PET compared with SPECT imaging.

Bone scans have been used clinically to help assess pain for decades. Bone scan activity is seen with numerous spinal pain generators such as osteoblastomas, osteoblastic metastases, stress reactions of the pars interarticularis region, compression fractures, and sacral insufficiency fractures (**Figs. 12** and **13**).[38] However, bone scan interpretation for characterization of degenerative-type axial pain generators remains challenging. Although initial studies suggested utility to identify a painful facet joint,[39,40] these had many limitations, including lack of cMBBs. Two recent prospective studies using cMBBs reported only moderate sensitivity and specificity.[41,42]

Further, facet joint activity is frequently found in locations without pain.[43]

Studies assessing the utility of ^{18}F-NaF PET/(MR imaging or CT) for spinal pain assessment are emerging. A pilot study of six patients with facetogenic LBP found a correlation between dynamic ^{18}F-NaF activity and the Oswestry Disability Index score.[44] Another study demonstrated that ^{18}F-NaF radiotracer uptake and Parthia grade of lumbar facet joint arthropathy on CT were only weakly correlated, demonstrating that bone scan activity provides different information than pure anatomic imaging.[45]

Fewer studies have assessed degenerative processes beyond the facet joints. One study found that bone scan activity has low sensitivity for SIJ pain.[46,47] A small series found that costovertebral joint activity did not predict response to local

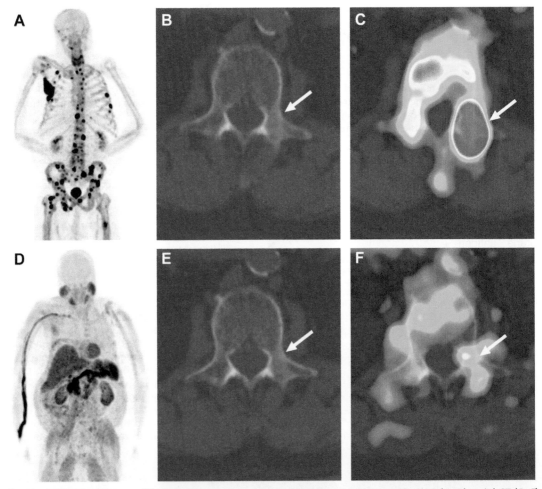

Fig. 12. A 82-year-old man with metastatic prostate cancer. Maximum intensity projection (*A*, *D*), axial CT (*B*, *E*), and fused PET/CT (*C*, *F*) images from ^{18}F-NaF (*A–C*) and ^{11}C-acetate (*D–F*) PET/CT examinations demonstrate more numerous skeletal metastases on ^{18}F-NaF compared with ^{11}C-acetate. Note the sclerotic metastasis in the left L1 pedicle (*arrow in B, E*), with greater uptake on ^{18}F-NaF (*C, arrow*) than ^{11}C-acetate (*F, arrow*).

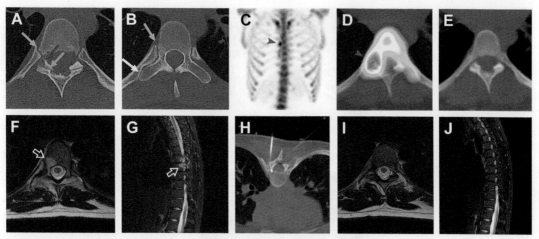

Fig. 13. (*A, B*) Axial non-contrast CT images in a 22-year-old woman demonstrate a 4-mm lytic lesion in the right superior articular facet of T7 (*red arrow*). These images also highlight the proximity of this lesion to the costovertebral (*blue arrow*), costotransverse (*yellow arrow*), and facet (*orange arrow*) joints. (*C–E*) MIP, fused, and CT images from a [99m]MDP SPECT/CT examination show uptake within the lesion (*arrowhead*), which is better localized with CT. Axial T2 (*F*) and sagittal T2 fat-saturated (*G*) MR images show prominent bone marrow edema around the lesion. Findings are compatible with osteoid osteoma, and the lesion was treated with percutaneous CT-guided cryoablation (*H*). Follow-up MR images approximately 8 months after treatment (*I, J*) demonstrate resolution of the bone marrow edema.

anesthetic and steroid injection.[48] Vertebral endplate activity is not entirely specific and can be seen with Modic changes, Schmorl's nodes, and osteophytes. Bone radiotracer activity can also be seen with pseudoarticulation of the lumbosacral junction, although this has not been well studied.[46]

Prostate-Specific Membrane Antigen Agents

Development of current prostate-specific membrane antigen (PSMA) agents has been a multifaceted endeavor requiring trial-and-error, serendipitous insights, and multidisciplinary collaboration (**Figs. 14** and **15**). Key developments include the establishment of a cancer cell line in 1983, PSMA gene cloning in 1993, FDA approval of indium-111 (^{111}In)-capromab pendetide in 1996 (which targeted the intracellular domain, limiting its use to dead or dying cells), report of strong homology to NAALADASE (for glutamate metabolism) in 1998, and development of the J591 antibody to the extracellular component in 1998.[49] A neuroradiologist studying NAALADASE, Martin Pomper, then collaborated with Alan Kozikowski over the next decade to produce the first PSMA PET agent, paving the way to the introduction of many others labeled with ^{68}Ga, ^{18}F, ^{177}Lu, or [225]Ac over the next 15 years. Despite the specificity for prostate cancer cells (which have 100–1000 times overexpression of PSMA compared with normal body tissue), receptor overexpression

is also found to varying degrees with other types of cancer and inflammatory cells.[37]

Although the rate of theranostic agent development is accelerating, the PSMA timeline demonstrates that the process of creating new agents may be more involved than radiologists might realize. In addition, optimization and repurposing of established agents for multiple indications and with multiple radiotracers has some practical advantages over creating new agents for each indication.

Other Radiotracers for Prostate Cancer Metastases

[11]C- or ^{18}F-choline and ^{11}C-acetate can also be used to image prostate cancer metastases with PET. Choline is a phospholipid precursor and contributes to proliferating cell membranes, whereas acetate is metabolized to acetyl coenzyme A, contributing to fatty acid metabolism (and the citric acid cycle in myocardial tissue). Prostate cancer metastases demonstrate inter- and intraindividual variability of PSMA overexpression and metabolic pathway alterations; thus, the activity of various MI probes can likewise vary. Although there is overlap in the detection of metastases with these various radiotracers, PSMA probes have shown higher sensitivity than carbon-11 (^{11}C)-acetate and ^{11}C-choline.[37,50]

The radiologist must be aware of the various other lesions that can demonstrate activity with

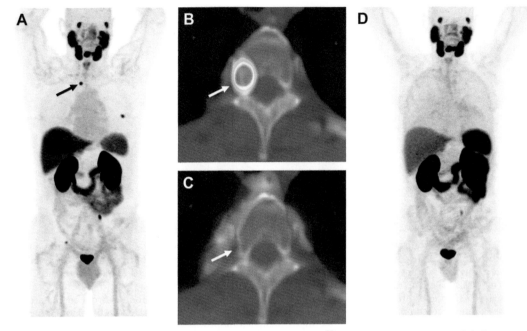

Fig. 14. A 72-year-old man with oligometastatic prostate cancer. 68Ga-PSMA PET MIP image (*A*) demonstrates multiple PSMA-avid skeletal metastases, including lesions in the right T3 vertebral body (*arrow*), a left rib, and the right acetabulum. Fused PET/CT image from the same study (*B*) demonstrates a PSMA-avid lesion in the right T3 vertebrae (*arrow*). The patient received targeted radiation therapy to all three lesions, with resolved PSMA uptake at T3 (*C, arrow*), and no evidence of residual radiotracer-avid osseous metastases on follow-up 68Ga-PSMA PET MIP (*D*).

any radiotracer used. For example, 11C-choline activity can be seen with some inflammatory lesions and fibrous dysplasia.[11,51] C-choline activity of the facet joints, SI joint, or vertebral endplates is uncommon in our experience, though there are little published data. 11C-acetate is also used to evaluate other tumors with low-grade proliferation, such as hepatocellular carcinoma or renal cell carcinoma, and can show incidental uptake with multiple myeloma.[52]

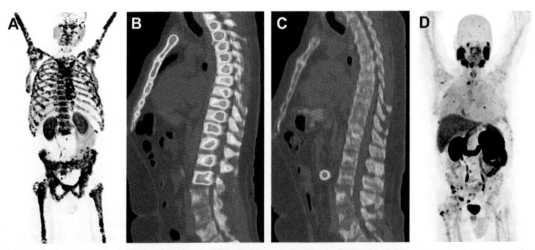

Fig. 15. A 66-year-old man with widely metastatic prostate cancer. Maximum intensity projection and sagittal fused 68Ga-PSMA PET/CT images before (*A, B*) and after (*C, D*) 177Lu-PSMA therapy demonstrates diffuse PSMA-avid osseous metastatic disease throughout the sternum, thoracic spine, and upper lumbar spine, with complete resolution of PSMA uptake on the posttreatment PET/CT.

Somatostatin Analogs

The radiolabeled peptide somatostatin analog octreotide was introduced in 1983 for imaging neuroendocrine tumors. More recently, DOTA-linker-based compounds with new-generation somatostatin analogs and ^{68}Ga have gained favor.[53] These have higher affinity for somatostatin receptors and are amenable to PET imaging, which has resulted in a paradigm shift in imaging patients with somatostatin-avid tumors away from planar and SPECT/CT imaging. One commonly used agent in this family, DOTATATE (1,4,7,10-tetraaza-cyclododecane-1,4,7,10-tetraacetic acid), is useful as it has high affinity for type 2 somatostatin receptors, which are abundant in neuroendocrine tumors and can be labeled with ^{177}Lu for treatment. Activity can be seen with either osteoblastic or inflammatory lesions.[53] In the spine, such activity can be seen with degenerative changes and fractures. Spinal meningiomas can also demonstrate DOTATATE activity.

SUMMARY

Clinical and anatomic imaging identification of spinal pain generators has numerous limitations. Nonanatomic imaging including FS MR imaging and nuclear medicine MI techniques may improve identification of degenerative, inflammatory, and oncologic pain generators; however, there are little data assessing nonanatomic imaging biomarkers to criterion standards. Pain pathway-specific imaging offers an enticing possibility but seems far from clinical implementation. Current MI techniques can characterize painful spinal metastases with increasing refinement, though radiologists should be aware of pitfalls. Theranostic techniques are emerging and can help assess and manage these metastases.

Imaging evaluation of spinal pain lies at the cross-roads of several specialties including clinical and interventional pain management, spine radiology, and MI. Optimal interpretation of imaging examinations and future study design requires consideration of key concepts in each of these areas.

CLINICS CARE POINTS

- Clinical findings do not reliably localize specific axial pain generators.
- Anatomic findings of "degenerative change" on imaging, such as osteophytes do not reliably identify pain generators, are seen commonly in asymptomatic individuals and show overlap with findings expected with normal aging.
- T2 hyperintensity and contrast enhancement on fat-suppressed MR imaging may facilitate identification of spine pain generators in some settings, but this topic needs further evaluation in the literature.
- Imaging findings of inflammation in the setting of a spondyloarthropathy have several unique features and can be more widespread compared with those seen with degenerative change.
- Numerous molecular imaging agents can help identify inflammatory or oncologic causes of spinal pain, but agents that target pain-specific molecular pathways remain in the early stages of evaluation.
- Theranostic agents can facilitate both evaluation and treatment of oncologic axial pain generators.

ACKNOWLEDGMENTS

The authors would like to thank Sonia Watson, PhD and Desiree Lanzino, PhD, for their assistance in editing the manuscript.

DISCLOSURE

None to declare for the authors.

SUPPLEMENTARY DATA

Supplementary data to this article can be found online at https://doi.org/10.1016/j.rcl.2023.09.005

REFERENCES

1. Hurley RW, Adams MCB, Barad M, et al. Consensus practice guidelines on interventions for cervical spine (facet) joint pain from a multispecialty international working group. Reg Anesth Pain Med 2022; 47(1):3–59.
2. DePalma MJ, Ketchum JM, Saullo T. What is the source of chronic low back pain and does age play a role? Pain Med 2011;12(2):224–33.
3. Manchikanti L, Manchikanti MV, Vanaparthy R, et al. Utilization Patterns of Sacroiliac Joint Injections from 2000 to 2018 in Fee-for-Service Medicare Population. Pain Physician 2020;23(5):439–50.
4. Manchikanti L, Sanapati MR, Pampati V, et al. Update of Utilization Patterns of Facet Joint Interventions in Managing Spinal Pain from 2000 to 2018 in the US Fee-for-Service Medicare Population. Pain Physician 2020;23(2):E133–49.

5. Bogduk N. Degenerative joint disease of the spine. Radiol Clin North Am 2012;50(4):613–28.

6. Krestin GP, Bernsen MR. Molecular imaging in radiology: the latest fad or the new frontier? Eur Radiol 2006;16(11):2383–5.

7. Bogduk N. ISIS practice guidelines for spinal diagnostic and treatment procedures. 2nd edition. San Francisco: International Spine Intervention Society; 2014.

8. Dreyfuss P, Henning T, Malladi N, et al. The ability of multi-site, multi-depth sacral lateral branch blocks to anesthetize the sacroiliac joint complex. Pain Med 2009;10(4):679–88.

9. Lorio M, Clerk-Lamalice O, Rivera M, et al. ISASS Policy Statement 2022: Literature Review of Intraosseous Basivertebral Nerve Ablation. Int J Spine Surg 2022;16(6):1084–94.

10. Schnapp W, Martiatu K, Delcroix GJ. Basivertebral Nerve Ablation for the Treatment of Chronic Low Back Pain: A Scoping Review of the Literature. Pain Physician 2022;25(4):E551–62.

11. Weissleder R, Mahmood U. Molecular imaging. Radiology 2001;219(2):316–33.

12. Yoon D, Cipriano P, Carroll I, et al. Sigma-1 receptor PET/MRI for identifying nociceptive sources of radiating low back pain. J Nucl Med 2020;61(supplement 1):178.

13. Ravert HT, Bencherif B, Madar I, et al. PET imaging of opioid receptors in pain: progress and new directions. Curr Pharm Des 2004;10(7):759–68.

14. Shen B, Behera D, James ML, et al. Visualizing Nerve Injury in a Neuropathic Pain Model with [(18)F]FTC-146 PET/MRI. Theranostics 2017;7(11):2794–805.

15. Tranel J, Feng FY, James SS, et al. Effect of micro-distribution of alpha and beta-emitters in targeted radionuclide therapies on delivered absorbed dose in a GATE model of bone marrow. Phys Med Biol 2021;66(3):035016.

16. Birch GP, Campbell T, Bradley M, et al. Optical Molecular Imaging of Inflammatory Cells in Interventional Medicine-An Emerging Strategy. Front Oncol 2019;9:882.

17. Kimm MA, Shevtsov M, Werner C, et al. Gold Nanoparticle Mediated Multi-Modal CT Imaging of Hsp70 Membrane-Positive Tumors. Cancers 2020;12(5).

18. Maus TP, Aprill CN. Lumbar diskogenic pain, provocation diskography, and imaging correlates. Radiol Clin North Am 2012;50(4):681–704.

19. Czervionke LF, Fenton DS. Fat-saturated MR imaging in the detection of inflammatory facet arthropathy (facet synovitis) in the lumbar spine. Pain Med 2008;9(4):400–6.

20. Friedrich KM, Nemec S, Peloschek P, et al. The prevalence of lumbar facet joint edema in patients with low back pain. Skeletal Radiol 2007;36(8):755–60.

21. Lehman VT, Wood CP, Hunt CH, et al. Facet joint signal change on MRI at levels of acute/subacute lumbar compression fractures. AJNR Am J Neuroradiol 2013;34(7):1468–73.

22. Nevalainen MT, Foran PJ, Roedl JB, et al. Cervical facet oedema: prevalence, correlation to symptoms, and follow-up imaging. Clin Radiol 2016;71(6):570–5.

23. Hermann KG, Baraliakos X, van der Heijde DM, et al. Descriptions of spinal MRI lesions and definition of a positive MRI of the spine in axial spondyloarthritis: a consensual approach by the ASAS/OMERACT MRI study group. Ann Rheum Dis 2012;71(8):1278–88.

24. Kang Y, Hong SH, Kim JY, et al. Unilateral Sacroiliitis: Differential Diagnosis Between Infectious Sacroiliitis and Spondyloarthritis Based on MRI Findings. AJR Am J Roentgenol 2015;205(5):1048–55.

25. Min JJ. Molecular Pain Imaging by Nuclear Medicine: Where Does It Stand and Where Is It Going? Nucl Med Mol Imaging 2016;50(4):273–4.

26. Wu C, Li F, Niu G, et al. PET imaging of inflammation biomarkers. Theranostics 2013;3(7):448–66.

27. Cho IY, Park SY, Park JH, et al. MRI findings of lumbar spine instability in degenerative spondylolisthesis. J Orthop Surg 2017;25(2). 2309499017718907.

28. Sambuceti G, Cossu V, Bauckneht M, et al. 18)F-fluoro-2-deoxy-d-glucose (FDG) uptake. What are we looking at? Eur J Nucl Med Mol Imaging 2021;48(5):1278–86.

29. Rosen RS, Fayad L, Wahl RL. Increased 18F-FDG uptake in degenerative disease of the spine: Characterization with 18F-FDG PET/CT. J Nucl Med 2006;47(8):1274–80.

30. Sawicki LM, Schaarschmidt BM, Heusch P, et al. Value of (18) F-FDG PET/MRI for the outcome of CT-guided facet block therapy in cervical facet syndrome: initial results. J Med Imaging Radiat Oncol 2017;61(3):327–33.

31. Lehman VT, Diehn FE, Broski SM, et al. Comparison of [(18)F] FDG-PET/MRI and Clinical Findings for Assessment of Suspected Lumbar Facet Joint Pain: A Prospective Study to Characterize Candidate Nonanatomic Imaging Biomarkers and Potential Impact on Management. AJNR Am J Neuroradiol 2019;40(10):1779–85.

32. Fosse P, Kaiser MJ, Namur G, et al. 18)F- FDG PET/CT joint assessment of early therapeutic response in rheumatoid arthritis patients treated with rituximab. Eur J Hybrid Imaging 2018;2(1):6.

33. Nguyen BJ, Burt A, Baldassarre RL, et al. The prognostic and diagnostic value of 18F-FDG PET/CT for assessment of symptomatic osteoarthritis. Nucl Med Commun 2018;39(7):699–706.

34. Kogan F, Fan AP, McWalter EJ, et al. PET/MRI of metabolic activity in osteoarthritis: A feasibility study. J Magn Reson Imaging 2017;45(6):1736–45.

35. Cipriano PW, Yoon D, Carroll I, et al. 18F-FDG PET/MRI of patients with chronic pain alters management. J Nucl Med 2019;60(supplement 1):93.

36. Kawada K, Iwamoto M, Sakai Y. Mechanisms underlying (18)F-fluorodeoxyglucose accumulation in colorectal cancer. World J Radiol 2016;8(11):880–6.

37. Regula N, Kostaras V, Johansson S, et al. Comparison of (68)Ga-PSMA-11 PET/CT with (11)C-acetate PET/CT in re-staging of prostate cancer relapse. Sci Rep 2020;10(1):4993.

38. Huang Z, Fang T, Si Z, et al. Imaging algorithm and multimodality evaluation of spinal osteoblastoma. BMC Muscoskel Disord 2020;21(1):240.

39. Dolan AL, Ryan PJ, Arden NK, et al. The value of SPECT scans in identifying back pain likely to benefit from facet joint injection. Br J Rheumatol 1996; 35(12):1269–73.

40. Pneumaticos SG, Chatziioannou SN, Hipp JA, et al. Low back pain: prediction of short-term outcome of facet joint injection with bone scintigraphy. Radiology 2006;238(2):693–8.

41. Freiermuth D, Kretzschmar M, Bilecen D, et al. Correlation of 99m Tc-DPD SPECT/CT Scan Findings and Diagnostic Blockades of Lumbar Medial Branches in Patients with Unspecific Low Back Pain in a Randomized-Controlled Trial. Pain Med 2015;16(10):1916–22.

42. Jain A, Jain S, Agarwal A, et al. Evaluation of Efficacy of Bone Scan With SPECT/CT in the Management of Low Back Pain: A Study Supported by Differential Diagnostic Local Anesthetic Blocks. Clin J Pain 2015;31(12):1054–9.

43. Lehman VT, Murphy RC, Kaufmann TJ, et al. Frequency of discordance between facet joint activity on technetium Tc99m methylene diphosphonate SPECT/CT and selection for percutaneous treatment at a large multispecialty institution. AJNR Am J Neuroradiol 2014;35(3):609–14.

44. Jenkins NW, Talbott JF, Shah V, et al. [(18)F]-Sodium Fluoride PET MR-Based Localization and Quantification of Bone Turnover as a Biomarker for Facet Joint-Induced Disability. AJNR Am J Neuroradiol 2017; 38(10):2028–31.

45. Mabray MC, Brus-Ramer M, Behr SC, et al. (18)F-Sodium Fluoride PET-CT Hybrid Imaging of the Lumbar Facet Joints: Tracer Uptake and Degree of Correlation to CT-graded Arthropathy. World J Nucl Med 2016;15(2):85–90.

46. Lehman VT, Murphy RC, Maus TP. 99mTc-MDP SPECT/CT of the spine and sacrum at a multispecialty institution: clinical use, findings, and impact on patient management. Nucl Med Commun 2013; 34(11):1097–106.

47. Slipman CW, Sterenfeld EB, Chou LH, et al. The value of radionuclide imaging in the diagnosis of sacroiliac joint syndrome. Spine 1996;21(19): 2251–4.

48. Verdoorn JT, Lehman VT, Diehn FE, et al. Increased 99mTc MDP activity in the costovertebral and costotransverse joints on SPECT-CT: is it predictive of associated back pain or response to percutaneous treatment? Diagn Interv Radiol 2015;21(4):342–7.

49. O'Keefe DS, Bacich DJ, Huang SS, et al. A Perspective on the Evolving Story of PSMA Biology, PSMA-Based Imaging, and Endoradiotherapeutic Strategies. J Nucl Med 2018;59(7):1007–13.

50. Schwenck J, Rempp H, Reischl G, et al. Comparison of (68)Ga-labelled PSMA-11 and (11)C-choline in the detection of prostate cancer metastases by PET/CT. Eur J Nucl Med Mol Imaging 2017;44(1): 92–101.

51. Gu CN, Hunt CH, Lehman VT, et al. Benign fibrous dysplasia on [(11)C]choline PET: a potential mimicker of disease in patients with biochemical recurrence of prostate cancer. Ann Nucl Med 2012; 26(7):599–602.

52. Grassi I, Nanni C, Allegri V, et al. The clinical use of PET with (11)C-acetate. Am J Nucl Med Mol Imaging 2012;2(1):33–47.

53. Hofmann UK, Keller RL, Walter C, et al. Predictability of the effects of facet joint infiltration in the degenerate lumbar spine when assessing MRI scans. J Orthop Surg Res 2017;12(1):180.

Functional Anatomy of the Spinal Cord

Allison Grayev, MD

KEYWORDS

• Spinal cord • Anatomy • Tracts • MR imaging

KEY POINTS

- Knowledge of spinal cord anatomy is key for understanding clinical presentation of different pathologies.
- Dividing the white matter tracts by location can help localize a level of spinal cord pathology.
- Central gray matter pathologies can affect motor and/or sensory neurons.

INTRODUCTION

Basic knowledge of spinal cord anatomy is critical to understand pathologies, which can often be difficult to localize based on clinical symptoms. Similar to the brain, the spinal cord contains both gray and white matter maintained in somatotopic organization as both originate from the neural tube. Although the spinal cord only extends to the level of L1/L2 generally, there are spinal cord segments corresponding to all lumbar and sacral levels; thus, spinal cord levels do not always correlate with vertebral body levels. Embryologically, this makes sense as the neural tube extends to the level of the coccyx and slowly ascends as there is differential growth of the vertebral column (ectodermal origin).[1]

IMAGING TECHNIQUES

When imaging the spinal cord, a combination of T1- and T2-weighted sequences is needed and the use of sagittal short-tau inversion recovery sequence in the sagittal plane is recommended as it is often critical in the assessment of cord edema. Both sagittal and axial imaging planes should be performed with additional consideration of coronal or oblique planes depending on the clinical history. The use of diffusion-weighted imaging (DWI) may be helpful, but as will be discussed, not all restricted diffusion in the cord represents infarct; cord contusion, infection (particularly intramedullary abscess) and demyelination can all result in restricted diffusion and decreased anisotropy on diffusion tensor imaging.[2–4] Contrast administration may be helpful to evaluate for breakdown of the blood–spinal cord border in neoplasm, infection, and inflammation. Future directions to explore include the use of diffusion tensor imaging, perfusion, and magnetization transfer.[5–7]

It is important to recognize the presence of truncation artifact, which can simulate T2 hyperintensity in the cord. This results from the contrast between cerebrospinal fluid and spinal cord signal and is exacerbated by cerebrospinal fluid pulsation, respiratory motion, and the heterogeneity of the magnetic field.[8] Ways to decrease or eliminate truncation artifact include increasing the phase-encoding steps, swapping the phase- and frequency-encoding directions, and decreasing view.[9]

NORMAL ANATOMY
Gray Matter

The gray matter of the spinal cord is located centrally and contains the neuronal cell bodies. The gray matter can be primarily divided into three horns: ventral (contains motor neuron cell bodies), dorsal (contains sensory neuron cell bodies), and lateral (autonomic nervous system: sympathetic from T1–L2 and parasympathetic S2–S4). A cross section of the spinal cord at the level of the cervical and lumbar enlargements demonstrates increased gray matter relating to the innervation of the limbs.[10]

Department of Radiology, University of Wisconsin School of Medicine and Public Health, E1/318, 600 Highland Avenue, Madison, WI 53792-3252, USA
E-mail address: agrayev@uwhealth.org

Radiol Clin N Am 62 (2024) 263–272
https://doi.org/10.1016/j.rcl.2023.09.001

The gray matter can be further divided into nine layers (Rexed lamina) with the commissure labeled as layer 10[11] (**Fig. 1**). The dorsal horn contains laminae 1 to 6 and the ventral horn contains laminae 7 to 9. Lamina 9 deserves special mention as it consists of medial, central, and lateral motor columns embedded within laminae 7 and 8. The medial column innervates the trunk, neck, and back muscles, the central motor column contains C1–C5 accessory nucleus, C3–C5 phrenic nucleus, and L2–S1 lumbosacral nucleus, and the lateral nucleus is present only in the cervical and lumbar enlargements providing innervation to the limbs.[12]

White Matter

The white matter of the spinal cord is located peripherally and can be divided into ascending and descending pathways (**Fig. 2**). Alternatively, the white matter can be divided based on location with three identified columns/funiculi: ventral, dorsal, and lateral (mirroring the divisions for the gray matter).[13] There are additional propriospinal pathways that connect gray matter interneurons within the spinal cord that although numerous, do not necessarily have the same clinical impact as the other white matter tracts.

Descending tracts: The largest descending tract of the spinal cord is the lateral corticospinal tract, which is located in the lateral column, and connects the axons from the motor and premotor cortex (upper motor neurons) to the lower motor neurons in the ventral horns. The lateral corticospinal tract decussates at the medulla and descends contralaterally and is critical in limb movement and fine motor control. The lateral column also contains the rubrospinal tract that connects the red nucleus to the ventral horn interneurons and assists with motor control. The ventral column contains the anterior corticospinal, reticulospinal, tectospinal, and vestibulospinal tracts. The anterior corticospinal tract is an uncrossed tract connecting the motor and premotor cortex to the ventral horn cells and is responsible for posture and movement of the trunk and neck. The reticulospinal tract extends from the reticular formations within the pons and medulla to the ventral and dorsal horns and functions in modulation of sensory transmission and spinal reflexes. The tectospinal tract connects the midbrain to the cervical ventral horn interneurons and controls reflexive head turning. The vestibulospinal tract originates in the vestibular nuclei and terminates in the ventral interneurons and motor neurons and modulates postural reflexes.[14]

Ascending tracts: The dorsal columns convey sensory information regarding fine touch, proprioception, and two-point discrimination. There is a somatotopic organization with the fasciculus gracilis medially carrying information from the lower extremities and the lateral fasciculus cuneatus conveying information from the upper extremities. The lateral column contains the dorsal and ventral

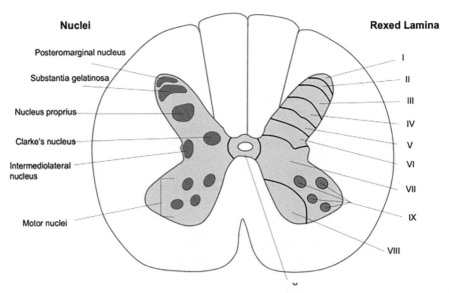

Fig. 1. Central gray matter, divided into Rexed lamina. (*Reproduced* with permission *from* Laureen D. Hachem, Ali Moghaddamjou, Michael G. Fehlings, Chapter 1 - Anatomy, Editor(s): Michael G. Fehlings, Brian K. Kwon, Alexander R. Vaccaro, F. Cumhur Oner, Neural Repair and Regeneration After Spinal Cord Injury and Spine Trauma, Academic Press, 2022, Pages 1 to 12, ISBN 9780128198353, https://doi.org/10.1016/B978-0-12-819835-3.00026-5.)

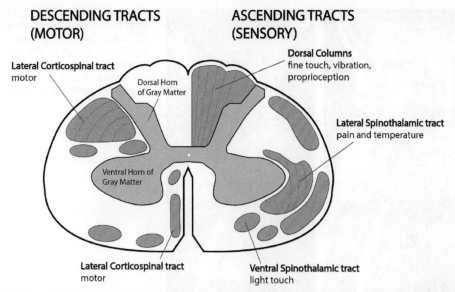

DESCENDING TRACTS (MOTOR)

ASCENDING TRACTS (SENSORY)

Lateral Corticospinal tract
motor

Dorsal Horn of Gray Matter

Dorsal Columns
fine touch, vibration, proprioception

Lateral Spinothalamic tract
pain and temperature

Ventral Horn of Gray Matter

Lateral Corticospinal tract
motor

Ventral Spinothalamic tract
light touch

Fig. 2. Ascending and descending white matter tracts. (*Reproduced* with permission *from* Shamik Bhattacharyya, Spinal Cord Disorders: Myelopathy, The American Journal of Medicine, Volume 131, Issue 11, 2018, Pages 1293 to 1297, ISSN 0002 to 9343, https://doi.org/10.1016/j.amjmed.2018.03.009.)

spinocerebellar tracts, which transmit information to the cerebellum regarding movement and position. The ventral column contains the spinothalamic tracts and spinoreticular pathway. The lateral spinothalamic tract transmits information regarding pain and temperature, and the anterior spinothalamic tract transmits crude touch.[15] Both terminate in the dorsal horn with second-order neurons projecting to the contralateral thalamus. The spinoreticular pathway connects the spinal cord to the reticular formation of the brainstem and functions in the modulation of pain; interestingly, there is no clear somatotopic organization of the spinoreticular pathway.[16]

CLINICAL CASES

Using the normal anatomy as a starting point, different pathologies can be better elucidated by application of this knowledge. Certain cases, such as complete cord transection can be easily identified by the loss of function below the level of spinal cord injury. However, for most other cases, the diagnosis can be more challenging as most abnormalities present with T2 hyperintensity within the cord. When considering patients presenting with a transverse myelopathy pattern of involvement, the radiologist's first job is to exclude compression of the spinal cord as a cause of the patient's symptoms. Beyond that, combining the imaging findings with the patient presentation and additional clinical history elements is needed to arrive at a differential diagnosis.[17] For the

purposes of the clinical cases, there are four key tracts that are implicated most often in patient presentations, which this article focuses on: descending tract—lateral corticospinal tract and ascending tracts—dorsal columns, spinocerebellar tracts, and spinothalamic tracts.

Cord Contusion/Transection

Often in the trauma setting, there is not a diagnostic dilemma regarding cord injury based on clinical examination and imaging findings. It is important to remember that ongoing compression from a translocation injury can mask underlying cord injury secondary to compression. For example, **Fig. 3**A demonstrates a patient status post a motorcycle accident presenting with subluxation at the C6–C7 level (arrow). Although there is T2 hyperintensity seen within the cord, it is not until the patient's spine is reduced (**Fig. 3**B), when the true extent of cord injury is seen (dotted circle). Note also the presence of blood products within the cord, a poor prognostic indicator for functional recovery.[18]

Central Cord

The central cord can be involved in several different pathologies, most often in patients with syrinx. Patients present with the loss of pain and temperature at the affected level secondary to involvement of the spinothalamic tracts. Although these tracts usually decussate on entering the cord, sometimes the axons will travel cephalad

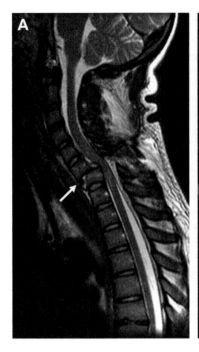
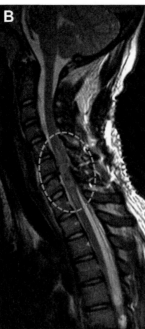

Fig. 3. (*A*) Sagittal T2 image of the cervical cord with subluxation at the C6–C7 level (*arrow*).(*B*) Post reduction sagittal T2 image of the cervical cord with increased T2 hyperintensity in the cord and central T2 hypointensity, consistent with hemorrhage (*dotted circle*).

to the next spinal level, which can make the presentation discordant. Vibration and position sense are maintained as the dorsal columns are spared.[19] Motor impairment is variable, but patients can present with lower motor neuron signs secondary to involvement of the ventral horns.[20]

Although syrinx can occur as the result of prior trauma or intramedullary tumor, a common etiology is Chiari I malformation.[21] As shown in **Fig. 4** on sagittal T2-weighted images, a patient presented with low-lying cerebellar tonsils with a peg-like configuration, resulting in a decreased flow of cerebrospinal fluid at the foramen magnum and syrinx formation with cord expansion (**Fig. 4**A, dotted circle). **Fig. 4**B demonstrates postoperative changes of occipital craniectomy and resection of the posterior arch of C1 (arrow) with decreased crowding at the foramen magnum and subsequent reduction in syrinx size and cord expansion (dotted circle).

Ventral Cord

Ventral cord syndromes present with motor impairment, which can be attributed to either upper or lower motor neurons and sometimes both depending on the extent of the cord involvement. Differentiating upper from lower motor neuron involvement can be done based on the clinical examination. Upper motor neuron processes present with spasticity, mild muscle atrophy, and hyperreflexia, whereas lower motor neuron diseases

present with hypotonia, severe muscle atrophy, hyporeflexia, and fasciculations. In addition, these patients may have associated loss of pain and temperature secondary to the involvement of decussation of the spinothalamic tracts.[22]

Cord infarct is most common in the ventral cord due to the single anterior spinal artery; cord infarcts can occur in the dorsal cord, but this is less likely secondary to the paired posterior spinal arteries. As in brain infarct, the key with cord infarct is the sudden onset of symptoms. A classic case presentation would be a patient awakening from aortic surgery with new onset paraplegia due to occlusion of the great anterior radiculomedullary artery. Restricted diffusion may be seen within the cord associated with an area of T2 hyperintensity as shown in **Fig. 5** (dotted circle). An additional finding that may help to make the diagnosis is an associated posterior vertebral body infarct as the blood supply to the vertebral body is from the anterior radiculomedullary arteries[23] (**Fig. 5**, arrow).

It is important to differentiate cord infarct from dural arteriovenous fistula, as there is significant overlap in the patient population—both are more likely to occur in males in their 5th to 6th decade.[24] However, although cord infarct patients present with the acute onset of symptoms, patients with dural arteriovenous fistula generally manifest slowly progressive symptoms secondary to the development of venous hypertension. As shown in **Fig. 6**, long-segment T2 hyperintensity is seen within the

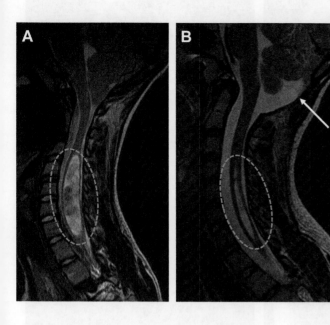

Fig. 4. (A) Sagittal T2 image of the cervical cord with low-lying cerebellar tonsils with central cord fluid collection and expansion (*dotted circle*). (B) Sagittal T2 image of the cervical cord with postoperative changes of decompression (*arrow*) with decreased cord fluid and expansion (*dotted circle*).

thoracic cord (arrow in **Fig. 6**A) with dilated intradural vessels seen on the parasagittal image (dotted circle in **Fig. 6**B). Dynamic contrast-enhanced magnetic resonance angiography was performed, demonstrating a dural arteriovenous fistula (dotted arrow in **Fig. 6**C). Early diagnosis is

important as the overall prognosis is based on the duration of symptoms before embolization.[25]

The other disease entity that often affects the ventral cord is viral infections. Diagnosis often requires confirmation with blood or cerebrospinal fluid testing. Enterovirus is one of the most common

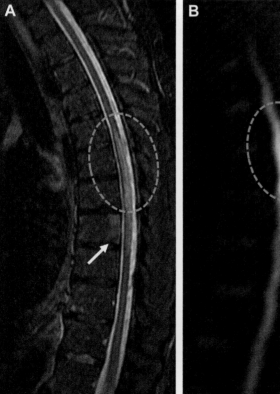
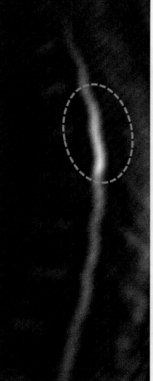

Fig. 5. (A) Sagittal T2 image of the thoracic cord with long-segment hyperintensity (*dotted circle*) and associated vertebral body infarct (*arrow*). (B) Sagittal DWI image of the thoracic cord with restricted diffusion (*dotted circle*).

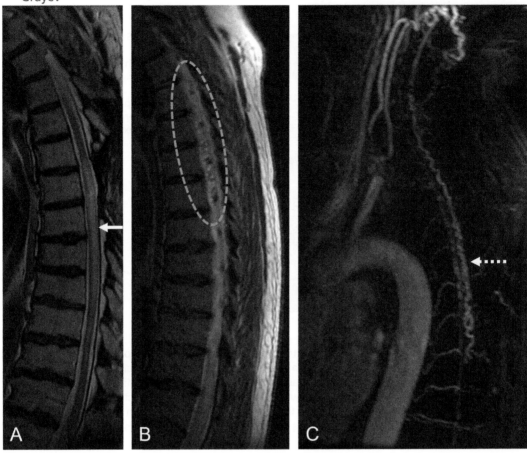

Fig. 6. (*A*) Sagittal T2 image of the thoracic cord with long-segment hyperintensity (*arrow*). (*B*) Parasagittal T2 image of the thoracic spine with dilated intradural vessels (*dotted circle*). (*B*) Single phase sagittal image of the cervicothoracic region from dynamic contrast-enhanced magnetic resonance angiography demonstrating tangle of vessels (*dotted arrow*).

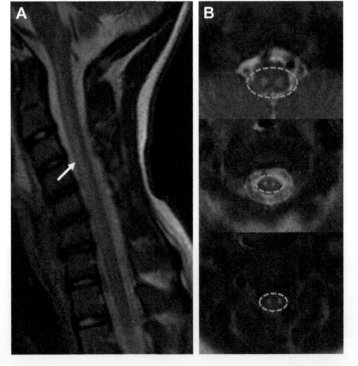

Fig. 7. (*A*) Sagittal T2 image of the cervical cord with long-segment ventral cord hyperintensity (*arrow*). (*B*) Serial axial T2 images of the cervical cord demonstrate involvement of ventral horns (*dotted circle*).

viruses to affect the ventral horn, and the acute flaccid myelitis outbreak of 2018 to 2019 was associated with enterovirus D68.[26] **Fig. 7** demonstrates long-segment ventral cord T2 hyperintensity (arrow in **Fig. 7A**) in a pediatric patient presenting with flaccid tetraplegia; the axial images (dotted circles in **Fig. 7B**) demonstrate preferential involvement of the ventral horns. Unfortunately, treatment is generally supportive with variable recovery.

Dorsal Cord

There are many different processes that affect the dorsal cord, ranging from toxic/metabolic to infectious. Dorsal cord abnormalities present with the loss of vibration and position sense due to dorsal column involvement. There may be sensory ataxia present if the dorsal spinocerebellar tracts are also involved. The classic metabolic derangement that presents with dorsal cord involvement is vitamin B12 deficiency, known as subacute combined degeneration. Vitamin B12 is a coenzyme needed for the metabolism of methylmalonic acid, and in its absence, methylmalonic acid build up can lead to myelin toxicity. Historically, this was associated with pernicious anemia leading to malabsorption or nitrous oxide toxicity; however, there is an increasing incidence in patients following a vegan or vegetarian diet secondary to inadequate intake.[27,28] Additional metabolic abnormalities that can lead to dorsal column involvement include copper and vitamin E deficiency. Infectious causes for dorsal column abnormalities include HIV vacuolar myelopathy and tabes dorsalis (tertiary syphilis). Paraneoplastic syndromes, toxic exposures (organophosphates, heroin, and chemotherapy) and spinocerebellar ataxia are additional causes for dorsal cord abnormalities. It is important to note that the appearance of these entities may be impossible to differentiate on imaging. For example, both patients A and B in **Fig. 8** have long-segment cord T2 hyperintensity (arrows) with involvement of the dorsal columns (dotted circles). Patient A had subacute combined degeneration, whereas patient B had copper deficiency; copper deficiency is more likely to present with peripheral neuropathy, which may be helpful in diagnosis.[29,30]

Hemicord Syndrome

This is a rare syndrome in which patients present with loss of all tracts secondary to a hemicord insult, often traumatic, but can be seen in demyelinating diseases such as multiple sclerosis or rarely in sulcal artery syndrome.[31] Patients present with ipsilateral paralysis, ipsilateral loss of vibration and position sense (dorsal columns), and contralateral loss of pain and temperature (spinothalamic tracts).

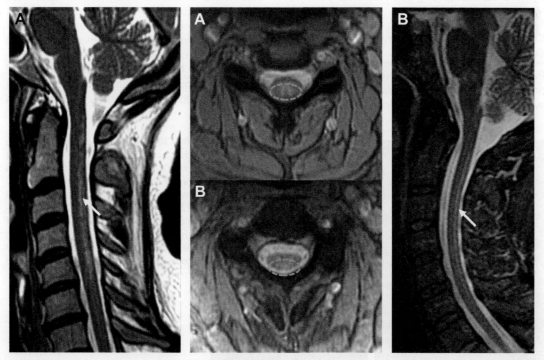

Fig. 8. (*A*) Sagittal and axial T2 images of the cervical cord with long-segment hyperintensity (*arrow*) and dorsal column involvement (*dotted circle*). (*B*) Sagittal and axial T2 images of the cervical cord with long segment hyperintensity (*arrow*) and dorsal column involvement (*dotted* circle).

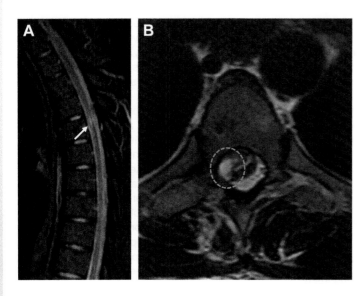

Fig. 9. (*A*) Sagittal T2 image of the thoracic cord with short-segment hyperintense lesion (*arrow*). (*B*) Axial T2 image of the thoracic cord with right hemicord hyperintensity (*dotted circle*).

Patients will often have upper motor neuron signs below the level of the lesion secondary to involvement of the lateral corticospinal tract with lower motor neuron signs at the level of the lesion secondary to lower motor neuron involvement in the ventral horns. **Fig. 9** demonstrates a patient status post stabbing injury with a short-segment T2 hyperintense cord lesion at T5 (arrow in **Fig. 9**A). Axial image (**Fig. 9**B) illustrates right hemicord injury with T2 hyperintensity (dotted circle).

Conus Medullaris Syndrome Versus Cauda Equina Syndrome

Patients presenting with conus medullaris syndrome are often confused for having cauda equina syndrome given that both groups can present with saddle anesthesia. The role of imaging in this patient group is to identify potentially compression lesions of the cord or nerve roots. There are differences that can be helpful in differentiating the two entities: conus medullaris syndrome generally presents with mixed upper and lower motor neuron weakness with early involvement of the urinary and anal sphincters[32], whereas in cauda equina syndrome, weakness tends to be more asymmetric and more dramatic and there is an early loss of reflexes at the ankle and knee.[33] **Fig. 10** demonstrates a patient with an enhancing intradural extramedullary mass at the level of the conus (arrow in **Fig. 10**A, sagittal T1 post-contrast). Note the anterior displacement of the conus with normal appearance of the nerve roots of the cauda equina below the level of the mass

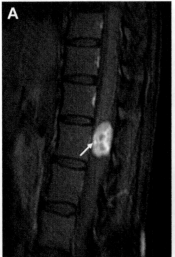
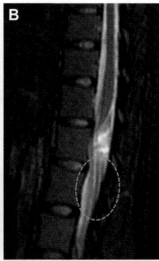

Fig. 10. (*A*) Sagittal T1 image of the thoracolumbar junction following contrast administration with enhancing intradural extramedullary mass at the conus (*arrow*). (*B*) Sagittal T2 image of the thoracolumbar junction with anterior displacement of the conus by T2 hyperintense mass with normal appearance of the nerve roots of the cauda equina (*dotted circle*).

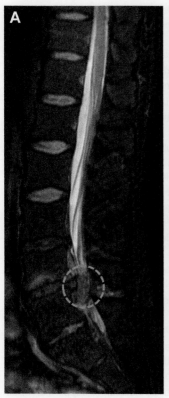
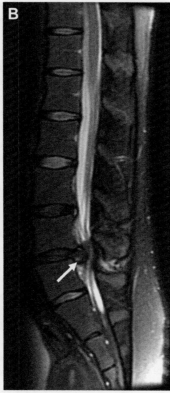

Fig. 11. (*A*) Sagittal T2 image of the lumbar spine with L4–L5 disc protrusion and epidural hematoma (*dotted circle*). (*B*) Sagittal T2 image of the lumbar spine with L4–L5 disc protrusion (*arrow*).

(dotted circle in **Fig. 10**B, sagittal T2). This is in distinction to the two patients presented in **Fig. 11.** Both patients have disc protrusions at L4–L5 (sagittal T2 images); patient A has additional epidural hematoma (dotted circle), whereas patient B has significant disc material (arrow), both leading to severe spinal canal narrowing.

SUMMARY

Knowledge of the intrinsic spinal cord anatomy is imperative in assessing patients presenting with a wide variety of symptoms. Although there may be a significant overlap in imaging findings, combining the MR imaging with clinical information and laboratory values in the patient chart can help narrow the differential diagnosis.

CLINICS CARE POINTS

- Knowledge of spinal cord anatomy is key for understanding clinical presentation of different pathologies.
- Cord lesions may result in either upper or lower motor neuron symptoms.

- Sensory testing may help to narrow a spinal cord level based on tract decussation.
- As most cord pathologies present with T2 hyperintensity, using information elicited from the patient's chart can be critical in narrowing the differential diagnosis.

DISCLOSURE

The author receives royalties from McGraw-Hill publishing.

REFERENCES

1. Elshazzly M, Lopez MJ, Reddy V, et al. Embryology, Central Nervous System. In: StatPearls. Treasure Island (FL: StatPearls Publishing; 2022. PMID: 30252280.
2. Rutman AM, Peterson DJ, Cohen WA, et al. Diffusion Tensor Imaging of the Spinal Cord: Clinical Value, Investigational Applications, and Technical Limitations. Curr Probl Diagn Radiol 2018;47:257–69.
3. Ali M, Safriel Y, Sohi J, et al. West Nile Virus Infection: MR Imaging Findings in the Nervous System. Am J Neuroradiol 2005;26:289–97.
4. Cohen-Adad J, El Mendili M-M, Lehéricy S, et al. Demyelination and degeneration in the injured

human spinal cord detected with diffusion and magnetization transfer MRI. Neuroimage 2011;55: 1024–33.

5. Martin AR, Tetreault L, Nouri A, et al. Imaging and Electrophysiology for Degenerative Cervical Myelopathy. Global Spine J 2022;12:130S–46S.

6. David G, Mohammadi S, Martin AR, et al. Traumatic and Nontraumatic Spinal Cord Injury: Pathological Insights from Neuroimaging. Nat Rev Neurol 2019; 15:718–31.

7. Martin AR, Aleksanderek I, Cohen-Adad J, et al. Translating State-of-the-art Spinal Cord MRI Techniques to Clinical Use: A Systematic Review of Clinical Studies Utilizing DTI, MT, MWF, MRS and fMRI. NeuroImage:Clinical 2016;10:192–238.

8. Lee MJ, Aronberg R, Manganaro MS, et al. Diagnostic Approach to Intrinsic Abnormality of Spinal Cord Signal Intensity. Radiographics 2019;39: 1824–39.

9. Taber KH, Herrick RC, Weathers SW, et al. Pitfalls and artifacts encountered in clinical MR imaging of the spine. Radiographics 1998;18:1499–521.

10. Leonard RJ. Human gross anatomy : an outline text. Incorporated: Oxford University Press; 1995.

11. Rexed B. A cytoarchitectomic atlas of the spinal cord in the cat. J Comp Neurol 1954;100:297–379.

12. Diaz E, Morales H. Spinal cord anatomy and clinical syndromes. Semin Ultrasound CT MRI 2016;37: 360–71.

13. Tan S, Faull RLM, Curtis MA. The Tracts, Cytoarchitecture, and Neurochemistry of the Spinal Cord. Anat Rec 2023;306:777–819.

14. Sabharwal S. Essentials of spinal cord medicine. Incorporated: Springer Publishing Company; 2014.

15. Willis WD, Westlund KN. Neuroanatomy of the Pain System and of the Pathways that Modulate Pain. J Clin Neurophysiol 1997;14:2–31.

16. Webb CM, Steeds CE. The Anatomy and Physiology of Pain. Clin Integrated Care 2022;14:10015.

17. Hardy TA. Spinal Cord Anatomy and Localization. Continuum 2021;271:12–29.

18. Bozzo A, Marcoux J, Radhakrishna M, et al. The Role of Magnetic Resonance Imaging in the Management of Acute Spinal Cord Injury. J Neurotrauma 2011;28: 1401–11.

19. Leclerc A, Matveeff L, Emery E. Syringomyelia and Hydromyelia: Current Understanding and Neurosurgical Management. Rev Neurol 2021;177:498–507.

20. Ciaramitaro P, Massimi L, Bertuccio A, et al. Diagnosis and Treatment of Chiari Malformation and Syringomyelia in Adults: International Consensus Document. Neuro Sci 2022;43:1327–42.

21. Holly LT, Batzdorf U. Chiari Malformation and Syringomyelia. J Neurosurg Spine 2019;31:619–28.

22. Santana JA, Dalal K. Ventral Cord Syndrome. In: StatPearls. Treasure Island (FL: StatPearls Publishing; 2022. PMID: 31082055.

23. Thron AK. Vascular anatomy of the spinal cord: radioanatomy as the key to diagnosis and treatment. New York, NY; Heidelberg, Germany; Basingstoke, UK: Springer International Publishing, Incorporated; 2016.

24. Muralidharan R, Saladino A, Lanzino G, et al. The Clinical and Radiological Presentation of Spinal Dural Arteriovenous Fistula. Spine 2011;36:E1641–7.

25. Krings T, Geibprasert S. "Spinal Dural Arteriovenous Fistulas". Am J Neuroradiol 2009;30:639–48.

26. Murphy OC, Messacar K, Benson L, et al. "Acute Flaccid Myelitis: Cause, Diagnosis, and Management". Lancet 2021;397:334–46.

27. De Rosa A, Rossi F, Lieto M, et al. Subacute Combined Degeneration of the Spinal Cord in a Vegan. Clin Neuro Neurosurg 2012;114:1000–2.

28. Rafailia Bakaloudi D, Halloran A, Rippin HL, et al. Intake and Adequacy of the Vegan Diet. A Systematic Review of the Evidence. Clin Nutr 2021;40: 3503–21.

29. Qureshi A, Bergbower E, Patel J. Copper Deficiency Myeloneuropathy with a History of Malabsorption: A Tale of Two Cases. J Community Hosp Intern Med Perspect 2021;11:152–5.

30. Altarelli M, Ben-Hamouda N, Schneider A, et al. Copper Deficiency: Causes, Manifestations, and Treatment. Nutr Clin Pract 2019;34:504–13.

31. Tan Y-J, Ng G-J, Yexian J, et al. Sulcal Artery Syndrome: A Three-patient Series and Review of Literature. J Clin Neurosci 2021;88:45–51.

32. Kunam VK, Velayudhan V, Chaudhry ZA, et al. Incomplete Cord Syndromes: Clinical and Imaging Review. Radiographics 2018;38:1201–22.

33. Ko H-K. Management and rehabilitation of spinal cord injuries. New York, NY; Heidelberg, Germany; Basingstoke, UK: Springer Publishing Company, Incorporated; 2022.

Diffusion Imaging of the Spinal Cord
Clinical Applications

Jason F. Talbott, MD, PhD[a,b,*], Vinil Shah, MD[c], Allen Q. Ye, MD, PhD[a,c]

KEYWORDS

- MR imaging • Spinal cord • Diffusion tensor imaging (DTI) • Tractography • Spinal cord injury
- Multiple sclerosis • FA

KEY POINTS

- The highly anisotropic and coherently oriented structure of white matter in the spinal cord is ideally suited for interrogating tissue integrity with diffusion imaging techniques.
- The spine and its surrounding anatomy present unique challenges to high-quality diffusion imaging of the spinal cord, thus familiarity with technical advancements for image optimization are key to successful incorporation of diffusion imaging in clinical spine protocols.
- Diffusion imaging offers promise for increasing sensitivity and specificity for diagnosis of many spinal cord pathologic conditions; however, more well-designed, prospective clinical studies are needed to further validate its routine utilization in many clinical settings.

INTRODUCTION

It has been nearly 200 years since the botanist Robert Brown first observed and reported on the random microscopic motions of pollen grains and dust particles in solution, thus introducing the phenomenon of microscopic diffusion to the world.[1] After further refinement by Fick,[2] Einstein[3] and others over subsequent decades, it was Edwin Hahn[4] who first recognized that this same diffusion principle contributed to decay of the spin-echo MR signal in the presence of an inhomogeneous magnetic field. From these fundamental observations, the mathematical framework for modern diffusion imaging was introduced by Carr and Purcell,[5] Stejskal and Tanner,[6] Le Bihan,[7] Basser,[8] and others. The highly anisotropic organization of tissue architecture in the central nervous system, particularly the spinal cord, presents predictable barriers to free water diffusion, thus making it ideally suited for probing both normal and pathologic states with diffusion-sensitive techniques.

This article is specifically devoted to the role of diffusion imaging for the evaluation of spinal cord pathologic conditions. For the brain, diffusion-weighted imaging (DWI) is a conventional and indispensable sequence integral to nearly every brain MR imaging protocol. Although incorporation of DWI sequences in spine MR imaging protocols has become increasingly common during the past decade, the added benefits and precise role for DWI in spinal cord imaging remains to be defined. DWI and associated more advanced water diffusion modeling techniques, such as diffusion tensor imaging (DTI) and diffusion tensor tractography (DTT) remain in the realm of "advanced" or supplemental sequences when

[a] Department of Radiology and Biomedical Imaging, Zuckerberg San Francisco General Hospital and Trauma Center, 1001 Potrero Avenue, Room 1X57, San Francisco, CA 94110, USA; [b] Brain and Spinal Injury Center, Zuckerberg San Francisco General Hospital; [c] Department of Radiology and Biomedical Imaging, Neuroradiology Division, University of California San Francisco, 505 Parnassus Avenue, #M-391, San Francisco, CA 94143, USA
* Corresponding author. Department of Radiology and Biomedical Imaging, Zuckerberg San Francisco General Hospital and Trauma Center, 1001 Potrero Avenue, Room 1X57C, San Francisco, CA 94110.
E-mail address: Jason.talbott@ucsf.edu

Radiol Clin N Am 62 (2024) 273–285
https://doi.org/10.1016/j.rcl.2023.10.002
0033-8389/24/© 2023 Elsevier Inc. All rights reserved.

compared to more conventional T1-weighted (T1-w) and T2-weighted (T2-w) sequences of the spinal cord. In this review, the basic principles of diffusion imaging will be summarized. Challenges that the complex spinal anatomy presents for diffusion imaging and techniques for mitigating the most common encountered artifacts will be reviewed. Both the promises and shortcomings of spinal cord diffusion imaging will then be explored in the context of several clinical applications for which diffusion imaging has been evaluated.

DIFFUSION IMAGING: FROM BASIC TO ADVANCED

Magnetic gradients are used in DWI to probe the thermal molecular motions of water molecules in tissue.[9] It is the Brownian motion of water that contributes directly to the attenuation of the MR signal in the presence of a bipolar diffusion-weighted magnetic field gradient. The first gradient pulse dephases the precessing water protons that contribute to MR imaging signal. If there is limited water diffusion, a second gradient pulse equal in amplitude but opposite in direction will near completely rephase the spins with negligible diffusion gradient-related signal loss. In contrast, if diffusion of water is high, the bipolar diffusion gradients more significantly attenuate signal as a function of water displacement magnitude. The MR parameters dictating the amplitude and duration of the diffusion gradients along with time interval between paired gradients are reflected by the "b-value." The b-value, coupled with the amount of water diffusion in tissue, dictates the measured diffusion-weighted signal.

Anisotropy refers to the directional dependence of water diffusion in tissue. In the spinal cord, highly anisotropic, longitudinally oriented white matter tracts composed predominantly of parallel axons and their myelin membranes are located peripherally, whereas the butterfly-shaped gray matter, composed primarily of more isotropic neuronal cell bodies, are located centrally. When a diffusion gradient is applied in an orientation parallel to peripheral white matter tracts of the spinal cord, there will be a relative loss of white matter signal in the diffusion-weighted image due to the near uninhibited free diffusion of extracellular water parallel to axonal and myelin membranes[10] (**Fig. 1**). If a diffusion-weighting gradient is applied perpendicular to the peripheral white matter tracts, relatively less attenuation of signal is noted due to the hindered diffusion of water perpendicular to axons and their myelin membranes (see **Fig. 1**). Thus, the highly anisotropic geometry of healthy white

matter compared to gray matter results in diffusion-weighted images with much higher gray–white matter tissue contrast when compared to conventional T2-w imaging, reflecting differences in gray and white matter tissue structure[10] (see **Fig. 1**).

The b-value and signal attenuation resulting from diffusion gradient application can be used to calculate quantitative apparent diffusion coefficient (ADC) values of spinal cord tissue. A baseline T2-w signal, which is obtained in the absence of a diffusion-sensitizing gradient and referred to as "b-zero (b0)" or "b-naught," is used to compare with the diffusion signal for ADC calculations[7] (**Fig. 2**). Signal intensity for each voxel of an ADC map is directly proportional to the ADC value. Thus, areas of hindered diffusion that are bright on the diffusion-weighted image will be dark on the corresponding ADC map and vice versa. In some cases, the underlying bright b0 T2-signal of tissue outweighs the diffusion-associated signal attenuation on a diffusion-weighted image, and the ADC value is high, a phenomenon known as "T2-Shine through." Therefore, one must always review the ADC map to truly infer diffusivity of tissue.

Diffusion Tensor Imaging and Tractography

At the most basic level of clinical diffusion imaging, diffusion gradients applied along 3 orthogonal axes of the magnetic field and a b0 image are sufficient to derive an average diffusion-weighted image and ADC map. However, given the highly anisotropic nature of spinal cord tissue, this ADC value may differ depending on the orientation of the patient in the scanner. More advanced diffusion modeling techniques are needed to ameliorate the limitations of tissue orientation dependence. To more accurately reflect water diffusion in tissues with anisotropic geometry without depending on a priori knowledge of tissue orientation relative to the magnetic field, DTI was developed.[7,8] With DTI, a minimum of 6 noncollinear diffusion-encoding gradients are applied, and the rotationally invariant directionality of Gaussian water motion can be modeled as an ellipse.[7,8] From the tensor model, quantitative scalar metrics reflecting diffusion properties serve as potential biomarkers of tissue organization.[8] DTI parameters include fractional anisotropy (FA), which is a unitless scalar metric ranging from 0 to 1 quantifying the fraction of the tensor that can be assigned to anisotropic water diffusion within a voxel. With the theoretic upper limit FA value of 1, all diffusion in a voxel is limited to a straight line, whereas an FA value of 0 represents equal

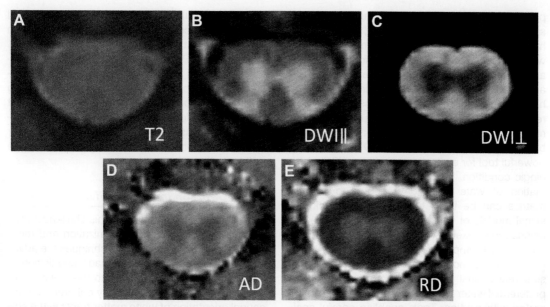

Fig. 1. Diffusion imaging increases gray–white matter contrast in the spinal cord compared with T2-w imaging. MR imaging of a normal rodent spinal cord demonstrates limited contrast between gray and white matter on T2-w sequence (*A*). Diffusion-weighted images with gradients applied parallel (*B*) and perpendicular (*C*) to the spinal cord provide high gray–white matter contrast due to highly anisotropic white matter tracts in the spinal cord periphery. Diffusion tensor-derived AD maps reflect the high diffusivity of water in white matter and corresponding hyperintense white matter signal (*D*) compared to hindered diffusion with relatively hypointense signal of white matter on RD maps (*E*).

spherical isotropic diffusion in all directions. The trace of the diffusion tensor is the sum of the 3 orthogonal axis, or eigenvalues, of the ellipse. The trace/3 provides the mean diffusivity (MD), which represents the magnitude of diffusivity averaged over the 3 orthogonal axis of the tensor ellipse. Compared to ADC values calculated from simple 3-direction DWI, tensor-derived MD is a more accurate measure of average diffusivity in all directions, because it is rotationally invariant,[11] meaning the orientation of the spinal cord within the scanner does not alter the MD values.

Additional DTI parameters include axial diffusivity (AD), sometimes referred to as longitudinal diffusivity or $\lambda_{\parallel}$ (see **Fig. 1**). AD is a measurement of diffusivity along the long axis or primary eigenvector of the diffusion tensor ellipse. Radial diffusivity (RD), sometimes also referred to as transverse diffusivity or the symbol $\lambda_{\perp}$, is the averaged diffusivity along the 2 minor axes of the tensor ellipse (see **Fig. 1**). AD reflects the relatively unimpeded motion of extracellular water traveling parallel to white matter bundles, whereas RD reflects the more hindered motion of water

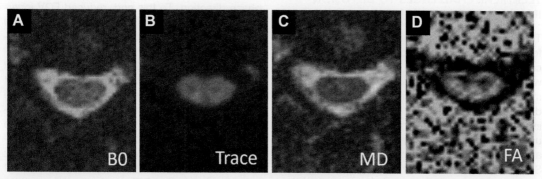

Fig. 2. DTI of the normal cervical spinal cord in human. Initial B0 image (*A*) is obtained, which lacks diffusion sensitization. All diffusion-sensitized acquisitions are summed to produce a trace map (*B*). Rotationally invariant and quantitative scalar maps for MD (*C*) and FA (*D*) are derived from the raw diffusion data.

perpendicular to axons.[7] In preclinical models of spinal cord pathologic condition, AD and RD have been shown to correlate with microstructural white matter pathologic conditions including axonal injury and demyelination, respectively,[12–14] although their specificity for these injury subtypes has been challenged.[15] Nevertheless, the relatively regular and parallel orientation of functionally significant ascending and descending white matter bundles in the spinal cord, makes DTI a potentially powerful tool for evaluating spinal cord (SC) pathologic condition.[16,17] With DTT, directional information of water diffusion reflected by tensor metrics can be used to approximate 3-dimensional models of white matter bundles by linking neighboring voxels, which share similar features (Fig. 3). It is important to recognize that these reconstructed models do not necessarily represent real axonal tracts but simply pathways of preferential water diffusion and thus must be interpreted with caution. Tools enabling careful analysis of quantitative spinal cord imaging data have historically been lacking. The Spinal Cord Toolbox (SCT) is a free open-source program, which has emerged as an important software platform for automated spinal cord segmentation, template registration and atlas-based quantitative regional analysis of diffusion metrics[18] (see Fig. 3).

Beyond DTI, several more complex multicompartmental water diffusion models have been developed to more accurately represent water diffusion, especially in tissues where there are crossing or otherwise nonuniform orientation of axons within a voxel. These techniques include diffusion kurtosis imaging (DKI),[19] neurite orientation dispersion and density imaging (NODDI),[20] and Q-space imaging (QSI)[21] among others. Experience with these techniques in the spine is primarily limited to preclinical and ex vivo studies due to their long acquisition times.

TECHNICAL CHALLENGES TO DIFFUSION IMAGING OF THE SPINAL CORD

There are numerous technical challenges to performing high-quality diffusion imaging of the spinal cord. Spinal anatomy is a primary consideration with the small caliber of the spinal cord, only measuring up to 12 to 15 mm in maximal transaxial dimension for adults. The segmented bone and intervertebral disc configuration of the spinal column as well as bone–cerebrospinal fluid (CSF) and bone–air interfaces in close proximity to the SC creates significant magnetic field inhomogeneities, contributing to off resonance geometric shifting and image warping.[22] The most used pulse sequence for DWI is single-shot echo-planar imaging (ss-EPI), which is rapid and therefore ideal for diffusion acquisitions given multiple diffusion directions must be obtained in a timely manner. However, ss-EPI is particularly susceptible to geometric warping from magnetic field inhomogeneities, making the spine a particularly challenging environment for this technique. Motion artifact related to swallowing, breathing, cardiac contraction as well as CSF pulsation also all further contribute to phase errors and associated image artifact in the spine.

Spinal Diffusion Imaging Artifact Mitigation

To mitigate artifacts related to this challenging imaging environment, study optimization and more recently developed diffusion techniques are advocated for the spinal cord.[23] Image acquisition in the axial plane (perpendicular to the spinal cord) takes advantage of the relatively coherent craniocaudal orientation of white matter tracts in the spinal cord and allows for thick slices (up to 5 mm), thus maximizing signal-to-noise ratio (SNR).[24] However, axial imaging is recommended when only a specific segment of the spinal cord needs imaging because it is too time consuming and impractical for total spine imaging in most clinical settings. Positioning of the patient with the spine as straight as possible is important to minimize partial-volume artifact with adjacent CSF and reduce tissue inhomogeneity within the shim volume. The imaging field-of view (FOV) should be rotated to align with the segment of spinal cord being imaged in both the sagittal and coronal planes. To maximize image signal, b-values for spinal cord DWI are generally lower than for brain imaging, typically 800 s/mm^2, compared with 1000 s/mm^2 typically used for adult clinical brain imaging.[24]

Susceptibility-related distortions are best reduced by minimizing the FOV to focus on the spinal cord and exclude nontarget outer tissues, which contribute to artifact, particularly in the phase direction. To this end, reduced FOV inner-excitation techniques such as zonally magnified oblique multislice EPI use spatially selective excitation in the slice select and phase-encoding directions to enhance SNR for the small spinal cord anatomy and reduce susceptibility artifact from nonexcited nontarget tissues and improve image quality.[25] Segmented readout EPI techniques such as RESOLVE allow for shorter echo spacing by filling k-space with a series of concatenated segments in the readout direction, thus further reducing geometric distortions. In attempt to better standardize DTI parameters for quantitative metric extraction and comparison across sites and MR imaging vendors, Cohen-adad and

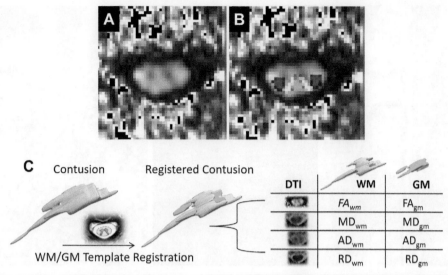

Fig. 3. Segmentation tools such as the SCT aid in atlas-based DTI analysis. FA map of the normal cervical spinal cord (*A*) reflecting high anisotropic differences between gray and white matter tissue in the spinal cord with hyperintense white matter peripherally and relatively hypointense gray matter frontal horns centrally. Following registration with available spinal atlases in the SCT, specific subregions of the spinal cord can be mapped on the FA map (*B, corticospinal tract in red and fasciculus cuneatus in yellow*). (*C*) A schematic for potential atlas-based workflow for quantitative DTI analysis of a segmented spinal cord contusion injury where DTI metrics can be uniquely extracted from specific regions of the spinal cord (white matter in yellow and gray matter in green in this example).

colleagues[24] recently published a recommended generic spine DTI protocol at 3 T.

CLINICAL APPLICATIONS
Traumatic Spinal Cord Injury

T2-w imaging of the spinal cord is the gold standard imaging technique for both diagnosis and neuroprognostication in acute traumatic spinal cord injury (tSCI).[26] For more than 2 decades, diffusion MR imaging techniques have promised improved diagnostic and prognostic capabilities for patients suffering from devastating complications of tSCI. A brief summary of the literature highlights both advances and limitations of DWI and DTI for tSCI patient triage, management, and neuroprognostication. Sagiuchi and colleagues[27] were the first to use 3-direction DWI obtained within 2 hours of acute high cervical SCI to demonstrate a reduction in ADC values at the injury epicenter in a single case report. In a larger study of 14 acute tSCI patients, Tsuchiya and colleagues[28] found DWI signal hyperintensity and subjectively reduced ADC signal intensity in 9 patients with acute tSCI. Although a trend toward significant ADC reductions was observed, this underpowered study did not show a statistically significant reduction in ADC values compared with normal appearing spinal cord.[28] Statistically significant reduced ADC values at the injury epicenter were reported by Zhang and Huan in a study of 20 patients with acute tSCI.[29] These differences were limited, however, to 10 patients with evidence of spinal cord contusion but no hemorrhage on T2-w imaging.[29] In a small retrospective cohort of 7 patients, Pauw and colleagues[30] showed a similar sensitivity for detecting cord injury with DWI and T2-w sequences when performed within the first 24 hours of injury. Collectively, the results from these studies show that acute SCI is usually associated with an initial DWI hyperintensity and reduction in spinal cord ADC values compared with normal spinal cord (**Fig. 4**). Presently, there is insufficient evidence to support DWI-derived ADC correlations with injury severity or outcome.[31] Although the precise molecular mechanisms of reduced ADC values in acute SCI are not completely understood,[32] the progression of injuries with low ADC values to cystic myelomalacia on follow-up MR imaging suggests some component of cytotoxic edema and irreversible tissue injury while preserved or increased ADC values more likely relate to vasogenic edema.[33]

In an early study applying DTI in acute SCI, Shanmuganathan and colleagues[34] found significantly lower MD, FA, and AD values at the injury site compared with values of the whole cervical spinal

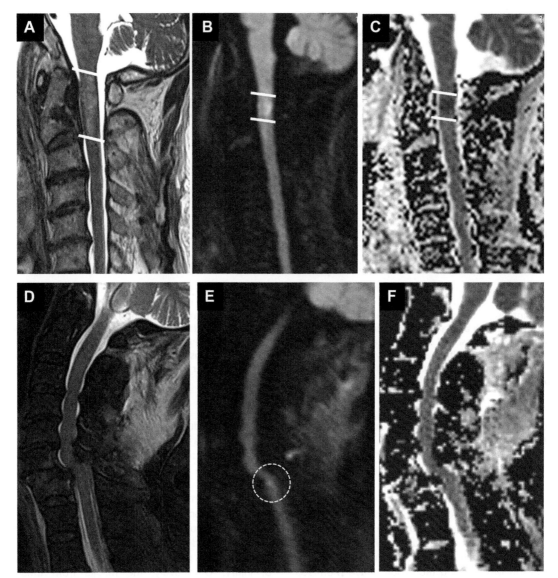

Fig. 4. DWI for the detection of acute tSCI. Sagittal T2-w image (A) of the cervical spinal cord in an 87-year-old female patient with quadriplegia after fall shows expansile cord contusion centered at the C1-C2 levels. Sagittal DWI (B) and corresponding ADC image (C) reveals central area of abnormal reduced diffusion, which are delimited by white lines in (B) and (C), suggesting cytotoxic edema and some component of irreversible injury. Sagittal T2-w image (D) in a different patient with bilateral upper extremity paresthesias and normal motor examination shows anterolisthesis of the spine at C6-C7 with severe canal stenosis and mild cord compression but without appreciable intramedullary T2 signal abnormality. Sagittal DWI (E) and ADC (F) images from the same patient show small focus of DWI hyperintensity (dotted circle in E) without corresponding reduced ADC signal, suggesting mild vasogenic edema and potentially reversible injury.

cord obtained from controls. In a follow-up study with 25 SCI patients, Cheran and colleagues[35] similarly demonstrated significant reductions in FA and AD values between SCI and controls. Further, in patients with nonhemorrhagic contusion, MD, FA, AD, and RD measures at the injury epicenter all correlated with initial injury severity as assessed with American Spinal Injury Association (ASIA) motor scores.[35] Shanmuganathan and colleagues prospectively correlated normalized DTI metrics from acute MR imaging with ASIA Impairment Scale (AIS) grade. The authors found AD as the most robust DTI parameter for predicting neurologic and functional outcomes. In another important prospective clinical study of DTI in tSCI, Poplawski and colleagues[36] determined the accuracy of DTI for predicting neurologic recovery in 23 patients with acute tSCI. By analyzing DTI metrics of the spinal cord at and away from the injury epicenter, the authors importantly showed that clinically relevant DTI metric alterations were identified rostral to the injury epicenter.[36] DTI analysis may therefore be useful, even in patients with spinal instrumentation, where metallic artifact often precludes evaluation of the injury epicenter (**Fig. 5**). In summary, these studies suggest an important diagnostic and prognostic role for DTI in tSCI. However, conspicuous by its absence throughout the literature is comparison of DTI metrics with more conventional T2-w MR classifications schemes such as the lesion length, sagittal grade, and the Brain and Injury Spinal Injury Center score. This may in part explain why a recent appraisal of clinical practice guidelines for imaging in tSCI found little evidence to support DTI in tSCI.[37] Advantages of DTI over conventional T2-w imaging for tSCI remain to be demonstrated so that the added image acquisition and processing time can be justified for routine clinical use.

Filtered double diffusion encoded imaging filtered DWI has more recently been demonstrated as a promising diffusion technique in clinical studies of acute tSCI.[38] Although reductions in the DTI metric AD have been proposed to represent hindered water diffusion parallel to traumatically injured axonal tracts secondary to axonal beading and traumatic disruption, overlapping acute tissue injury responses including vasogenic edema and hemorrhage confound AD measurements. By application of a "filter" diffusion gradient perpendicular to the long axis of the spinal cord, isotropic diffusion signal from vasogenic edema is suppressed, whereas signal from a "probing" diffusion gradient oriented along the spinal cord longitudinal axis more accurately reflects AD independent of filtered vasogenic edema. FDWI thus diminishes the impact of vasogenic edema on masking AD reductions and increases specificity for axonal injury in the acute phase of injury. Murphy and colleagues[38] recently demonstrated, in a cohort of patients with acute tSCI, that fDWI showed greater sensitivity to acute white matter damage at the spinal cord contusion epicenter compared with standard DTI metrics. Future larger cohort prospective studies are needed to validate these promising results.

Spinal Cord Infarct

Acute SC infarct is a clinical emergency occurring more frequently in women, with an average age of onset of 56 years.[39] There are several factors that increase the risk for SC infarct including recent aortic surgery, vasculitis, aortic dissection, and hypotension. The spinal cord arterial supply includes a complex arterial network of collateralization between a single anterior spinal artery and paired posterior spinal arteries. The dominant radicular artery of Adamkiewicz provides anterior spinal arterial supply to the lower spinal card with relatively limited collaterals, accounting for the more common incidence of lower thoracic anterior SC infarcts.[39]

Clinical diagnosis of acute cord infarction is challenging because patients often present with nonspecific symptoms including acute onset weakness, sensory changes, and bowel and bladder dysfunction. MR imaging is the gold standard imaging modality for diagnosis, and DWI plays a critical role in helping distinguish T2 hyperintensity in the spinal cord from vast number of other acute noncompressive myelopathies that may seem similar to infarct on conventional MR imaging sequences and present with overlapping clinical symptoms. Anterior spinal artery territory infarcts are the most common and present with T2 hyperintensity primarily involving gray matter frontal horns, referred to as the "owl's eye" sign.[40] However, more confluent centromedullary T2 hyperintensity may also be observed (**Fig. 6**). Frontal horn predominant T2 signal hyperintensity can also be seen with several nonischemic infectious, inflammatory, and compressive myelopathies.[41,42] Therefore, demonstrating abnormal reduced diffusion corresponding to areas of T2 hyperintensity can greatly increase the specificity of diagnosis of spinal cord infarct in the appropriate clinical setting. More advanced diffusion imaging techniques including DTI and DTT have not shown significant benefit in diagnosis or characterization of acute spinal cord infarct.

Compressive Spondylotic Myelopathy

Degenerative compressive spondylotic myelopathy (CSM) is the most common cause of spinal cord injury. MR imaging is the gold-standard imaging technique for characterizing morphologic changes related to degenerative spine disease, including spinal canal compromise, spinal cord compression, and intramedullary spinal cord T2 signal abnormality. Correlation between these morphologic changes on conventional MR imaging and patient's clinical symptoms as well as response to surgical decompression, however, are limited.[43] For example, in the asymptomatic population, the literature cites a range from 4.9% to 7.6% of individuals with cervical cord compression on MR imaging.[44,45]

DTI has emerged as a diagnostic tool with potential for increased sensitivity and specificity for

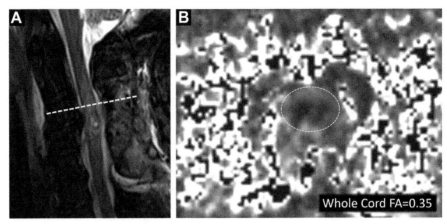

Fig. 5. FA maps from DTI can be used for characterizing tissue injury in acute tSCI. Sagittal T2-w image (*A*) in a 75-year-old man obtained following posterior decompression for tSCI shows spinal cord contusion spanning the lower C2 to C4 vertebral levels with central cystic change. Axial FA map (*B*) obtained along the cranial aspect of the contusion injury reveals markedly decreased whole cord FA values (0.35) compared with expected values of 0.65 to 0.7 at this level in the uninjured spinal cord. Dashed white line in A corresponds to the axial level for FA map image in B. Approximate margins for spinal cord FA measurement indicated by dashed oval in (*B*).

diagnosis and treatment planning in patients with CSM. Similar to other spinal cord pathologic conditions that disrupt the normal highly anisotropic structure of spinal cord tissue, CSM is associated with an increase in MD and a decrease in FA.[46] A recent meta-analysis of 10 studies involving 495 cervical spinal cord compression patients found

that there was an overall reduction in spinal cord FA for patients with CSM.[47] This finding is in keeping with the current hypotheses where compression and subsequent disruption to the spinal cord leads to damage to intercellular and intracellular barriers resulting in less organized diffusion of water molecules in the cord. Recent studies have

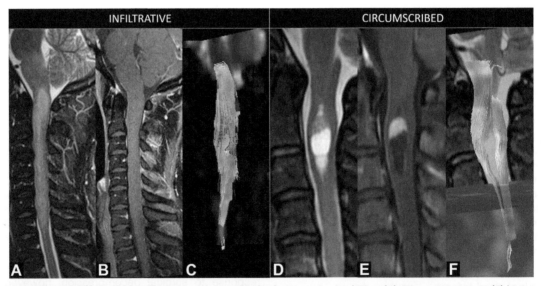

Fig. 6. DTT can differentiate infiltrative and circumscribed tumors. Sagittal T2-w (*A*), T1-w postcontrast (*B*) images show a longitudinally extensive expansile astrocytoma spanning virtually the entire cervical spinal cord. DTT (*C*) reveals complete encasement of white matter fibers reflecting the highly infiltrative nature of tumor. In a different patient, sagittal T2-w (*D*) and T1-w postcontrast (*E*) images of the cervical spine show a solid and cystic spinal cord ependymoma with nodular enhancement superiorly.. DTT (*F*) reveals lateral displacement of modeled white matter tracts without any appreciable encasement of axons by tumor, reflecting the circumscribed nature of this tumor.

also found that decreases in FA both at the site of compression and in segments above the level of compression are observed prior to the onset of clinical symptoms and could be an early biomarker of future myelopathy.[48,49]

In addition to diagnosis, DTI also holds promise for prognostication in the setting of CSM. Maki and colleagues[50] showed that prospective analysis of DTI in 26 patients with CSM had predictive value on the Japanese Orthopaedia Association (JOA) score 6 months after decompressive surgery. The primary biomarkers were FA and MD and change and recovery rate of JOA score was moderately correlated with FA. In a longitudinal study of nonoperative patients, Ellingson and colleagues[51] demonstrated that quantitative DTI measurements FA and MD were significantly correlated with a modified JOA (mJOA) score with direct relationship of FA to JOA and an inverse relationship between MD and mJOA. Rao and colleagues[52] noted that preoperative FA correlated inversely with recovery throughout the postoperative period most significantly at the 12-month time period. A statistically significant threshold (FA <0.55) when measuring at the level of maximal cord compression was presented. Patients with FA below that cutoff improved more after surgery than those above, as measured on the mJOA. As with other spinal pathologic conditions, larger prospective and randomized trials for CSM are needed to validate these results and solidify a role for DTI in assessing injury severity, predicting outcome, and potentially aiding in selection of ideal surgical candidates.

Inflammatory Myelopathy

Multiple sclerosis (MS) is the most common inflammatory myelopathy. MS is a complex autoimmune disorder with a variety of pathologic subtypes characterized by inflammatory demyelination. Conventional MR imaging demonstrates relatively short-segment lesions with predominant peripheral spinal cord location, gadolinium contrast enhancement, and T2 hyperintensity during the acute active phase of disease. Nonenhancing T2 hyperintense plaques with volume loss are noted in the more chronic phase of injury. Spinal cord involvement with MS is observed in approximately 50% to 90% of patients with known disease.[53] Overlapping inflammation and edema associated with white matter tissue disruption in MS results in predictable pattern of DTI alterations, namely decreased FA and increased MD values,[54] rather nonspecific features of pathologic white matter injury as has been noted in other myelopathies described in

this review. RD has been proposed as a more specific biomarker of demyelination due to increased water diffusivity perpendicular to demyelinated white matter tracts.[55,56] However, the specificity of RD for myelin disruption has not been convincingly demonstrated.[15,57] Although DTI metrics have not been shown to convincingly disambiguate unique pathoanatomic entities such as demyelination, axonal disruption, edema, and inflammation, they do offer increased sensitivity to clinically important white matter pathologic condition in MS compared with conventional T2 imaging by detecting alterations in normal appearing white matter (NAWM).[58,59] Given the relatively poor correlation between T2 injury burden and neurologic disability in MS, DTI promises to enhance prediction of clinical course and monitoring of disease progression for routine treatment and clinical trials.

To further increase sensitivity to pathologic condition and advance pathoanatomic characterization of injury in MS, more recent studies have applied advanced diffusion techniques to the spinal cord. With QSI, instead of assuming a Gaussian diffusion of water molecules via the Einstein–Smoluchowski equation, a probability density map of water molecules in one voxel is generated to determine a true diffusion evaluation. Early studies noted high sensitivity of QSI metrics to MS lesions in the brain.[21] More recent studies evaluating the spinal cord in patients with MS have shown increases in the QSI-derived perpendicular diffusivity despite normal spinal cord volumes, suggesting QSI's increased sensitivity to white matter perturbations in MS.[60] NODDI is a biophysical model of diffusion that presumes a microstructural model and fits diffusion data to the improved representation of the neuronal configuration including a component of neurite density. NODDI assumes 3 compartments: a free water (CSF) component, an intraneurite component, and an extraneurite component. The respective percentage of each component can be estimated. Additionally, the orientation of structures within the voxel is also calculated via the orientation dispersion.[20] In 28 patients with relapsing remitting MS, Collorone and colleagues[61] showed that the presence of reduced neurite density in the cervical spinal cord was associated with higher disability. NODDI metrics have also been shown to have increased contrast between NAWM and lesion in patients with MS when compared with DKI and DTI.[62] Although such results are promising, QSI and NODDI require additional imaging time to acquire more diffusion directions and often, multiple b-values, thus challenging clinical feasibility for routine spinal cord

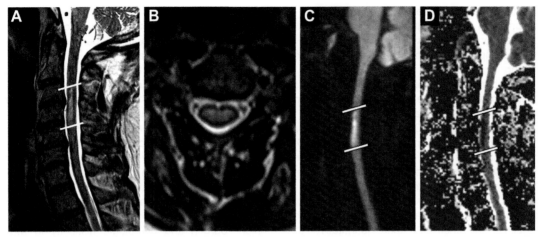

Fig. 7. Diffusion imaging aids in diagnosis of acute spinal cord infarct. Sagittal (A) and axial (B) T2-w images show abnormal central spinal cord T2-hyperintensity in a 60-year-old man with hypertension, diabetes mellitus, and hyperlipidemia presenting with 1-day history of progressive weakness, bowel and bladder dysfunction, and hyperreflexia. Central cord signal T2 hyperintensity is delimited by horizontal white lines in A. Sagittal diffusion weighted (C) and corresponding ADC map (D) from the same patient clearly demonstrate abnormal reduced diffusion in the anterior spinal cord, confirming clinically suspected diagnosis of acute cord infarct, despite rather nonspecific T2-w pattern of cord signal abnormality.

imaging and accounting for the relatively limited clinical translation.

With respect to inflammatory myelopathies other than MS, DTI has been shown useful in monitoring severity and treatment response of patients with imaging features of transverse myelitis. Lee and colleagues[63] demonstrated decreased FA at the lesion epicenter and distal to the lesion in normal appearing spinal cord of patients with idiopathic transverse myelitis with a moderate correlation between decreased FA at those 2 levels and increasing clinical severity of symptoms. In a cohort of patients with heterogenous inflammatory myelopathies, Renoux and colleagues[64] found similar trend of decreased FA values in the setting of transverse myelitis.

Neoplastic Pathologic Condition of the Spinal Cord

There is tremendous variability in the imaging appearance of intramedullary spinal cord masses, including primary and metastatic tumors.[65] Primary spinal cord neoplasms observed with highest frequency include ependymomas, astrocytomas, and hemangioblastomas. Spinal cord metastases are fortunately rare and typically expansile and induce prominent surrounding edema.[65]

At the most basic level, spinal cord masses can be characterized as circumscribed or infiltrative (Fig. 7). This distinction is key to clinical management as the goal for circumscribed tumors is

complete surgical resection while more infiltrative tumors require primary noninvasive treatments such as radiotherapy and chemotherapy. The presence of an intramedullary tumor has predictable impact on the diffusion metrics of the normal highly anisotropic tissue of the spinal cord, namely significant reduction in FA due to the more isotropic diffusion of water in the tumor environment and interruption of normal anisotropic white matter tracts. Highly cellular and infiltrative tumors such as lymphoma and high-grade gliomas are expected to have relatively lower ADC values compared with more "watery" less cellular tumors such as ependymomas. In a cohort of 40 patients with expansile tumefactive spinal cord lesions, Hohenhaus and colleagues[66] demonstrated that DTI metrics were able to differentiate between inflammatory and neoplastic lesions, although differentiation of specific tumor subtypes was not feasible. Setzer and colleagues[67] used DTI to predict resectability of intramedullary spinal tumors. In this small pilot study of 13 patients, intramedullary tumors were classified into 3 subtypes: (1) no passing fibers through tumor on tractography, (2) majority of lesion volume lacks passing fibers on tractography, and (3) complete tumoral encasement of passing fibers. The authors presented high interrater reliability for this DTT-based classification scheme and reliable differentiation between resectable and unresectable tumors using this schema. At least one subsequent small retrospective study found similar results.[68] Although larger prospective studies are needed to validate these findings, they demonstrate the potential for DTT in characterization of tumor infiltration and guidance of surgical management.

SUMMARY

MR imaging is the established gold standard imaging modality for evaluating the spinal cord. DTI holds promise for overcoming limitations of conventional MR imaging techniques with respect to more sensitively and specifically diagnosing and characterizing the nature of tissue injury and predicting outcome but requires further validation for most clinical applications. Many of the limitations related to lack of specificity of T2-w alterations in the spinal cord for injury classification also apply to DTI, where decreased FA and increased MD metrics are observed in a wide variety of cord pathologic conditions because of white matter disruption, regardless of the mechanism of injury. More advanced diffusion modeling techniques including QSI, NODDI, and DKI may add sensitivity and specificity for spinal cord pathologic condition but face practical challenges in routine clinical implementation. Validation of DTI application in standardized, high-quality clinical trials with long-term neurologic and functional outcome data is still lacking for most spinal diseases.

CLINICS CARE POINTS

- When performing diffusion imaging of the spinal cord to target a specific level of injury, acquisition in the axial plane with b-value of 800 s/mm^2 and slice thickness of 5 mm is recommended.

- Utilization of reduced field-of-view or readout segmented EPI diffusion techniques for the spinal cord will enhance image quality by reducing distortion and warping artifact.

- Alterations in spinal cord DTI metrics, especially FA and AD, are quite sensitive for the detection of pathologic white matter disruption, although nonspecific with respect to cause.

DISCLOSURES

The authors have no disclosures of commercial or financial conflict of interest.

REFERENCES

1. Brown R. A brief account of microscopical observations made in the months of June, July, August, 1827 on the particles contained in the pollen of plants; and on the general existence of active molecules in organic and inorganic bodies. Phil Mag 1828; 4(1828):161–73.

2. Fick A. Concerns diffusion and concentration gradient. Ann Phys Lpz 1855;170:59.

3. Einstein A. Investigations on the theory of the brownian movement. New York: Dover Publications; 1926.

4. Hahn H. Spin Echoes. Phys Rev 1950;80:580–94.

5. Carr HYPE. Effects of diffusion on free precession in nuclear magnetic resonance experiments. Phys Rev 1954;94(3):630–8.

6. Stejskal EOTJ. Use of spin echoes in a pulsed magnetic-field gradient to study anisotropic, restricted diffusion and flow. J Chem Phys 1965; 42(1):288–92.

7. Le Bihan D, Mangin JF, Poupon C, et al. Diffusion tensor imaging: concepts and applications. J Magn Reson Imaging 2001;13(4):534–46.

8. Basser PJ, Mattiello J, LeBihan D. Estimation of the effective self-diffusion tensor from the NMR spin echo. J Magn Reson B 1994;103(3):247–54.

9. Le Bihan D, Breton E, Lallemand D, et al. MR imaging of intravoxel incoherent motions: application to diffusion and perfusion in neurologic disorders. Radiology 1986;161(2):401–7.

10. Holder CA, Muthupillai R, Mukundan S Jr, et al. Diffusion-weighted MR imaging of the normal human spinal cord in vivo. AJNR Am J Neuroradiol 2000; 21(10):1799–806.

11. Iima M, Le Bihan D. Clinical Intravoxel Incoherent Motion and Diffusion MR Imaging: Past, Present, and Future. Radiology 2016;278(1):13–32.

12. Budde MD, Kim JH, Liang HF, et al. Axonal injury detected by in vivo diffusion tensor imaging correlates with neurological disability in a mouse model of multiple sclerosis. NMR Biomed 2008;21(6):589–97.

13. Budde MD, Kim JH, Liang HF, et al. Toward accurate diagnosis of white matter pathology using diffusion tensor imaging. *Magnetic resonance in medicine : official journal of the Society of Magnetic Resonance in Medicine/Society of Magnetic Resonance in Medicine.* Magn Reson Med 2007;57(4):688–95.

14. Budde MD, Xie M, Cross AH, et al. Axial diffusivity is the primary correlate of axonal injury in the experimental autoimmune encephalomyelitis spinal cord: a quantitative pixelwise analysis. J Neurosci 2009; 29(9):2805–13.

15. Talbott JF, Nout-Lomas YS, Wendland MF, et al. Diffusion-Weighted Magnetic Resonance Imaging Characterization of White Matter Injury Produced by Axon-Sparing Demyelination and Severe Contusion Spinal Cord Injury in Rats. J Neurotrauma 2016;33(10):929–42.

16. Facon D, Ozanne A, Fillard P, et al. MR diffusion tensor imaging and fiber tracking in spinal cord

compression. AJNR Am J Neuroradiol 2005;26(6): 1587–94.

17. Vedantam A, Eckardt G, Wang MC, et al. Clinical correlates of high cervical fractional anisotropy in acute cervical spinal cord injury. World neurosurgery 2015;83(5):824–8.

18. De Leener B, Fonov VS, Collins DL, et al. PAM50: Unbiased multimodal template of the brainstem and spinal cord aligned with the ICBM152 space. Neuroimage 2018;165:170–9.

19. Wu EX, Cheung MM. MR diffusion kurtosis imaging for neural tissue characterization. NMR Biomed 2010;23(7):836–48.

20. Zhang H, Schneider T, Wheeler-Kingshott CA, et al. NODDI: practical in vivo neurite orientation dispersion and density imaging of the human brain. Neuroimage 2012;61(4):1000–16.

21. Assaf Y, Ben-Bashat D, Chapman J, et al. High b-value q-space analyzed diffusion-weighted MRI: application to multiple sclerosis. Magn Reson Med 2002;47(1):115–26.

22. Rutman AM, Peterson DJ, Cohen WA, et al. Diffusion Tensor Imaging of the Spinal Cord: Clinical Value, Investigational Applications, and Technical Limitations. Curr Probl Diagn Radiol 2018;47(4):257–69.

23. Martin Noguerol T, Barousse R, Amrhein TJ, et al. Optimizing Diffusion-Tensor Imaging Acquisition for Spinal Cord Assessment: Physical Basis and Technical Adjustments. Radiographics 2020;40(2): 403–27.

24. Cohen-Adad J, Alonso-Ortiz E, Abramovic M, et al. Generic acquisition protocol for quantitative MRI of the spinal cord. Nat Protoc 2021;16(10):4611–32.

25. Alizadeh M, Poplawski MM, Fisher J, et al. Zonally Magnified Oblique Multislice and Non-Zonally Magnified Oblique Multislice DWI of the Cervical Spinal Cord. AJNR Am J Neuroradiol 2018;39(8): 1555–61.

26. Talbott JF, Huie JR, Ferguson AR, et al. MR Imaging for Assessing Injury Severity and Prognosis in Acute Traumatic Spinal Cord Injury. Radiol Clin 2019;57(2): 319–39.

27. Sagiuchi T, Tachibana S, Endo M, et al. Diffusion-weighted MRI of the cervical cord in acute spinal cord injury with type II odontoid fracture. J Comput Assist Tomogr 2002;26(4):654–6.

28. Tsuchiya K, Fujikawa A, Honya K, et al. Value of diffusion-weighted MR imaging in acute cervical cord injury as a predictor of outcome. Neuroradiology 2006;48(11):803–8.

29. Zhang JS, Huan Y. Multishot diffusion-weighted MR imaging features in acute trauma of spinal cord. Eur Radiol 2014;24(3):685–92.

30. Pouw MH, van der Vliet AM, van Kampen A, et al. Diffusion-weighted MR imaging within 24 h post-injury after traumatic spinal cord injury: a qualitative meta-analysis between T2-weighted imaging and diffusion-weighted MR imaging in 18 patients. Spinal Cord 2012;50(6):426–31.

31. Martin AR, Aleksanderek I, Cohen-Adad J, et al. Translating state-of-the-art spinal cord MRI techniques to clinical use: A systematic review of clinical studies utilizing DTI, MT, MWF, MRS, and fMRI. Neuroimage Clin 2016;10:192–238.

32. Budde MD, Skinner NP. Diffusion MRI in acute nervous system injury. J Magn Reson 2018;292:137–48.

33. Endo T, Suzuki S, Utsunomiya A, et al. Prediction of neurological recovery using apparent diffusion coefficient in cases of incomplete spinal cord injury. Neurosurgery 2011;68(2):329–36.

34. Shanmuganathan K, Gullapalli RP, Zhuo J, et al. Diffusion tensor MR imaging in cervical spine trauma. AJNR Am J Neuroradiol 2008;29(4):655–9.

35. Cheran S, Shanmuganathan K, Zhuo J, et al. Correlation of MR diffusion tensor imaging parameters with ASIA motor scores in hemorrhagic and nonhemorrhagic acute spinal cord injury. J Neurotrauma 2011;28(9):1881–92.

36. Poplawski MM, Alizadeh M, Oleson CV, et al. Application of Diffusion Tensor Imaging in Forecasting Neurological Injury and Recovery after Human Cervical Spinal Cord Injury. J Neurotrauma 2019; 36(21):3051–61.

37. Guan B, Li G, Zheng R, et al. A critical appraisal of clinical practice guidelines for diagnostic imaging in the spinal cord injury. Spine J 2023;23(8):1189–98.

38. Murphy SA, Furger R, Kurpad SN, et al. Filtered Diffusion-Weighted MRI of the Human Cervical Spinal Cord: Feasibility and Application to Traumatic Spinal Cord Injury. AJNR Am J Neuroradiol 2021;42(11): 2101–6.

39. McEntire CR, Dowd RS, Orru E, et al. Acute Myelopathy: Vascular and Infectious Diseases. Neurol Clin 2021;39(2):489–512.

40. Weidauer S, Nichtweiss M, Lanfermann H, et al. Spinal cord infarction: MR imaging and clinical features in 16 cases. Neuroradiology 2002;44(10):851–7.

41. Talbott JF, Narvid J, Chazen JL, et al. An Imaging-Based Approach to Spinal Cord Infection. Semin Ultrasound CT MR 2016;37(5):411–30.

42. Mathieu J, Talbott JF. Magnetic Resonance Imaging for Spine Emergencies. Magn Reson Imag Clin N Am 2022;30(3):383–407.

43. Wen CY, Cui JL, Liu HS, et al. Is diffusion anisotropy a biomarker for disease severity and surgical prognosis of cervical spondylotic myelopathy? Radiology 2014;270(1):197–204.

44. Lee MJ, Cassinelli EH, Riew KD. Prevalence of cervical spine stenosis. Anatomic study in cadavers. J Bone Joint Surg Am 2007;89(2):376–80.

45. Nouri A, Martin AR, Mikulis D, et al. Magnetic resonance imaging assessment of degenerative cervical myelopathy: a review of structural changes and measurement techniques. Neurosurg Focus 2016; 40(6):E5.

46. Cheng SJ, Tsai PH, Lee YT, et al. Diffusion Tensor Imaging of the Spinal Cord. Magn Reson Imag Clin N Am 2021;29(2):195–204.

47. Ouyang Z, Zhang N, Li M, et al. A meta-analysis of the role of diffusion tensor imaging in cervical spinal cord compression. J Neuroimaging 2023;33(4):493–500.

48. Grabher P, Mohammadi S, David G, et al. Neurodegeneration in the Spinal Ventral Horn Prior to Motor Impairment in Cervical Spondylotic Myelopathy. J Neurotrauma 2017;34(15):2329–34.

49. Kara B, Celik A, Karadereler S, et al. The role of DTI in early detection of cervical spondylotic myelopathy: a preliminary study with 3-T MRI. Neuroradiology 2011;53(8):609–16.

50. Maki S, Koda M, Kitamura M, et al. Diffusion tensor imaging can predict surgical outcomes of patients with cervical compression myelopathy. Eur Spine J 2017;26(9):2459–66.

51. Ellingson BM, Salamon N, Woodworth DC, et al. Reproducibility, temporal stability, and functional correlation of diffusion MR measurements within the spinal cord in patients with asymptomatic cervical stenosis or cervical myelopathy. J Neurosurg Spine 2018;28(5):472–80.

52. Rao A, Soliman H, Kaushal M, et al. Diffusion Tensor Imaging in a Large Longitudinal Series of Patients With Cervical Spondylotic Myelopathy Correlated With Long-Term Functional Outcome. Neurosurgery 2018;83(4):753–60.

53. Ikuta F, Zimmerman HM. Distribution of plaques in seventy autopsy cases of multiple sclerosis in the United States. Neurology 1976;26(6 PT 2):26–8.

54. Hori M, Maekawa T, Kamiya K, et al. Advanced Diffusion MR Imaging for Multiple Sclerosis in the Brain and Spinal Cord. Magn Reson Med Sci 2022;21(1):58–70.

55. Freund P, Wheeler-Kingshott C, Jackson J, et al. Recovery after spinal cord relapse in multiple sclerosis is predicted by radial diffusivity. Mult Scler 2010;16(10):1193–202.

56. Song SK, Yoshino J, Le TQ, et al. Demyelination increases radial diffusivity in corpus callosum of mouse brain. Neuroimage 2005;26(1):132–40.

57. Klawiter EC, Schmidt RE, Trinkaus K, et al. Radial diffusivity predicts demyelination in ex vivo multiple sclerosis spinal cords. Neuroimage 2011;55(4):1454–60.

58. Hesseltine SM, Law M, Babb J, et al. Diffusion tensor imaging in multiple sclerosis: assessment of regional differences in the axial plane within normal-appearing cervical spinal cord. AJNR Am J Neuroradiol 2006;27(6):1189–93.

59. Valsasina P, Rocca MA, Agosta F, et al. Mean diffusivity and fractional anisotropy histogram analysis of the cervical cord in MS patients. Neuroimage 2005;26(3):822–8.

60. Abdel-Aziz K, Schneider T, Solanky BS, et al. Evidence for early neurodegeneration in the cervical cord of patients with primary progressive multiple sclerosis. Brain 2015;138(Pt 6):1568–82.

61. Collorone S, Cawley N, Grussu F, et al. Reduced neurite density in the brain and cervical spinal cord in relapsing-remitting multiple sclerosis: A NODDI study. Mult Scler 2020;26(13):1647–57.

62. By S, Xu J, Box BA, et al. Application and evaluation of NODDI in the cervical spinal cord of multiple sclerosis patients. Neuroimage Clin 2017;15:333–42.

63. Lee JW, Park KS, Kim JH, et al. Diffusion tensor imaging in idiopathic acute transverse myelitis. AJR Am J Roentgenol 2008;191(2):W52–7.

64. Renoux J, Facon D, Fillard P, et al. MR diffusion tensor imaging and fiber tracking in inflammatory diseases of the spinal cord. AJNR Am J Neuroradiol 2006;27(9):1947–51.

65. Waldron JS, Cha S. Radiographic features of intramedullary spinal cord tumors. Neurosurg Clin 2006;17(1):13–9.

66. Hohenhaus M, Merz Y, Klingler JH, et al. Diffusion tensor imaging in unclear intramedullary tumor-suspected lesions allows separating tumors from inflammation. Spinal Cord 2022;60(7):655–63.

67. Setzer M, Murtagh RD, Murtagh FR, et al. Diffusion tensor imaging tractography in patients with intramedullary tumors: comparison with intraoperative findings and value for prediction of tumor resectability. J Neurosurg Spine 2010;13(3):371–80.

68. Korkmazer B, Kemerdere R, Bas G, et al. The efficacy of preoperative diffusion tensor tractography on surgical planning and outcomes in patients with intramedullary spinal tumor. Eur Spine J 2023. https://doi.org/10.1007/s00586-023-07872-5.

Dynamic Contrast Enhanced MR Perfusion and Diffusion-Weighted Imaging of Marrow-Replacing Disorders of the Spine
A Comprehensive Review

Onur Yildirim, MD[a],*, Kyung K. Peck, PhD[b], Atin Saha, MD, MS[a], Sasan Karimi, MD[a], Eric Lis, MD[a]

KEYWORDS

- Dynamic contrast-enhanced MR imaging • Diffusion-weighted imaging • Spinal metastases
- Hypervascular metastases • Hypovascular metastases
- Benign and malignant vertebral compression fractures
- Atypical hemangiomas (intraosseous venous malformations) • Chordoma

KEY POINTS

- Dynamic contrast-enhanced (DCE) MR imaging is a valuable tool for assessing spinal metastases because they typically exhibit elevated plasma volume (Vp) and permeability constant (Ktrans), indicating viable tumors.
- Decreased quantitative perfusion parameters may indicate treatment response and nonviable disease.
- Atypical hemangiomas (intraosseous venous malformations) do not display elevated perfusion levels when compared with spinal metastases.
- Vertebral body compression fractures accompanied by elevated Vp and Ktrans are likely to have pathologic origins.
- The prognostic value of DCE MR imaging in detecting early treatment response has the potential to enhance patient care and improve outcomes.
- Incorporating the emerging MR imaging sequence, diffusion-weighted imaging, into the standard MR imaging protocol for patients with cancer undergoing metastatic spinal evaluation holds potential as a reliable tool for distinguishing between benign and malignant vertebral marrow lesions.

INTRODUCTION

Significant advancements in cancer treatment have resulted in longer survival rates for patients. Improved chemotherapy regimens have revolutionized cancer care, offering more effective and targeted therapies. Enhanced radiotherapy techniques, such as image-guided radiation therapy and single fraction therapy, have improved treatment precision and minimized side effects. Moreover, advancements in interventional procedures have allowed for minimally invasive techniques,

a Department of Radiology, Memorial Sloan Kettering Cancer Center, 1275 York Avenue, New York, NY 10065, USA; b Department of Medical Physics
* Corresponding author.
E-mail address: yildirio@mskcc.org

Radiol Clin N Am 62 (2024) 287–302
https://doi.org/10.1016/j.rcl.2023.09.004

reducing patient discomfort and promoting faster recovery. These developments have collectively contributed to extended life spans and improved outcomes for patients with cancer.[1] Early detection and treatment are crucial for improving survival rates, and monitoring progress is critical for identifying treatment failure in metastatic cancer, which can be as challenging as treating primary cancer. Hence, it is crucial to detect spinal metastases and monitor the progress of treatment.[2]

Following the lungs and liver, the skeletal system emerges as the third most prevalent site for cancer metastasis, with the spine being the most frequently affected area. Approximately 5% to 10% of individuals with cancer experience spinal metastases, leading to notable morbidity.[3] MR imaging has emerged as the preferred and widely accepted imaging modality for detecting and evaluating spinal neoplasms. It is often considered the "gold standard" in this context.[4] Although T1-weighted and short-tau inversion recovery sequences (STIR) effectively detect spinal metastasis,[5] their utility for monitoring treatment progress is limited.[6,7]

Standard imaging methods (MR imaging, CT, PET, and bone scintigraphy), although valuable in detecting and evaluating spinal neoplasms, cannot provide physiologic information such as tumor vascularity and hemodynamics. New advanced imaging techniques incorporating diffusion, perfusion, and tumor microenvironment characteristics offer promising advantages. T1-weighted dynamic contrast enhancement (dynamic contrast-enhanced [DCE] MR imaging) is an emerging advanced MR imaging technique that enables the measurement of perfusion in the body.[8] Incorporating perfusion imaging of vertebral marrow can significantly enhance the diagnostic process, treatment assessment, and follow-up of patients with metastatic tumors. By assessing blood flow and tissue perfusion within the vertebral marrow, perfusion imaging offers valuable insights into tumor characteristics and response to treatment. This information can aid improving the management of metastatic spinal tumors.

DCE MR imaging and diffusion-weighted imaging (DWI) offer insights into tissue perfusion and permeability. Although their applications in body imaging are relatively limited compared with brain imaging, recent studies have demonstrated successful utilization in studying healthy bone marrow and detecting lesions. DWI holds promise in distinguishing between benign and malignant marrow lesions. Both techniques offer both nonquantitative and quantitative approaches for analysis. This review provides an overview of the principles and applications of DWI and DCE MR imaging.

DYNAMIC CONTRAST-ENHANCED MR IMAGING
Marrow Perfusion and Background

The distribution pattern of yellow and red marrows significantly influences bone marrow perfusion.[9] Distinct differences in vascular supply can be observed between red and yellow marrows, resulting in structural variations. Yellow marrow is predominantly composed of fat cells and exhibits a limited vascular network.[10] Following the administration of a contrast agent, only a slight and gradual increase in signal intensity is observed.[11] In contrast, red marrow differs significantly with its abundance of fenestrated vessels, large vascular pools and channels, and minimal presence of poorly vascularized fat. Enhancement is often inconspicuous due to fatty marrow's high inherent signal intensity, which hinders the visibility of enhancement. Nevertheless, by conducting meticulous signal intensity measurements, it is possible to detect enhancement.[12]

The enhancement of bone marrow significantly decreases with age and the conversion of marrow to fat, although there is notable variability among individuals.[8] Age-related arteriosclerosis can lead to changes in marrow perfusion and the occurrence of ischemic changes.[13] Chen and colleagues[13] demonstrated decreased perfusion with advancing age, particularly in women. Furthermore, studies have indicated a reduction in perfusion indexes in the vertebral body and paraspinal tissues that share the same arterial supply as bone mineral density declines, observed in both genders.[14]

DCE MR imaging is a novel perfusion MR imaging technique used for spinal tumor imaging. This method is particularly useful in evaluating spinal metastases due to its ability to quantitatively evaluate the tumor microvasculature. Spinal metastases can trigger the release of proangiogenic growth factors, which subsequently promote the formation of abnormal neoangiogenesis and increased vascular permeability.[15] DCE MR imaging effectively characterizes vascular changes and detects viable early diseases. It provides quantitative parameters such as plasma volume (Vp) and permeability constant (Ktrans), as well as semi-quantitative parameters such as area under the curve (AUC), for assessing spinal neoplasms. The noninvasive nature of DCE MR imaging has led to its widespread utilization in the assessment of intracranial neoplasms, and it is now being extended to the diagnosis and monitoring of spinal metastasis.[9,16]

Earlier studies have highlighted the usefulness of DCE perfusion MR imaging for assessing spinal lesions.[17–22] In the study titled "T1-Weighted

Dynamic Contrast-Enhanced MRI to Differentiate Non-neoplastic and Malignant Vertebral Body Lesions in the Spine" by Guan and colleagues, the researchers evaluated 100 patients with biopsy-proven vertebral body lesions. The study findings revealed that Vp was significantly lower in nonneoplastic lesions compared with malignant lesions, with respective values of 1.6 ± 1.3 and 4.2 ± 3.0 (P < .001). The sensitivity of Vp in distinguishing between nonneoplastic and malignant lesions was 93% (77 out of 83), with a 95% confidence interval (CI) of 85% to 97%. The specificity was found to be 78% (40 out of 51) with a 95% CI of 65% to 89%. The area under the curve was calculated as 0.88 (95% CI: 0.82–0.95), indicating a high accuracy of Vp in differentiation between these types of vertebral body lesions. These findings suggest that Vp imaging can be a valuable tool for distinguishing between malignant and nonmalignant spinal lesions in various primary cancers, including hypovascular types such as breast and prostate cancers.

Several earlier studies have reported on the usefulness of DCE perfusion in examining spinal metastases. Specifically, Chu and colleagues,[17] Kumar and colleagues,[18] and Lis and colleagues[19] all noted a significant decrease in Vp changes at varying time points after radiation therapy (RT) for spinal metastases. In a retrospective study conducted by Kumar and colleagues,[18] 30 patients with spinal metastases who underwent RT, the utility of DCE MR imaging in predicting tumor response to RT and local tumor recurrence (LR) was investigated. The study demonstrated that changes in perfusion parameters, particularly Vp, served as predictive indicators for both RT response and LR. Notably, DCE MR imaging exhibited the ability to predict LR during 6 months earlier than standard imaging, suggesting its potential clinical implications in guiding patient care.

In separate studies, Arevalo-Perez and colleagues[22] and Saha and colleagues[20] demonstrated the usefulness of DCE perfusion MR imaging in distinguishing between benign and pathologic spinal fractures, as well as differentiating between hypervascular and hypovascular spinal metastases. Furthermore, Morales and colleagues used Vp to distinguish atypical hemangiomas from metastatic vertebral lesions. Tumors acquire an enhanced blood supply through multiple mechanisms.[23] The presence of an abnormal vascular network within a metastatic lesion enables the accumulation of contrast agents, leading to an elevated Vp (plasma volume) on DCE perfusion MR imaging scans.

Perfusion studies have been used to examine the response of bone marrow neoplasms to chemotherapy. It is anticipated that cytotoxic drugs would influence angiogenesis, resulting in a reduction of contrast medium uptake within the bone marrow.[24] Moreover, quantitative analysis of DCE MR imaging data has been used to explore angiogenesis and blood vessel permeability induced by myeloma, focusing on microcirculation variables. This approach has been suggested as a prognostic marker for event-free survival in cases of progressive multiple myeloma.[25]

IMAGING PROTOCOLS
Gadolinium Diethylene Triamine Pentaacetic Acid Contrast Agent

DCE MR imaging perfusion imaging technique involves the rapid intravenous administration of gadolinium diethylene triamine pentaacetic acid (Gd-DTPA), followed by the acquisition of dynamic T1-weighted imaging sequences. The administration rate for gadolinium during MR imaging perfusion using a power injector is typically around 2 to 3 mL/s. Quantitative estimation of vascular properties can be achieved by analyzing the temporal changes in signal intensity through the utilization of pharmacokinetic modeling of contrast agent uptake (ΔSI). This protocol has been extensively used for perfusion assessment in the brain, heart, and various neoplasms.[26] Furthermore, it has been validated for investigating bone perfusion in both healthy bone and areas affected by infiltration.[27]

DCE MR imaging uses the contrast agent Gd-DTPA to enhance perfusion measurements, surpassing endogenous contrast techniques such as arterial spin labeling. This enables the detection of heightened tumor permeability by analyzing the accumulation of the contrast agent. Postcontrast T1-weighted sequences provide superior lesion visualization compared with preinjection images. In the brain, dynamic susceptibility contrast (DSC) MR imaging quantifies relative cerebral blood volume to assess tumor diagnosis and progression.[28,29] However, this technique is not without limitations, including the context-dependency of perfusion measurements, low spatial resolution of images, and inconsistent analysis techniques.

TWO COMPARTMENT MODEL

DCE MR imaging is a real-time imaging technique that uses a contrast agent to analyze tissue perfusion and vascular permeability. It uses the extended pharmacokinetic 2-compartment model to estimate quantitative parameters such as permeability (Ktrans) and fractional plasma volume

(Vp), providing information about vascularity. The 2-compartment kinetic model evaluates blood vessel compartment (Vp) and vessel permeability (Ktrans) by fitting a mathematical model to dynamic contrast concentration curves.[30]

In quantitative analysis of spinal perfusion, accurately detecting the arterial input function (AIF) is vital. Typically, a major artery such as the aorta is chosen to obtain the AIF, offering valuable insights into blood flow characteristics in the specific region of interest. To ensure precision, pixels showing significant changes in signal intensity, rapid transition after contrast injection, and early peak intensity are often selected to represent the AIF curve. Certain software packages even provide automated methods to identify appropriate arteries for generating the AIF curve.

Semiquantitative analysis of DCE MR imaging involves examining time–intensity curves (TICs) to evaluate MR signal intensity changes during contrast accumulation in a specific region of interest (ROI). The TIC provides 3 derived parameters: peak enhancement signal percentage change, wash-in enhancement slope, and AUC. This approach offers advantages such as not requiring the measurement of the AIF and being relatively unaffected by contrast injection protocols. However, limitations include the lack of direct physiologic correlations and sensitivity to acquisition protocol variations. Chen and colleagues proposed a categorical system classifying TIC morphologies into 5 types: Type A (nearly flat), Type B (gradual enhancement), Type C (rapid wash-in plateau), Type D (rapid wash-in followed by wash-out), and Type E (rapid wash-in with a slower second enhancement).[31]

SPINE MR IMAGING ACQUISITION PROTOCOL

One commonly used approach for acquiring DCE MR imaging data is the 3D T1-weighted spoiled gradient recalled echo technique. However, a more recent method called 3D volume Differential Subsampling with Cartesian Ordering (DISCO) has emerged as a promising alternative, demonstrating the ability to maintain spatial resolution while achieving an effective temporal resolution of 3 to 4 seconds for capturing contrast kinetics. In DISCO, postcontrast 3D T1-weighted images are acquired at intervals of approximately 4 to 5 seconds to construct the contrast concentration-TIC. To assess the signal change induced by the contrast agent, low flip angles ranging from 15° to 25° can be used. Additionally, using a short echo time helps mitigate the T2* effect of the contrast, whereas a shorter repetition time enhances scan efficiency.[32]

CLINICAL APPLICATIONS
Identifying the Vascularity of Healthy Bone Marrow and Tumors

DCE MR imaging has demonstrated promising outcomes in the diagnosis of spinal metastases. In a study by Khadem and colleagues, a retrospective analysis was conducted on 26 patients with spinal metastases. The study revealed that by examining overall TIC morphologies, DCE MR imaging was capable of distinguishing between healthy bone marrow and spinal metastases.[33] In healthy subjects, minimal to no contrast enhancement was observed, whereas spinal metastases displayed contrast enhancement above the baseline, characterized by a "flat" type of TIC (**Fig. 1**). Moreover, DCE MR imaging can differentiate between newly formed spinal metastases and previously treated ones, even when they seem similar on conventional MR imaging scans. This distinction becomes effortless by using Vp maps and analyzing TIC patterns, enabling differentiation between new and treated metastases as well as normal bone marrow.

Furthermore, DCE MR imaging provides the capability to differentiate between hypervascular and hypovascular metastases, a distinction that conventional MR imaging techniques are unable to achieve. Khadem and colleagues observed that the conventional MR signal intensity percentage changes between preinjection and postinjection of Gd-DTPA did not exhibit a significant difference between hypervascular and hypovascular spinal metastases.[31] DCE MR imaging effectively differentiated between 2 groups by analyzing quantitative parameters. Hypervascular metastases exhibited significantly higher average wash-in enhancement slope and peak enhancement signal percentage change compared with hypovascular metastases ($P < .01$). These findings indicate that DCE MR imaging can offer valuable insights for differentiating between hypervascular and hypovascular spinal metastases.

Mazura and colleagues demonstrated that DCE MR imaging could serve as a noninvasive alternative to spinal catheter angiography for evaluating tumor perfusion. This highlights the potential of DCE MR imaging as a valuable tool in assessing and characterizing the vascularity of spinal tumors without the need for invasive procedures.[34]

DCE MR imaging enables the noninvasive identification of hypervascularity, guiding preoperative tumor embolization. Accurate characterization of spinal tumor vascularity helps identify hypervascular lesions that can benefit from preoperative embolization. This proactive approach reduces

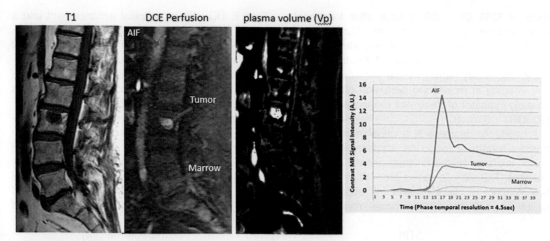

Fig. 1. Differentiating healthy bone marrow from tumor tissue. **Fig. 1** presents a side-by-side comparison of imaging findings highlighting the vascularity of healthy bone marrow and tumor tissue in a patient with prostate cancer. The images were obtained using MR imaging with dynamic contrast-enhanced sequences. The image emphasizes the intricate network of sinusoidal vessels in healthy bone marrow and the aberrant vascular features associated with tumor development. This comparative illustration underscores the importance of assessing vascularity to differentiate between healthy and pathologic tissues, facilitating accurate diagnosis and tailored treatment strategies for patients with cancer. (AIF, arterial input function).

intraoperative blood loss and improves surgical outcomes by optimizing surgical preparation.

Although spinal catheter angiography is considered as "gold standard" for assessing tumor vascularity, it is an invasive and expensive procedure. Conversely, DCE MR imaging has gained recognition as a noninvasive and cost-effective alternative. By providing valuable insights into tumor vascularity, DCE MR imaging offers a safer and more affordable approach for evaluating vascular characteristics in spinal tumors, minimizing the requirement for invasive techniques such as spinal catheter angiography.[34]

DCE MR imaging plays a crucial role in surgical procedures by detecting hypervascularity, allowing for targeted approaches. This helps reduce intraoperative blood loss and optimize surgical interventions including preoperative tumor embolization. Additionally, DCE MR imaging shows promise in evaluating the response to antiangiogenic therapy, providing valuable information on its effectiveness in inhibiting tumor growth and reducing blood supply.

Evaluating the Response to Radiation Therapy

DCE MR imaging has the potential to be valuable in monitoring the posttreatment responses of patients who have undergone RT. RT induces alterations in the microvasculature of tumors, resulting in reduced blood flow due to various factors such as thrombosis, fibrosis, and apoptosis.[35]

Recent studies have indicated that DCE MR imaging can detect hemodynamic changes shortly

after treatment, allowing for the identification of treatment response in spinal metastases following high-dose RT.[17,36] Chu and colleagues conducted a study involving a cohort of 19 spinal bone metastases treated with RT and observed that changes in Vp served as the most reliable indicator of treatment response. Among the successfully treated lesions, a decrease in Vp was consistently observed. In contrast, the 2 treatment failures exhibited a significant increase in Vp, indicating a lack of favorable response to the therapy. This finding underscores the potential of Vp as a predictive parameter for assessing treatment efficacy in spinal bone metastases following RT.[17]

In a study by Spratt and colleagues, a homogeneous cohort of 12 patients with sarcoma metastases to the spine underwent stereotactic body radiation therapy (SBRT). The findings showed that changes in perfusion parameters, specifically Ktrans and Vp, achieved a remarkable accuracy in predicting local control outcomes. This predictive capability outperformed conventional size measurements and subjective neuroradiology impressions. With only one instance of local failure observed, the study highlights the strong predictive value of perfusion parameters in assessing treatment response and local control in sarcoma metastases treated with SBRT.[36]

Lis and colleagues conducted a study that demonstrated the capability of DCE MR imaging to detect decreased perfusion levels 1 hour after high-dose image-guided radiation therapy (HD-IGRT), indicating a favorable treatment response. The quantitative metric Vp exhibited a significant drop of 65% (*P* < .05) 1 hour after treatment compared with pretreatment levels. Furthermore, the follow-up imaging consistently showed low Vp values, suggesting sustained treatment efficacy. This study highlights the potential of DCE MR imaging in monitoring perfusion changes as an early indicator of treatment response following HD-IGRT[19] (**Fig. 2**).

An early Vp decrease is a valuable indicator of positive treatment response, surpassing conventional imaging methods that assess structural changes. TIC analysis shows promise as a qualitative measure to classify treatment response after radiotherapy. Successful outcomes often exhibit a Type E TIC with rapid initial enhancement and a slower second increase, whereas unsuccessful responses typically display a Type D TIC with rapid wash-in followed by wash-out. Combining quantitative and qualitative metrics is crucial for evaluating treatment response and monitoring contrast enhancement changes during radiotherapy.[17]

Moreover, DCE MR imaging has shown its potential in the early detection of local spinal metastatic recurrence, providing valuable information several months ahead of conventional MR imaging. By assessing parameters such as Vp and Ktrans, DCE MR imaging can identify elevated values in these metrics, serving as an indicator of

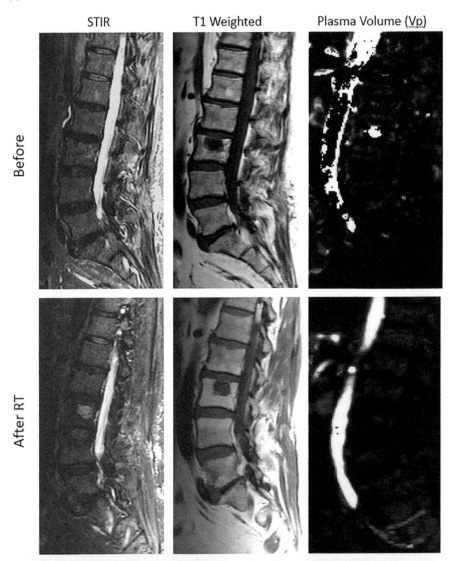

Fig. 2. RT response assessment in DCE. **Fig. 2** provides a representation of the RT response assessment in a 68-year-old male patient with prostate cancer and solitary L3 bone metastasis. L3 metastasis is treated with RT 27GY in 3 fractions. The figure demonstrates the pre-RT scan and the 1-year post-RT scan, highlighting the evolution of vascularity in the treated L3 metastasis. These findings contribute to our understanding of treatment outcomes and guide future clinical decision-making for similar patients.

recurrent disease. This early detection capability enables prompt intervention and timely adjustments to the treatment plan, potentially leading to improved patient outcomes.[18]

Detecting Benign and Pathologic Compression Fractures

Accurate differentiation between benign and malignant compression fractures is of utmost importance in patients with cancer because it significantly influences disease staging. Although benign fractures are common among the elderly and linked to conditions such as osteoporosis, patients with cancer may experience pathologic fractures. Distinguishing between the 2 can be challenging due to overlapping clinical presentations. A precise diagnosis is vital for making appropriate management decisions for patients with cancer with compression fractures.[37] Cancer treatments, including RT, steroids, hormone therapy, and chemotherapy, can contribute to nonmalignant compression fractures.[38]

Conventional MR imaging cannot frequently differentiate between malignant and benign fractures.[39] In contrast, DCE MR imaging has shown promise in distinguishing between benign and malignant fractures by using perfusion metrics.

Arevalo-Perez and colleagues conducted a study demonstrating that pathologic fractures exhibited higher values of Vp, Ktrans, peak enhancement, and wash-in slope in comparison to nonmalignant fractures ($P < .01$) (**Fig. 3**). Moreover, DCE MR imaging has shown sensitivity in distinguishing between acute and chronic vertebral body fractures. These findings underscore the potential of DCE MR imaging as a valuable tool for differentiating types of fractures, enabling accurate diagnosis and characterization of spinal lesions.[22]

Geith and colleagues[40] conducted a study that revealed significantly higher quantitative perfusion parameters such as interstitial volume, extracellular volume, and extraction flow in regions with high plasma flow in acute osteoporotic vertebral fractures when compared with acute malignant vertebral fractures. Furthermore, the study observed that the mean values of Ktrans, plasma flow, and Vp tended to be higher in areas with increased plasma flow in malignant fractures when compared with osteoporotic fractures, although no statistically significant differences were detected. These findings indicate that DCE MR imaging can provide valuable insights into the perfusion characteristics of different types of fractures. However, further research is necessary to establish more definitive distinctions between benign and malignant fractures based on these perfusion parameters.

Chordomas

Chordoma is an uncommon cancer originating from persistent or ectopic remnants of the notochord, often located in the clivus, spine, and sacrum. Despite their low-grade histology, chordomas exhibit local invasiveness, aggressiveness, and a high likelihood of recurrence. As a result, patients experience clinical progression similar to that of malignant neoplasms. Chordomas pose challenges in evaluating treatment response using conventional imaging methods due to their nature and propensity for recurrence.[41] Their slow growth, followed by rapid progression, further complicates the assessment.[41] The utilization of DCE MR imaging has become increasingly valuable in differentiating between successful treatment responses and failures. Specifically, the analysis of lower quantitative perfusion metrics such as Vp and Ktrans has proven effective in this regard.[42] Additionally, chordomas exhibit a distinctive Type E TIC pattern on DCE MR imaging, characterized by a rapid initial contrast enhancement followed by a slower increase, aiding in their differentiation from other spinal lesions.[42]

Santos and colleagues[42] found that changes in Vp and vascular permeability can be used to monitor chordoma growth and treatment response. In their study, following treatment, both quantitative and semiquantitative DCE parameters, including Vp, Ktrans, and AUC, exhibited a significant decrease. This decrease reflects the degree of vascular damage caused by RT. They also discovered that the dynamic MR signal intensity–time curve of chordomas could help differentiate them from other spinal lesions. Overall, these findings highlight the ability of DCE-MR imaging to effectively capture changes in tumor physiology in response to therapy.

Atypical Hemangiomas (Intraosseous Venous Malformations)

Atypical hemangiomas (intraosseous venous malformations) can seem like neoplastic lesions or spinal metastases on conventional MR imaging due to their similar signal characteristics, increased vascularity, and low-fat content.[43] Diagnosing atypical hemangiomas is currently based on classic radiographic appearance and long-term stability. However, identifying the vertical trabecular appearance can be difficult, adding further complexity to the diagnostic process.[43] Occasionally, atypical hemangiomas may exhibit "aggressive" behavior and leads to potential confusion with malignancies.

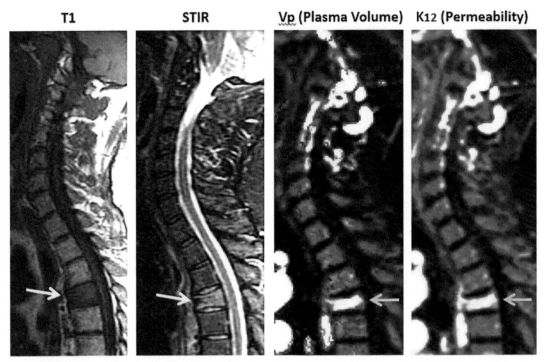

Fig. 3. Pathologic vertebral compression fracture. Fig. 3 exhibits sagittal T1-weighted and STIR MR images, accompanied by corresponding Vp and Ktrans maps, displaying pathologic vertebral fractures (indicated by *arrows*). The absence of paraspinal or epidural soft tissue involvement, as well as the lack of convexity in the posterior cortex, suggests that these fractures can simulate an acute benign fracture, deviating from the typical characteristics of a pathologic fracture.

Concurrent occurrence of metastatic disease from primary malignancies such as colon adenocarcinoma[44] and thyroid cancer[45] has been reported, adding to the challenge of distinguishing atypical hemangiomas from metastatic disease.

Differentiating between hemangiomas and cancerous lesions has been attempted using DWI, apparent diffusion coefficient (ADC), and quantitative chemical shift MR imaging.[46,47] However, DCE MR imaging quantitative metrics have been shown by Morales and colleagues[21] to effectively distinguish spinal metastases from atypical hemangiomas. Analysis of DCE MR imaging TIC revealed distinct differences in signal intensity and morphology between metastases and atypical hemangiomas, indicating the potential for qualitative differentiation. Qualitative analysis of the TIC revealed that spinal metastases exhibited higher signal intensities and a characteristic curve morphology of Type D TIC. However, atypical vertebral hemangiomas typically displayed a curve morphology of closely resembling Type C TIC.[21] Furthermore, quantitative assessment of perfusion parameters Vp and Ktrans demonstrated significantly higher values in metastatic lesions compared with atypical hemangiomas ($P < .01$)[21] (**Figs. 4** and **5**).

Practical Uses in Clinical Settings

DCE MR imaging has become an integral part of our practice, representing a significant portion of our MR imaging spine volume. Perfusion imaging accounts for approximately 35% to 40% of our daily studies, equivalent to 7 to 10 cases per day. The demand for advanced spine imaging is primarily to assess treatment response or failure when standard MR imaging sequences are insufficient. As a leading cancer institution, our commitment lies in the advancement of innovative therapies. The inclusion of DCE MR imaging in the assessment of viable spinal disease and treatment response allows us to promptly adapt treatment strategies for improved patient outcomes. Many of our patients have undergone multiple lines of treatment including RT and/or surgery for spinal metastases, presenting difficulties in assessing viable disease and treatment efficacy solely through anatomic imaging. DCE MR imaging effectively characterizes treated areas and noninvasively identifies viable tumors, offering valuable insights in this regard.

Fast T1 sequences in DCE MR imaging add minimal scan time (only 3–4 minutes). We use software packages to analyze perfusion data and overlay it

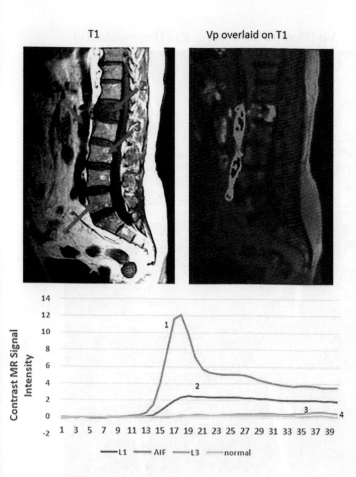

T1   **Vp overlaid on T1**

Fig. 4. Spinal metastasis and atypical hemangioma. **Fig. 4** presents representative sagittal T1-weighted image, Vp and dynamic images obtained from DCE MR imaging, highlighting atypical hemangioma at L3 and spinal metastasis at L1. The L1 metastasis exhibits an evident increase in Vp, whereas the L3 atypical hemangioma does not show any signs of increased Vp. The lower panel of the figure displays the MR imaging signal enhancement curve for each lesion, illustrating the changes in signal intensity during different phases (time).

on anatomic T1-weighted images. This integrated approach enables our radiologists to provide comprehensive assessments for informed decision-making by referring physicians.

However, DCE MR imaging has certain limitations that should be considered. In our current practice, as well as in other institutions, we rely on software specifically designed for brain analysis to assess spinal imaging. However, this approach presents certain challenges. Notably, the perfusion in the brain is significantly higher compared with the spine. Additionally, it takes a longer duration for blood, including the contrast agent used in our DCE method, to reach the area of interest in the spine compared with the brain. Consequently, if we solely use software optimized for the brain, it may lead to an underestimation of spine perfusion. One significant limitation is the accuracy of measuring the AIF, which is necessary for the pharmacokinetic 2-compartment model.[19] To mitigate this issue, we need to introduce a delay or phase shift in the AIF to ensure alignment with the acquired data. This adjustment is crucial in accurately evaluating spinal perfusion and ensuring reliable results. The temporal resolution of DCE MR imaging can be compromised due to factors such as the need for high spatial resolution and a wide field-of-view (FOV). Consequently, this can lead to inaccuracies in measuring the AIF and saturation effects during the initial contrast agent influx. Furthermore, the assumptions underlying the pharmacokinetic model used in DCE MR imaging may not universally apply to all tissue types or tumor characteristics, thereby introducing potential unreliability in the obtained outcomes. The physiologic basis of semiquantitative parameters such as peak enhancement and AUC is not fully understood, and the mechanisms underlying perfusion differences before and after RT remain unclear.[19]

Notwithstanding these constraints, the utilization of DCE MR imaging has exhibited promising potential in the management of spinal metastases. However, to further enhance our understanding of its clinical applications and overcome these limitations, it is imperative to conduct comprehensive studies involving larger cohorts of patients encompassing diverse pathologic conditions. Such investigations will enable us to gather additional insights and refine the utilization of DCE MR imaging in the management of spinal metastases.

T1   **Vp (Plasma Volume)**   **K12 (Permeability)**

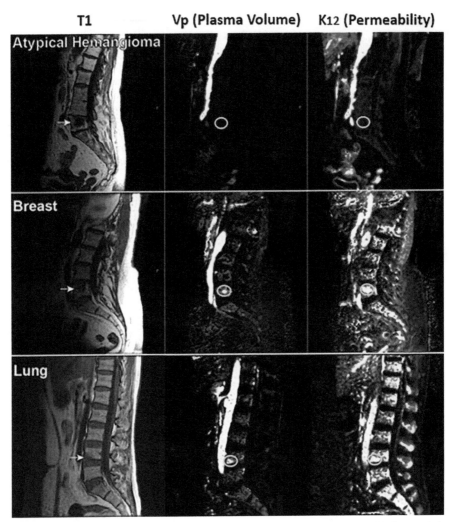

Fig. 5. Spinal metastases and atypical hemangioma. Fig. 5 presents representative sagittal T1-weighted images and dynamic images derived from DCE MR imaging, illustrating atypical hemangiomas and spinal lesions originating from primary breast and lung carcinoma. The corresponding bottom panel displays the MR imaging signal enhancement curve, depicting the temporal changes in signal intensity for each depicted representative lesion.

Diffusion-Weighted Imaging

DWI is an advanced MR imaging technique that extends beyond stroke imaging and now contributes to tumor assessment. It provides an in vivo representation of water mobility, providing valuable information about the cellular environment. This allows for the characterization of tissue microstructure and provides insights into tumor properties and behavior.[48]

DWI can be evaluated qualitatively using techniques such as bull's eye imaging or quantitatively by analyzing the ADC.[49,50] This sequence provides functional information about tissues. Metastatic lesions characterized by densely packed cells and cytotoxic edema display lower ADC values than normal bone marrow.[51,52] The quantification of

signal contrast in DWI using apparent diffusion coefficient maps serves as a valuable tool for evaluating treatment response and assessing the progression of the disease. However, there is conflicting research regarding the use of DWI for imaging the marrow, and its interpretation should be combined with routine marrow sequences.[51–53] In clinical practice, DWI of the spine has several applications, including differentiating between benign and pathologic fractures,[54] distinguishing between infective and degenerative sub-endplate changes,[55] and monitoring the treatment response of neoplastic marrow lesions.[56]

Tumors show restricted diffusion due to increased cellularity. By converting DWI into an ADC map, the amount of diffusion in each voxel can be quantified. Lower ADC values indicate higher cellularity, with tumors appearing hypointense on ADC maps.[57] DWI is a commonly used MR imaging sequence that can effectively differentiate between malignant and nonneoplastic lesions.[58,59] Studies by Xing and colleagues[58] and Lee and colleagues[59] have demonstrated the ability to distinguish between metastases and myeloma, as well as differentiate Schmorl nodes from metastases, respectively. Receiver operating characteristic curves were used, with Xing and colleagues achieving a range of 0.7 and Lee and colleagues attaining a value of 0.94.

MR Imaging Acquisition

DWI scans are obtained using a single-shot echo planar imaging protocol at multiple b-values, typically in a T2-weighted sequence. The b-value plays a critical role in determining the level of diffusion weighting. Higher b-values enhance sensitivity to diffusion properties, allowing for better detection of diffusion-related information. Conversely, lower b-values optimize the signal-to-noise ratio, resulting in clearer and more reliable images.[60]

DWI offers the advantage of rapid image acquisition, making it a time-efficient imaging modality. Moreover, unlike perfusion MR imaging, DWI does not necessitate the use of intravenous contrast agents. This renders it a safe option for patients with contraindications such as allergies, compromised renal function, or pregnancy, who need to avoid the administration of contrast agents.

The Use of Diffusion-Weighted Imaging in Diagnostic Imaging

Pathologic fractures, characterized by the presence of tumor cells, exhibit reduced water mobility due to the narrowing of interstitial spaces. As a result, they seem as areas of higher signal intensity compared with normal bone marrow on DWI. However, benign fractures, which are associated with conditions such as osteoporosis or trauma, show increased water mobility due to expanded interstitial spaces caused by edema or hemorrhage. Consequently, they seem as areas of lower signal intensity on DWI.[61] To mitigate potential misinterpretation caused by T2 shine-through effects, studies by Zidan and Elghazaly[62] and Padhani and colleagues[56] highlight the significance of correlating high b-value DWI with the corresponding ADC values. This approach helps improve the accuracy and interpretation of DWI findings in spinal lesions.

After the study of Baur and colleagues[63] highlighted the excellent differentiation capability of DWI between benign and malignant compression fractures, subsequent research has further supported its promising findings. Sung and colleagues[64] demonstrated that the addition of qualitative and quantitative axial DWI to a standard MR imaging protocol significantly improved diagnostic accuracy in distinguishing between acute malignant and nonmalignant compression fractures at 3.0 T. According to a meta-analysis performed by Suh and colleagues, ADC demonstrated the ability to distinguish between benign and malignant vertebral bone marrow lesions with a sensitivity of 89% and specificity of 87%. Additionally, ADC proved to be effective in discriminating between benign and malignant compression fractures, achieving a sensitivity of 92% and specificity of 91%.[65] Numerous studies have consistently demonstrated that spinal metastases have lower ADC values than normal bone marrow, and malignant fractures show lower ADC values than benign fractures. Additionally, spinal metastases exhibit lower ADC values than typical and atypical vertebral hemangiomas.[66–69] However, it should be noted that Pozzi and colleagues found that DWI is not effective in differentiating between malignant primary spinal tumors and spinal metastases.[68]

Earlier studies by Padhani and colleagues[56] and Zidan and Elghazaly[62] have shown a significant difference in ADC values between malignant and inflammatory/infective lesions, with a P-value of less than .05. Nevertheless, there remains some similarity in signal intensity between these entities, despite their discernible differences.

The application of DWI to bone marrow malignancies outside of the vertebral column has been limited in terms of research. Nonquantitative whole-body DWI has demonstrated high sensitivity in detecting malignant bone-marrow lesions.[70,71] Furthermore, DWI has proven effective in the detection of malignant lymphoma involvement in the bone marrow[72] and for localizing malignant lesions in the cranial bone marrow.[73]

The Use of Diffusion-Weighted Imaging in Monitoring Treatment Response

DWI proves to be a valuable tool for evaluating treatment responses in spinal metastases, as evidenced by the observed increase in ADC values in successfully treated cases. Conversely, unsuccessful treatments are associated with a sustained decrease in ADC values, noticeable as early as 1 month following RT.[74] Notably, these changes may not be apparent in conventional MR imaging sequences. Therefore, DWI provides additional information regarding treatment response (Fig. 6).

T1   DWI

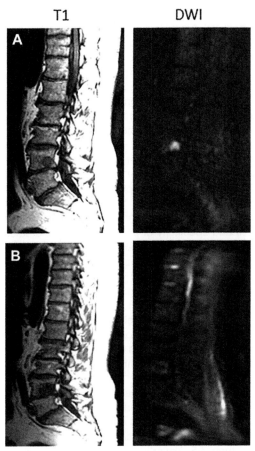

Fig. 6. RT response assessment in DWI. The preradiation therapy Sagittal T1 and diffusion-weighted MR images with a high b value (A) reveal elevated DWI signal intensity in the metastatic lesion at L4 vertebral body, whereas the postradiation therapy diffusion-weighted MR image with a high b value (B) exhibit decreased signal intensity in the metastatic lesion at L4 vertebral body. The corresponding ADC maps obtained after radiation therapy exhibited increased signal intensity. After treatment, DCE MR imaging of the same patient revealed a reduction in Vp and Ktrans values.

DWI can also evaluate treatment response to androgen withdrawal therapy. Resichauer and colleagues reported a notable increase in ADC values at 1, 2, and 3 months after successful treatment of pelvic metastases.[75] DWI proves useful in evaluating treatment efficacy and tracking tumor cellularity over time. Its application extends to assessing treatment responses in spinal metastases and evaluating therapeutic interventions such as RT and androgen withdrawal therapy.

Limitations of Diffusion-Weighted Imaging

Despite the clinical value of DWI, there are certain limitations associated with its use. One challenge is the difficulty in establishing a precise ADC value threshold for different diagnoses because ADC values are influenced by factors such as the MR imaging scanner's field strength and the specific b-value used in diffusion-sensitive gradients.[76] Consequently, it becomes impractical to rely on a universal cutoff for distinguishing between various pathologic conditions.

Another limitation originates from the unsuitability of DWI in evaluating sclerotic lesions, which have low water content.[77] This characteristic can lead to false-negative results because the restricted diffusion of water may not be adequately captured by DWI in such cases. Furthermore, certain conditions such as infections, blood products, and abscess formations can cause decreased ADC values, potentially resulting in false-positive interpretations.[78] In the detection of spinal metastases, DWI may not offer significant advantages over conventional MR imaging, as noted by Castillo and colleagues.[53] This observation may be attributed to the T2 shine-through effect in DWI, where the influence of T2-weighted signal intensity can hinder the specificity of DWI findings in detecting spinal metastases.

The assessment of treatment response using DWI can be challenging due to the heterogeneity of tumors and the intricate changes that occur because of therapy. Tumor heterogeneity can lead to varying ADC values, with both increases and decreases observed within the tumor. This complexity poses a challenge when interpreting mean ADC analysis for evaluating treatment response.[79]

Considering these limitations, it is important to approach DWI findings with caution and to complement DWI with other imaging modalities to enhance diagnostic accuracy and the evaluation of treatment response.

SUMMARY

Dynamic perfusion MR imaging and diffusion MR imaging have emerged as promising modalities in the diagnosis and monitoring of spinal metastases, offering valuable information beyond routine MR imaging protocols. The combination of DWI and DCE MR imaging provides insights into microstructural changes, bone marrow pathologic conditions, and perfusion characteristics. By using these techniques, we can effectively identify treatment failure, detect viable tumors, and enhance patient care. Ongoing development and integration of these advanced imaging methods are essential for optimizing clinical outcomes in the management of spinal metastases.

CLINICS CARE POINTS

- DCE MR imaging is a valuable tool for assessing spinal metastases because they typically exhibit elevated Vp and permeability constant (Ktrans), indicating viable tumors.

- Decreased quantitative perfusion parameters may indicate treatment response and nonviable disease.

- Hypervascular metastases typically exhibit higher perfusion parameters compared with hypovascular metastases.

- Atypical hemangiomas (intraosseous venous malformations) do not display elevated perfusion levels when compared with spinal metastases.

- Vertebral body compression fractures accompanied by elevated Vp and Ktrans are likely to have pathologic origins.

- The prognostic value of DCE MR imaging in detecting early treatment response has the potential to enhance patient care and improve outcomes.

- Incorporating the emerging MR imaging sequence, DWI, into the standard MR imaging protocol for patients with cancer undergoing metastatic spinal evaluation holds potential as a reliable tool for distinguishing between benign and malignant vertebral marrow lesions.

DISCLOSURE

The authors have nothing to disclose.

REFERENCES

1. Coughlin SS. Surviving cancer or other serious illness: a review of individual and community resources. CA Cancer J. Clin. 2008;58:60–4.
2. Hutton B, Addison C, Mazzarello S, et al. De-escalated administration of bone-targeted agents in patients with breast and prostate cancer-A survey of Canadian oncologists. J. Bone Oncol. 2013;2:77–83.
3. Togawa D, Lewandrowski K-U. The pathophysiology of spinal metastases. In: McLain RF, editor. Cancer in the spine. 17–23. . Humana Press; 2006. https://doi.org/10.1007/978-1-59259-971-4_3.
4. Traill Z, Richards MA, Moore NR. Magnetic resonance imaging of metastatic bone disease. Clin Orthop Relat Res 1995;76–88.
5. Biffar A, Dietrich O, Sourbron S, et al. Diffusion and perfusion imaging of bone marrow. Eur J Radiol 2010;76:323–8.
6. Yankelevitz DF, Henschke CI, Knapp PH, et al. Effect of radiation therapy on thoracic and lumbar bone marrow: evaluation with MR imaging. AJR Am J Roentgenol 1991;157:87–92.
7. Otake S, Mayr NA, Ueda T, et al. Radiation-induced changes in MR signal intensity and contrast enhancement of lumbosacral vertebrae: do changes occur only inside the radiation therapy field? Radiology 2002;222:179–83.
8. Montazel J-L, Divine M, Lepage E, et al. Normal spinal bone marrow in adults: dynamic gadolinium-enhanced MR imaging. Radiology 2003;229:703–9.
9. Vande Berg BC, Malghem J, Lecouvet FE, et al. Magnetic resonance imaging of the normal bone marrow. Skeletal Radiol 1998;27:471–83.
10. Vogler JB, Murphy WA. Bone marrow imaging. Radiology 1988;168:679–93.
11. Erlemann R, Reiser MF, Peters PE, et al. Musculoskeletal neoplasms: static and dynamic Gd-DTPA–enhanced MR imaging. Radiology 1989;171:767–73.
12. Vande Berg BC, Malghem J, Lecouvet FE, et al. Magnetic resonance imaging of normal bone marrow. Eur Radiol 1998;8:1327–34.
13. Chen WT, Shih TT, Chen RC, et al. Vertebral bone marrow perfusion evaluated with dynamic contrast-enhanced MR imaging: significance of aging and sex. Radiology 2001;220:213–8.
14. Griffith JF, Yeung DKW, Antonio GE, et al. Vertebral marrow fat content and diffusion and perfusion indexes in women with varying bone density: MR evaluation. Radiology 2006;241:831–8.
15. Sze G, Krol G, Zimmerman RD, et al. Intramedullary disease of the spine: diagnosis using gadolinium-DTPA-enhanced MR imaging. AJR Am J Roentgenol 1988;151:1193–204.
16. Beltran J, Chandnani V, McGhee RA, et al. Gadopentetate dimeglumine-enhanced MR imaging of the musculoskeletal system. AJR Am J Roentgenol 1991;156:457–66.
17. Chu S, Karimi S, Peck KK, et al. Measurement of blood perfusion in spinal metastases with dynamic contrast-enhanced magnetic resonance imaging: evaluation of tumor response to radiation therapy. Spine 2013;38:E1418–24.
18. Kumar KA, Peck KK, Karimi S, et al. A Pilot Study Evaluating the Use of Dynamic Contrast-Enhanced Perfusion MRI to Predict Local Recurrence After Radiosurgery on Spinal Metastases. Technol Cancer Res Treat 2017;16:857–65.
19. Lis E, Saha A, Peck KK, et al. Dynamic contrast-enhanced magnetic resonance imaging of osseous spine metastasis before and 1 hour after high-dose image-guided radiation therapy. Neurosurg Focus 2017;42:E9.
20. Saha A, Peck KK, Lis E, et al. Magnetic resonance perfusion characteristics of hypervascular renal

and hypovascular prostate spinal metastases: clinical utilities and implications. Spine 2014;39: E1433–40.

21. Morales KA, Arevalo-Perez J, Peck KK, et al. Differentiating Atypical Hemangiomas and Metastatic Vertebral Lesions: The Role of T1-Weighted Dynamic Contrast-Enhanced MRI. AJNR Am J Neuroradiol 2018;39:968–73.

22. Arevalo-Perez J, Peck KK, Lyo JK, et al. Differentiating benign from malignant vertebral fractures using T1-weighted dynamic contrast-enhanced MRI. J Magn Reson Imag 2015;42:1039–47.

23. Carmeliet P, Jain RK. Molecular mechanisms and clinical applications of angiogenesis. Nature 2011; 473:298–307.

24. Moehler TM, Hawighorst H, Neben K, et al. Bone marrow microcirculation analysis in multiple myeloma by contrast-enhanced dynamic magnetic resonance imaging. Int J Cancer 2001;93:862–8.

25. Nosàs-Garcia S, Moehler T, Wasser K, et al. Dynamic contrast-enhanced MRI for assessing the disease activity of multiple myeloma: a comparative study with histology and clinical markers. J Magn Reson Imag 2005;22:154–62.

26. Pauliah M, Saxena V, Haris M, et al. Improved T(1)-weighted dynamic contrast-enhanced MRI to probe microvascularity and heterogeneity of human glioma. Magn Reson Imaging 2007;25:1292–9.

27. Northam M, de Campos ROP, Ramalho M, et al. Bone metastases: evaluation of acuity of lesions using dynamic gadolinium-chelate enhancement, preliminary results. J Magn Reson Imag 2011;34: 120–7.

28. Barajas RF, Chang JS, Sneed PK, et al. Distinguishing recurrent intra-axial metastatic tumor from radiation necrosis following gamma knife radiosurgery using dynamic susceptibility-weighted contrast-enhanced perfusion MR imaging. AJNR Am J Neuroradiol 2009;30:367–72.

29. Hatzoglou V, Ulaner GA, Zhang Z, et al. Comparison of the effectiveness of MRI perfusion and fluorine-18 FDG PET-CT for differentiating radiation injury from viable brain tumor: a preliminary retrospective analysis with pathologic correlation in all patients. Clin Imag 2013;37:451–7.

30. Tofts PS, Brix G, Buckley DL, et al. Estimating kinetic parameters from dynamic contrast-enhanced t1-weighted MRI of a diffusable tracer: Standardized quantities and symbols. J Magn Reson Imag 1999; 10:223–32.

31. Chen W-T, Shih TTF, Chen RC, et al. Blood perfusion of vertebral lesions evaluated with gadolinium-enhanced dynamic MRI: in comparison with compression fracture and metastasis. J Magn Reson Imag 2002;15:308–14.

32. Saranathan M, Rettmann DW, Hargreaves BA, et al. DIfferential Subsampling with Cartesian Ordering (DISCO): a high spatio-temporal resolution Dixon imaging sequence for multiphasic contrast enhanced abdominal imaging. J Magn Reson Imag 2012;35: 1484–92.

33. Khadem NR, Karimi S, Peck KK, et al. Characterizing hypervascular and hypovascular metastases and normal bone marrow of the spine using dynamic contrast-enhanced MR imaging. AJNR Am J Neuroradiol 2012;33:2178–85.

34. Mazura JC, Karimi S, Pauliah M, et al. Dynamic contrast-enhanced magnetic resonance perfusion compared with digital subtraction angiography for the evaluation of extradural spinal metastases: a pilot study. Spine 2014;39:E950–4.

35. Barker HE, Paget JTE, Khan AA, et al. The tumour microenvironment after radiotherapy: mechanisms of resistance and recurrence. Nat Rev Cancer 2015;15:409–25.

36. Spratt DE, Arevalo-Perez J, Leeman JE, et al. Early magnetic resonance imaging biomarkers to predict local control after high dose stereotactic body radiotherapy for patients with sarcoma spine metastases. Spine J 2016;16:291–8.

37. Jung H-S, Jee W-H, McCauley TR, et al. Discrimination of metastatic from acute osteoporotic compression spinal fractures with MR imaging. Radiographics 2003;23:179–87.

38. Croarkin E. Osteopenia in the patient with cancer. Phys Ther 1999;79:196–201.

39. Verstraete KL, Van der Woude HJ, Hogendoorn PC, et al. Dynamic contrast-enhanced MR imaging of musculoskeletal tumors: basic principles and clinical applications. J Magn Reson Imag 1996;6: 311–21.

40. Geith T, Biffar A, Schmidt G, et al. Quantitative analysis of acute benign and malignant vertebral body fractures using dynamic contrast-enhanced MRI. AJR Am J Roentgenol 2013;200:W635–43.

41. Walcott BP, Nahed BV, Mohyeldin A, et al. Chordoma: current concepts, management, and future directions. Lancet Oncol 2012;13:e69–76.

42. Santos P, Peck KK, Arevalo-Perez J, et al. T1-Weighted Dynamic Contrast-Enhanced MR Perfusion Imaging Characterizes Tumor Response to Radiation Therapy in Chordoma. AJNR Am J Neuroradiol 2017; 38:2210–6.

43. Gaudino S, Martucci M, Colantonio R, et al. A systematic approach to vertebral hemangioma. Skeletal Radiol 2015;44:25–36.

44. Zapałowicz K, Bierzyńska-Macyszyn G, Stasiów B, et al. Vertebral hemangioma coincident with metastasis of colon adenocarcinoma. J Neurosurg Spine 2016;24:506–9.

45. Laguna R, Silva F, Vazquez-Sellés J, et al. Vertebral hemangioma mimicking a metastatic bone lesion in well-differentiated thyroid carcinoma. Clin Nucl Med 2000;25:611–3.

46. Leeds NE, Kumar AJ, Zhou XJ, et al. Magnetic resonance imaging of benign spinal lesions simulating metastasis: role of diffusion-weighted imaging. Top Magn Reson Imag 2000;11:224–34.

47. Zajick DC, Morrison WB, Schweitzer ME, et al. Benign and malignant processes: normal values and differentiation with chemical shift MR imaging in vertebral marrow. Radiology 2005;237:590–6.

48. White NS, McDonald C, McDonald CR, et al. Diffusion-weighted imaging in cancer: physical foundations and applications of restriction spectrum imaging. Cancer Res 2014;74:4638–52.

49. Lichy MP, Aschoff P, Plathow C, et al. Tumor detection by diffusion-weighted MRI and ADC-mapping–initial clinical experiences in comparison to PET-CT. Invest Radiol 2007;42:605–13.

50. Costa FM, Ferreira EC, Vianna EM. Diffusion-weighted magnetic resonance imaging for the evaluation of musculoskeletal tumors. Magn Reson Imag Clin N Am 2011;19:159–80.

51. Baur A, Huber A, Dürr HR, et al. Differentiation of benign osteoporotic and neoplastic vertebral compression fractures with a diffusion-weighted, steady-state free precession sequence. Röfo 2002; 174:70–5.

52. Biffar A, Baur-Melnyk A, Schmidt GP, et al. Multiparameter MRI assessment of normal-appearing and diseased vertebral bone marrow. Eur Radiol 2010; 20:2679–89.

53. Castillo M, Arbelaez A, Smith JK, et al. Diffusion-weighted MR imaging offers no advantage over routine noncontrast MR imaging in the detection of vertebral metastases. AJNR Am J Neuroradiol 2000;21:948–53.

54. Karchevsky M, Babb JS, Schweitzer ME. Can diffusion-weighted imaging be used to differentiate benign from pathologic fractures? A meta-analysis. Skeletal Radiol 2008;37:791–5.

55. Eguchi Y, Ohtori S, Yamashita M, et al. Diffusion magnetic resonance imaging to differentiate degenerative from infectious endplate abnormalities in the lumbar spine. Spine 2011;36:E198–202.

56. Padhani AR, Koh D-M, Collins DJ. Whole-body diffusion-weighted MR imaging in cancer: current status and research directions. Radiology 2011; 261:700–18.

57. Baur A, Stäbler A, Bartl R, et al. MRI gadolinium enhancement of bone marrow: age-related changes in normals and in diffuse neoplastic infiltration. Skeletal Radiol 1997;26:414–8.

58. Xing X, Zhang J, Chen Y, et al. Application of mono-exponential, biexponential, and stretched-exponential models of diffusion-weighted magnetic resonance imaging in the differential diagnosis of metastases and myeloma in the spine-Univariate and multivariate analysis of related parameters. Br J Radiol 2020;93:20190891.

59. Lee JH, Park S. Differentiation of schmorl nodes from bone metastases of the spine: use of apparent diffusion coefficient derived from DWI and fat fraction derived from a dixon sequence. AJR Am J Roentgenol 2019;213:W228–35.

60. Khoo MMY, Tyler PA, Saifuddin A, et al. Diffusion-weighted imaging (DWI) in musculoskeletal MRI: a critical review. Skeletal Radiol 2011;40:665–81.

61. Mubarak F, Akhtar W. Acute vertebral compression fracture: differentiation of malignant and benign causes by diffusion weighted magnetic resonance imaging. J Pakistan Med Assoc 2011;61:555–8.

62. Zidan DZ, Elghazaly HA. Can unenhanced multiparametric MRI substitute gadolinium-enhanced MRI in the characterization of vertebral marrow infiltrative lesions? The Egyptian Journal of Radiology and Nuclear Medicine 2014;45:443–53.

63. Baur A, Stäbler A, Brüning R, et al. Diffusion-weighted MR imaging of bone marrow: differentiation of benign versus pathologic compression fractures. Radiology 1998;207:349–56.

64. Sung JK, Jee WH, Jung JY, et al. Differentiation of acute osteoporotic and malignant compression fractures of the spine: use of additive qualitative and quantitative axial diffusion-weighted MR imaging to conventional MR imaging at 3.0 T. Radiology 2014; 271:488–98.

65. Suh CH, Yun SJ, Jin W, et al. ADC as a useful diagnostic tool for differentiating benign and malignant vertebral bone marrow lesions and compression fractures: a systematic review and meta-analysis. Eur Radiol 2018;28:2890–902.

66. Herneth AM, Philipp MO, Naude J, et al. Vertebral metastases: assessment with apparent diffusion coefficient. Radiology 2002;225:889–94.

67. Pozzi G, Albano D, Messina C, et al. Solid bone tumors of the spine: Diagnostic performance of apparent diffusion coefficient measured using diffusion-weighted MRI using histology as a reference standard. J Magn Reson Imag 2018;47:1034–42.

68. Pozzi G, Garcia Parra C, Stradiotti P, et al. Diffusion-weighted MR imaging in differentiation between osteoporotic and neoplastic vertebral fractures. Eur Spine J 2012;21(Suppl 1):S123–7.

69. Shi Y-J, Li XT, Zhang XY, et al. Differential diagnosis of hemangiomas from spinal osteolytic metastases using 3.0 T MRI: comparison of T1-weighted imaging, chemical-shift imaging, diffusion-weighted and contrast-enhanced imaging. Oncotarget 2017;8: 71095–104.

70. Kwee TC, Takahara T, Ochiai R, et al. Diffusion-weighted whole-body imaging with background body signal suppression (DWIBS): features and potential applications in oncology. Eur Radiol 2008;18: 1937–52.

71. Mürtz P, Krautmacher C, Träber F, et al. Diffusion-weighted whole-body MR imaging with background

body signal suppression: a feasibility study at 3.0 Tesla. Eur Radiol 2007;17:3031–7.

72. Yasumoto M, Nonomura Y, Yoshimura R, et al. MR detection of iliac bone marrow involvement by malignant lymphoma with various MR sequences including diffusion-weighted echo-planar imaging. Skeletal Radiol 2002;31:263–9.

73. Moon WJ, Lee MH, Chung EC. Diffusion-weighted imaging with sensitivity encoding (SENSE) for detecting cranial bone marrow metastases: comparison with T1-weighted images. Korean J Radiol 2007;8:185–91.

74. Cappabianca S, Capasso R, Urraro F, et al. Assessing Response to Radiation Therapy Treatment of Bone Metastases: Short-Term Followup of Radiation Therapy Treatment of Bone Metastases with Diffusion-Weighted Magnetic Resonance Imaging. Journal of Radiotherapy 2014;1–8.

75. Reischauer C, Froehlich JM, Koh DM, et al. Bone metastases from prostate cancer: assessing treatment response by using diffusion-weighted imaging and functional diffusion maps–initial observations. Radiology 2010;257:523–31.

76. Dale BM, Braithwaite AC, Boll DT, et al. Field strength and diffusion encoding technique affect the apparent diffusion coefficient measurements in diffusion-weighted imaging of the abdomen. Invest Radiol 2010;45:104–8.

77. Hackländer T, Scharwächter C, Golz R, et al. Value of diffusion-weighted imaging for diagnosing vertebral metastases due to prostate cancer in comparison to other primary tumors. Röfo 2006;178:416–24.

78. Subhawong TK, Jacobs MA, Fayad LM. Diffusion-weighted MR imaging for characterizing musculoskeletal lesions. Radiographics 2014;34:1163–77.

79. Messiou C, Collins DJ, Giles S, et al. Assessing response in bone metastases in prostate cancer with diffusion weighted MRI. Eur Radiol 2011;21:2169–77.

Essentials of Spinal Tumor Ablation

Anderanik Tomasian, MD[a], Jack W. Jennings, MD, PhD[b],*

KEYWORDS

- Spinal metastases • Thermal ablation • Vertebral augmentation • Thermal protection

KEY POINTS

- Percutaneous minimally invasive thermal ablation and vertebral augmentation offer a robust armamentarium for radiologists for management of patients with spinal metastases.
- Thermal ablation is safe, effective, and durable in management of selected patients with spinal metastases to achieve pain palliation and local tumor control.
- Thermal protection is important to ensure procedure safety.

INTRODUCTION

According to the American Cancer Society, approximately 1.96 million cases of new cancer diagnosis are expected in the United States in 2023. Most of these patients will develop metastases that in 40% of cases will involve the spinal column.[1] Skeletal-related events such as intractable pain due to direct vertebral osseous involvement by tumor, pathologic fracture with or without mechanical instability, metastatic epidural spinal cord compression, and neurologic compromise commonly unfavorably affect patient quality of life and functional independence.[2,3]

The limitations of external beam radiation therapy, as the reference standard for pain palliation and local tumor control of vertebral metastases, should be considered for each patient when multidisciplinary treatment decisions are rendered. The important limitations of radiation therapy include (1) limited efficacy in providing adequate and timely pain palliation in up to 75% of cases, (2) relatively radiation-resistant tumors affecting efficacy, and (3) cumulative tolerance of the spinal cord influencing further radiation treatment of tumor progression or recurrence.[4,5] In patients with spinal instability or neurologic compromise, surgical intervention is typically indicated; however, it is limited by morbidity and commonly not favored due to patients' frequent poor functional status. Additional limitations of alternative treatment options include inadequate response of spinal metastases to systemic therapies such as chemotherapy, hormonal therapy, immunotherapy, radiopharmaceuticals, and bisphosphonates as well as the common side effects and insufficient efficacy of opioids for many patients.[6]

Minimally invasive percutaneous image-guided thermal ablations, which are often combined with vertebral augmentation (VA), have proven safe, efficacious, and durable for management of subset of patients with spinal metastases in the past several years.[7–29] The goal of such interventions is to achieve pain palliation, local tumor control, or cure in conjunction with or supplemented by adjuvant radiation therapy, chemotherapy, or surgery. In light of these substantial benefits, the National Comprehensive Cancer Network (NCCN) and the American College of Radiology (ACR) have endorsed and incorporated thermal ablation and VA in treatment guidelines of patients with spinal metastases.[30,31]

In this review, the authors discuss the essentials of minimally invasive thermal ablation and VA in management of patients with spinal metastases.

PROCEDURE CONSIDERATIONS, INTERVENTION GOALS, AND PATIENT

Selection

A multidisciplinary approach is recommended to evaluate and select patients to undergo minimally

[a] University of California Irvine, 101 The City Dr S, Orange, CA, USA; [b] Mallinckrodt Institute of Radiology, 510 S Kingshighway Boulevard, Saint Louis, MO, USA
* Corresponding author.
E-mail address: jackwjennings@wustl.edu

Radiol Clin N Am 62 (2024) 303–309
https://doi.org/10.1016/j.rcl.2023.09.007
0033-8389/24/© 2023 Elsevier Inc. All rights reserved.

invasive percutaneous thermal ablation for management of spinal metastases to maximize patient benefits and establish a therapeutic plan. A multidisciplinary team of radiologists, radiation oncologists, medical oncologists, and oncologic surgeons typically reach a treatment consensus, which is followed by a pretreatment consultation visit reevaluate patient symptoms and perform a focused physical examination to reconfirm concordant focal tenderness and mechanical pain at the target site and determine potential neurologic deficits.

Pain palliation and local tumor control as well as cure (skeletal oligometastases; fewer than five lesions) are the treatment goals in patients with vertebral metastases[7–29]

The indications for percutaneous thermal ablation, commonly combined with VA for pathologic fracture stabilization or prevention, include (1) persistent pain or imaging evidence of tumor progression despite maximized radiation therapy, (2) contraindications to radiation therapy, (3) patient lack of desire for radiation treatment, or (4) inadequate therapeutic response to systemic therapies and analgesics/opioids. The patient factors guiding eligibility for percutaneous thermal ablation consist of pain, performance status, life expectancy, status of spinal stability and metastatic epidural spinal cord compression, and extent of visceral metastases.[7–9,11–19] Validated and clinically adopted Karnofsky Performance Status Scale is commonly used to determine patient performance status.[32] The NCCN has incorporated thermal ablation into guidelines for treatment of skeletal metastases.[30] The most recent NCCN guidelines for adult cancer pain (version 1.2023) indicate that thermal ablation may be considered for palliation of metastatic bone pain in the absence of oncologic emergency when chemotherapy is inadequate and radiation therapy is contraindicated or not desired by the patient.[30] The ACR Appropriateness Criteria offer the following guidelines for treatment of spinal metastases[31]: Thermal ablation and VA may be appropriate for treatment of asymptomatic pathologic vertebral fracture with or without edema on MR imaging and are usually appropriate for treatment of pathologic vertebral fracture with severe and progressive pain. The ACR Appropriateness Criteria also indicates that thermal ablation may be appropriate for treatment of pathologic vertebral fracture with spinal malalignment.[31]

Thermal ablation may be contraindicated in the presence of spinal instability depending on the severity, which is typically determined by the Spinal Instability Neoplastic Score (SINS).[33] Surgical consultation for potential tumor resection/debulking and stabilization is typically considered for SINS of 7 or higher.[33] Spinal metastases with central canal compromise are commonly managed surgically[34]; however, in the absence of spinal cord compression, thermal ablation may be alternatively performed when surgery is not an option. It is important to recognize that when central canal compromise is due to tumor alone, thermal ablation may lead to arrest or retraction of epidural tumor.[9] However, in the presence of bone retropulsion, thermal ablation will not result in alleviation of symptoms.

THERMAL ABLATION MODALITIES
Radiofrequency Ablation

The recent developments in radiofrequency ablation (RFA) technology, including navigational and bipolar electrodes, provide substantial advantages compared with traditional unipolar straight electrodes, which are important for patient safety and outcomes and advance treatment of spinal metastases in challenging sites.[7–10,14,17,27] Such advantages include electrode tip navigation, which can be articulated in different orientations through a single skin and osseous entry site, supporting treatment of challenging-to-access lesions along the posterior central vertebral body, creating larger ablation volumes, and improving efficiency. Precise real-time intraprocedural monitoring of ablation volume made possible by built-in thermocouples along electrode shaft, and bipolar technology eliminating the need for grounding pad application and risk of electrode-related skin thermal injury are additional advantages[7–10,14,17,27] (Fig. 1). In addition, simultaneous bipedicular vertebral ablations can be performed with such electrodes resulting in larger, confluent, and coalescent ablation volumes.[9,27] Intact vertebral cortex acts as a relative barrier against nontarget RF energy propagation, which is an important point to consider.[35] The primary indications for use of RFA for treatment of spinal metastases include (1) primarily osteolytic or mixed osteolytic–osteoblastic metastases, (2) geographic spinal metastases with no or small extraosseous components, and (3) challenging-to-access lesions such as tumors within the posterior central vertebral body where access is possible using navigational articulating electrodes (see Fig. 1). Densely osteoblastic metastases are typically not treated with RFA as the higher impedance of such tumors may render RFA ineffective.[36] In our practice, we recommend simultaneous bipedicular RFA for treatment of vertebral metastases aligned with consensus recommendations of the International Spine Radiosurgery Consortium, to treat the entire clinical target volume (CTV) to achieve

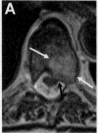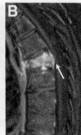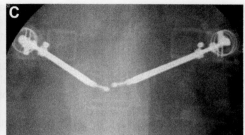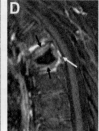

Fig. 1. 66-year-old woman with metastatic small-cell lung cancer and painful T6 lesion with tumor progression following radiation therapy. Axial fluid-sensitive MR imaging (*A*) and sagittal T1-weighted fat-saturated contrast-enhanced MR imaging (*B*) show bone marrow replacing metastatic lesion within T6 vertebral body (*A, white arrows*) with pathologic fracture and epidural tumor extension with deformation of the thecal sac and abutment of spinal cord by tumor (*A, black arrow* and *B, white arrow*). Radiofrequency ablation (RFA) was performed for pain palliation and local tumor control. Anterior–posterior fluoroscopic image during RFA (*C*) shows bipedicular placement of two bipolar navigational electrodes within T6 vertebral body and clinical target volume was treated with simultaneous ablations. Note medial articulation of the transpedicular electrode tips, which are in close proximity to generate confluent coalescent ablation zone. Thermal ablation was immediately followed by vertebral augmentation (not shown). Sagittal T1-weighted contrast-enhanced MR imaging obtained 3 months following treatment (*D*) shows local tumor control with enhancing granulation tissue along the periphery of ablation zone (*D, black arrows*). Note retraction of epidural tumor (*D, white arrow*). Note hypointense cement within T6 vertebral body (*D*).

improved local tumor control rates and more durable pain palliation[9,37] (see **Fig. 1**). CTV is defined as the gross tumor volume plus the surrounding abnormal bone marrow signal intensity on MR imaging to account for microscopic tumor invasion and the adjacent normal bone to account for subclinical tumor spread in marrow.[37] This translates into ablation of the entire vertebral body volume plus both pedicles with two confluent, coalescent, and overlapping ablation zones in close proximity minimizing convective cooling, risk of thermal injury, as well as tissue charring and impedance related issues (see **Fig. 1**).

The disadvantages of RFA include (1) CT-occult ablation zone, (2) convective cooling effect particularly with hypervascular metastases and cerebrospinal fluid as well as vertebral venous plexus flow, (3) relative ineffectiveness for ablation of densely osteoblastic lesions due to impedance, and (4) intraprocedural pain and at times, increased periprocedural pain.[7–10,14,17,27]

In the largest series published to date on RFA of spinal metastases,[27] investigators treated 266 vertebral metastases in 166 patients using navigational bipolar RF electrode system and reported statistically significant and durable pain palliation at 1-week, 1-month, 3-month, and 6-month post-treatment follow-up intervals with local tumor control rate of 78.9%. The authors reported a total complication rate of 3% (8/266) and major complication rate of 0.4% (1/266).[27] The single major complication included lower extremity weakness, difficulty in urination, and lack of erection as a result of a spinal cord venous infarct. The seven minor

complications included four cases of periprocedural transient radicular pain (common terminology criteria for adverse events [CTCAE] grade 2) requiring transforaminal steroid injections, one case of delayed secondary vertebral body fracture (CTCAE grade 2) requiring analgesics, and two cases of asymptomatic spinal cord edema on routine follow-up imaging (CTCAE grade 1).[27]

In a multicenter prospective study, the investigators treated 50 patients with spinal metastases using RFA (total of 69 ablations) and VA (96% of patients) and reported statistically significant pain palliation and improvement in functional status and quality of life with no complications.[8] In a multicenter prospective trial, the investigators used RFA for treatment of 100 patients with bone metastases, which included 87 patients with spinal tumors and reported statistically significant pain palliation and improvement in quality of life with adverse effects rate of 3%.[17]

Cryoablation

During cryoablation, an initial freezing cycle (commonly 10 minutes) is immediately followed by a thawing phase (commonly 5–8 minutes), a second freezing cycle (commonly 10 minutes), and a second thawing phase (commonly 5–8 minutes).[11,12,14,28] Reliable cell death is achieved at the temperature of −40°C or lower.[38] The hypoattenuating ice ball margin on CT corresponds to 0°C, and extension of ice ball beyond tumor margins by at least 3 to 5 mm is recommended to ensure sufficient treatment.[11,12,14,28] The latest generations of cryoprobes offer various ablation volumes which allow sculpting of desired ablation zones particularly in close proximity to critical structures, whereas the relatively small gauge of such cryoprobes allow optimal positioning.[11,12,14,28] Cryoablation is used primarily for treatment of spinal metastases with the following features: (1) large tumors with complex geometry, (2) spinal metastases with large soft-tissue components, (3) large tumors involving the posterior vertebral elements, (4) paravertebral soft-tissue metastases (**Fig. 2**), and (5) densely osteoblastic metastases. The advantages of cryoablation include (1) distinct visualization of hypoattenuating ice ball on CT, (2) concurrent use of several cryoprobes to generate additive overlapping ablation volumes, (3) less intraprocedural and immediate post-ablation pain compared with heating-based ablation modalities, and (4) availability of MR imaging-compatible cryoprobes. Disadvantages of cryoablation include (1) often lack of discrete visualization of ice ball within osteoblastic metastases (and at times relatively normal bone), (2) cost with use of several cryoprobes, (3) prolonged procedures in large tumors, and (4) delay in cementation to minimize interference with cement polymerization.

In a retrospective study, the investigators treated 105 spinal metastases in 74 patients (combined with cementation in 72.4% of tumors) with cryoablation[28] and documented statistically significant pain palliation at 1-day and 1-month post-procedural follow-up intervals as well as the last available posttreatment follow-up (mean of 14.7 months, median of 6 months). In a total of 53.1% of patients, pain-free status was reported at the last available follow-up. The local tumor control rate was reported at 82.1% (mean follow-up of 25.9 months, median of 16.5 months).[28] The total complication rate was 8.5% (nine patients including two major and seven minor complications).[28] The investigators treated 31 spinal metastases in 14 patients with cryoablation using thermal protection and documented 96.7% local tumor control, significant pain palliation, and decreased analgesics usage 1-week, 1-month, and 3-month intervals with no major complications.[11]

Microwave Ablation

Microwave ablation is most commonly used for treatment of spinal metastases with the following characteristics: (1) osteoblastic metastases and

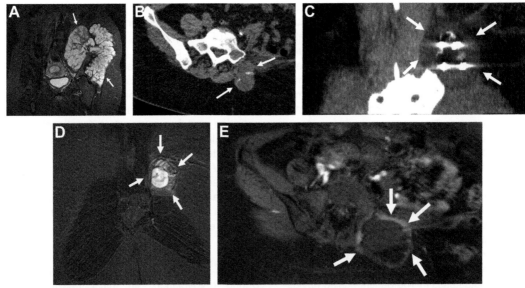

Fig. 2. 28-year-old woman with multiple hereditary exostoses and recurrent secondary chondrosarcoma. Coronal fat-saturated fluid-sensitive MR (*A*) shows large chondrosarcoma emanating from the left innominate bone and extending to the paraspinal region (*A, arrows*). The patient was managed by surgical resection and left internal hemipelvectomy. Axial CT image obtained 2 years following surgery (*B*) shows recurrent chondrosarcoma in the left L5–S1 paraspinal region (*B, arrows*) with no evidence of metastases on restaging imaging. Cryoablation was performed with curative intent. Coronal CT image during cryoablation (*C*) shows placement of four cryoprobes within the tumor with hypoattenuating ice ball encompassing the tumor and extending to surrounding soft tissues to ensure adequate treatment (*C, arrows*). Coronal fat-saturated fluid-sensitive MR (*D*) and axial T1-weighted fat-saturated contrast-enhanced MR imaging (*E*) obtained 2 months following cryoablation show local tumor control (curative ablation) with ablation zone extending beyond treated tumor boundaries (*D, E, arrows*) with enhancing granulation tissue at the periphery of the ablation zone (*E, arrows*).

(2) large paraspinal tumors with complex geometry. The advantages of microwave ablation include (1) less susceptibility to heat sink effect and variable tumor tissue impedance resulting in more uniform and larger ablation volumes as well as improved efficiency compared with RFA, (2) lack of need for grounding pad application, (3) concurrent use of several antennas to sculpt additive overlapping ablation zones, (4) lack of contraindication in patients with metallic implants, and (5) availability of articulating antennas allowing access to challenging vertebral tumor sites.[13,19,26,29] The disadvantages of microwave ablation are (1) largely CT-occult ablation zone, (2) less distinct ablation zone boundaries as compared with RFA and cryoablation, and (3) potential nontarget overheating due to rapid delivery of high-power output (up to 100 W).[13,19,26,29]

In a single-center retrospective study, the investigators treated 140 spinal metastases in 91 patients with microwave ablation (combined with VA) and reported statistically significant pain palliation and reduction in opioid usage up to 6 months following treatment with decreased disability scores as well as a local tumor control rate of 94.8% at 6-month follow-up.[29] In a retrospective study, the investigators reported successful treatment of 102 spinal tumors in 69 patients with statistically significant pain palliation at 2 to 4 week and 20 to 24 week postprocedural intervals as well as local tumor control rate of 97% at 20 to 24 weeks[20] with complications in two patients (S1 nerve thermal injury and skin burn).[13]

Vertebral Augmentation

VA is performed following thermal ablation in majority of patients with spinal metastases (in the absence of neurologic compromise or spinal instability) to minimize the possibility of post-ablation fracture and pathologic fracture stabilization[8–11,13,14,17,19,24,27,28] (see Fig. 1). VA may be performed as a standalone intervention for spinal metastases in patients with many osseous or visceral metastases.[21] In the cancer patient fracture evaluation (CAFÉ) randomized controlled trial, the investigators documented that VA provides pain palliation while improving the quality of life as a stand-alone intervention (134 treated patients).[39] The investigators treated 72 vertebral pathologic fractures with epidural tumor involvement in 51 patients and reported statistically significant pain palliation for 94%, 86%, and 92% of patients at 1-day, 1-month, and 1-year post-procedural intervals.[22] Balloon kyphoplasty may improve the quality of tumor filling in spinal metastases. However, in cases with low risk of cement

leakage, the use of balloon kyphoplasty may decrease cement interdigitation into the surrounding trabecular matrix, potentially compromising anchorage.[23] Kyphoplasty using a variety of implants have been used for management of pathologic compression fractures to restore vertebral body height, improve kyphosis, decrease osseous retropulsion, and improve central canal stenosis.[20] The investigators performed kyphoplasty with implants for 53 vertebral body fractures with posterior wall retropulsion (no neurologic compromise) in 51 patients and documented statistically significant reduction in mean posterior wall retropulsion and improved mean vertebral body height.[20] The authors reported three new fractures at treated levels (follow-up of 1–36 months) for which required no intervention.[20]

Thermal Protection

Undesired thermal injury to spinal cord, spinal nerve roots, torso vital organs, and skin are the major risk of vertebral thermal ablations. Several passive and active thermal protection approaches are available and may be used to minimize the risk of thermal injury.[7,9,11,14]

Passive thermal protection strategies include assessing patient biofeedback when ablating under conscious sedation (particularly heat-based ablations), real-time temperature monitoring by the application of thermocouples in the epidural space and neuroforamina, monitoring motor- and somatosensory-evoked potentials when ablating under general anesthesia, and electrostimulation of peripheral nerves for early detection of impending nerve injury.[7,9,11,14] Active thermal protection may be implemented prophylactically and is recommended when temperature reaches 45°C (heat) or 10°C (cold).[14,40] Active thermal protection is achieved by thermal modification, displacement of the structure at risk, or thermal insulation using pneumodissection with carbon dioxide insufflation as well as hydro-dissection with injection of warm or cool liquid surrounding the at-risk structure. Skin thermal protection is typically achieved by the precise assessment of ablation volume, active thermal protection of subcutaneous tissues, and skin surface application of warm saline during cryoablation.

SUMMARY

Minimally invasive percutaneous thermal ablation (combined with VA) offers an important arsenal for radiologists to deliver safe, durable, and efficacious treatment for a subset of patients with spinal metastases. Utilization of procedural safety measures is important to minimize adverse effects and improve outcomes.

CLINICS CARE POINTS

- Percutaneous minimally invasive thermal ablation and vertebral augmentation offer a robust armamentarium for radiologists for management of patients with spinal metastases.

- Thermal ablation is safe, effective, and durable in management of selected patients with spinal metastases to achieve pain palliation and local tumor control.

- Thermal protection is important to ensure procedure safety.

DISCLOSURE

All authors have no commercial or financial conflicts of interest and no funding sources.

REFERENCES

1. https://www.cancer.org/content/dam/cancer-org/research/cancer-facts-and-statistics/annual-cancer-facts-and-figures/2023/2023-cancer-facts-and-figures.pdf. Accessed June 24, 2023.
2. Macedo F, Ladeira K, Pinho F, et al. Bone metastases: an overview. Oncol Rev 2017;11:321.
3. Urch C. The pathophysiology of cancer-induced bone pain: current understanding. Palliat Med 2004; 18:267–74.
4. Strander H, Turesson I, Cavallin-Ståhl E. A systematic overview of radiation therapy effects in soft tissue sarcomas. Acta Oncol 2003;42:516–31.
5. van der Linden YM, Steenland E, van Houwelingen HC, et al. Dutch Bone Metastasis Study Group.Patients with a favourable prognosis are equally palliated with single and multiple fraction radiotherapy:results on survival in the Dutch Bone Metastasis Study. Radiother Oncol 2006;78:245–53.
6. Paice JA. Cancer pain management and the opioid crisis in America: How to preserve hard-earned gains in improving the quality of cancer pain management. Cancer 2018;124(12):2491–7.
7. Anchala PR, Irving WD, Hillen TJ, et al. Treatment of metastatic spinal lesions with a navigational bipolar radiofrequency ablation device: a multicenter retrospective study. Pain Physician 2014;17: 317–27.
8. Bagla S, Sayed D, Smirniotopoulos J, et al. Multicenter prospective clinical series evaluating radiofrequency ablation in the treatment of painful spine metastases. Cardiovasc Intervent Radiol 2016;39: 1289–97.
9. Tomasian A, Hillen TJ, Chang RO, et al. Simultaneous bipedicular radiofrequency ablation combined with vertebral augmentation for local tumor control of spinal metastases. AJNR 2018;39:1768–73.
10. Wallace AN, Tomasiana A, Vaswani D, et al. Radiographic local control of spinal metastases with percutaneous radiofrequency ablation and vertebral augmentation. AJNR 2016;37:759–65.
11. Tomasian A, Wallace A, Northrup B, et al. Spine cryoablation:pain palliation and local tumor control for vertebral metastases. AJNR 2016;37:189–95.
12. Auloge P, Cazzato RL, Rousseau C, et al. Complications of percutaneous bone tumor cryoablation:a 10-year experience. Radiology 2019;291:521–8.
13. Khan MA, Deib G, Deldar B, et al. Efficacy and safety of percutaneous microwave ablation and cementoplasty in the treatment of painful spinal metastases and myeloma. AJNR 2018;39:1376–83.
14. Tomasian A, Gangi A, Wallace AN, et al. Percutaneous thermal ablation of spinal metastases: recent advances and review. AJR 2018;210:142–52.
15. McMenomy BP, Kurup AN, Johnson GB, et al. Percutaneous cryoablation of musculoskeletal oligometastatic disease for complete remission. J Vasc Intervent Radiol 2013;24:207–13.
16. Cazzato RL, Auloge P, De Marini P, et al. Percutaneous image-guided ablation of bone metastases: local tumor control in oligometastatic patients. Int J Hyperthermia 2018;35:493–9.
17. Levy J, Hopkins T, Morris J, et al. Radiofrequency Ablation for the Palliative Treatment of Bone Metastases:Outcomes from the Multicenter OsteoCool Tumor Ablation Post-Market Study (OPuS One Study) in 100 Patients. J Vasc Intervent Radiol 2020; 31(11):1745–52.
18. Cazzato RL, Palussière J, Auloge P, et al. Complications Following Percutaneous Image-guided Radiofrequency Ablation of Bone Tumors:A 10-year. Dual-Center Experience Radiology 2020;296(1):227–35.
19. Pusceddu C, Sotgia B, Fele RM, et al. Combined Microwave Ablation and Cementoplasty in Patients with Painful Bone Metastases at High Risk of Fracture. Cardiovasc Intervent Radiol 2016;39:74–80.
20. Venier A, Roccatagliata L, Isalberti M, et al. Armed Kyphoplasty:An Indirect Central Canal Decompression Technique in Burst Fractures. Am J Neuroradiol 2019;40(11):1965–72.
21. Wallace AN, Robinson CG, Meyer J, et al. The Metastatic Spine Disease Multidisciplinary Working Group algorithms. Oncol 2015;20:1205–15.
22. Saliou G, Kocheida EM, Lehmann P, et al. Percutaneous vertebroplasty for pain management in malignant fractures of the spine with epidural involvement. Radiology 2010;254(3):882–90.
23. Dalton BE, Kohm AC, Miller LE, et al. Radiofrequency targeted vertebral augmentation versus traditional balloon kyphoplasty:radiographic and

morphologic outcomes of an ex vivo biomechanical pilot study. Clin Interv Aging 2012;7:525–31.

24. Wallace AN, Greenwood TJ, Jennings JW. Radiofrequency ablation and vertebral augmentation for palliation of painful spinal metastases. J Neuro Oncol 2015;124:111–8.

25. Tsoumakidou G, Koch G, Caudrelier J, et al. Image-guided spinal ablation: a review. Cardiovasc Intervent Radiol 2016;39:1229–38.

26. Kastler A, Alnassan H, Aubry S, et al. Microwave thermal ablation of spinal metastatic bone tumors. J Vasc Intervent Radiol 2014;25:1470–5.

27. Tomasian A, Marlow J, Hillen TJ, et al. Complications of Percutaneous Radiofrequency Ablation of Spinal Osseous Metastases: An 8-Year Single-Center Experience. AJR Am J Roentgenol 2021;216(6):1607–13.

28. Cazzato RL, Jennings JW, Autrusseau PA, et al. Percutaneous image-guided cryoablation of spinal metastases: over 10-year experience in two academic centersEuropean. Radiology 2022;32:4137–46.

29. Chen L, Hou G, Zhang K, et al. Percutaneous CT-Guided Microwave Ablation Combined with Vertebral Augmentation for Treatment of Painful Spinal Metastases. AJNR Am J Neuroradiol 2022;43(3):501–6.

30. National Comprehensive Cancer Network website.NCCN clinical practice guidelines in oncology: adult cancer pain,version 1.2023.www.nccn.org\

31. Shah LM, Jennings JW, Kirsch CFE, et al, Expert Panels on Neurological Imaging, Interventional Radiology, and Musculoskeletal Imaging. ACR Appropriateness Criteria: management of vertebral compression fractures. J Am Coll Radiol 2018;15(suppl 11):S347–64.

32. Schag CC, Heinrich RL, Ganz PA. Karnofsky performance status revisited:reliability,validity, and guidelines. J Clin Oncol 1984;2:187–93.

33. Fisher CG, DiPaola CP, Ryken TC, et al. A novel classification system for spinal instability in neoplastic disease:an evidence-based approach and expert consensus from the Spine Oncology Study Group. Spin 2010;35:E1221–9.

34. Patchell RA, Tibbs PA, Regine WF, et al. Direct decompressive surgical resection in the treatment of spinal cord compression caused by metastatic cancer:a randomised trial. Lancet 2005;366:643–8.

35. Dupuy DE, Hong R, Oliver B, et al. Radiofrequency ablation of spinal tumors: temperature distribution in the spinal canal. AJR 2000;175:1263–6.

36. Singh S, Saha S. Electrical properties of bone:a review. Clin Orthop Relat Res 1984;186:249–71.

37. Cox BW, Spratt DE, Lovelock M, et al. International Spine Radiosurgery Consortium consensus guidelines for target volume definition in spinal stereotactic radiosurgery. Int J Radiat Oncol Biol Phys 2012;83:e597–605.

38. Weld KJ, Landman J. Comparison of cryoablation,-radiofrequency ablation and high-intensity focused ultrasound for treating small renal tumours. BJU Int 2005;96:1224–9.

39. Berenson J, Pflugmacher R, Jarzem P, et al. Cancer Patient Fracture Evaluation (CAFE) Investigators. Balloon kyphoplasty versus non-surgical fracture management for treatment of painful vertebral body compression fractures in patients with cancer: a multicentre, randomised controlled trial. Lancet Oncol 2011;12(3):225–35.

40. Buy X, Tok CH, Szwarc D, et al. Thermal protection during percutaneous thermal ablation procedures: interest of carbon dioxide dissection and temperature monitoring. Cardiovasc Intervent Radiol 2009;32:529–34.

Spinal Cerebrospinal Fluid Leak Localization with Dynamic Computed Tomography Myelography
Tips, Tricks, and Pitfalls

William P. Dillon, MD

KEYWORDS

- Dynamic computed tomography myelography • Spontaneous intracranial hypotension
- Cerebrospinal fluid leak

KEY POINTS

- Decubitus dynamic myelography with or without CSF saline pressure augmentation and review of 0.625mm sections is essential to detect subtle CSF venous fistula.
- Careful attention to all sites is needed as CSF venous fistula may be multiple and or bilateral.
- CSF venous fistula may be present in up to 10% of patients with orthostatic headache syndromes and normal MR scans.
- Dynamic CT myelography may be helpful in localizing both type 1 and 2 CSF leaks as well as CSF venous fistulae, but requires attention to detail and the presence or absence of extradural CSF on fat saturated axial MR of the spine.

Locating spinal cerebrospinal fluid (CSF) leaks can be a diagnostic dilemma for clinicians and radiologists, as well as frustrating for patients. Digital subtraction dynamic myelogram for the detection of ventral osteophytic spinal leaks was first demonstrated by Hoxworth and colleagues[1] and adapted by others to assess both spinal leaks and cerebrospinal venous fistulas.[2]

Dynamic computed tomography myelography (dCTM) has emerged as a valuable tool in localizing spinal CSF leaks, aiding in accurate diagnosis, and guiding appropriate management.[3–5] This article aims to provide insights into the technique, tips, tricks, and potential pitfalls associated with dCTM for spinal CSF leak localization. By understanding the nuances of this procedure, clinicians can optimize the diagnostic process and improve patient outcomes.

SPINAL CEREBROSPINAL FLUID LEAK LOCALIZATION: IMPORTANCE AND CHALLENGES

Three major categories of spontaneous spinal CSF leaks have been described. Type 1 CSF leaks consist of a dural tear, either at the ventral dura (type 1A) or posterolateral dura (type 1B), usually from a herniated disc or osteophyte (**Figs. 1** and **2**). Type 2 CSF leaks are secondary to the rupture of a meningeal diverticulum. Both type 1 and 2 leaks result in CSF leakage into the epidural space, sometimes referred to as spinal longitudinal extradural CSF collection (SLEC) and are visible on T2-weighted fat-suppressed MRI scans and/or conventional computed tomography (CT) myelography. Type 3 leaks are abnormal connections between spinal CSF and an adjacent venous structure and are not usually associated with SLEC (**Fig. 3**). Finally, distal nerve root sleeve rents,

Department of Radiology and Biomedical Imaging, University of California, 505 Parnassus Avenue, Room M396A Box 0628, San Francisco, CA 94143-0628, USA
E-mail address: william.dillon@ucsf.edu

Radiol Clin N Am 62 (2024) 311–319
https://doi.org/10.1016/j.rcl.2023.09.002
0033-8389/24/© 2023 Elsevier Inc. All rights reserved.

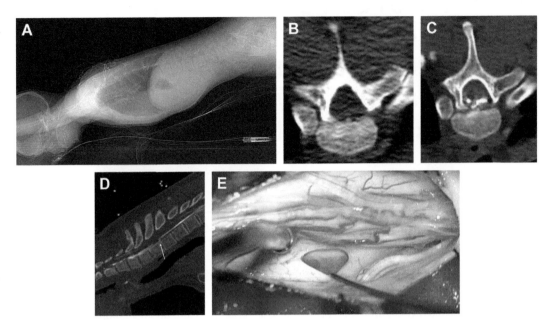

Fig. 1. Prone dynamic CT Myelogram performed using a wedge.(A) Patient positioned in prone Trendelenberg position on a wedge pillow.(B) Noncontrast CT demonstrates osteophyte.(C) Axial CT following intrathecal contrast demonstrates epidural contrast leaking at the site of the osteophyte, which is partially obscured by contrast material.(D) Sagittal reformation demonstrates extravasation of contrast material into ventral epidural space (E) The patient was taken to surgery and a ventral fistula was found and repaired. CT, computed tomography. (Operative photo *courtesy* of Dr. Wouter Scheivink.)

sometimes called type 4, may also give rise to spontaneous intracranial hypotension (SIH) and do not demonstrate SLEC. These lesions are usually solitary; however, in rare cases, both leaks and venous fistulas have been localized simultaneously in the same patient on dCTM.[6] Multiple simultaneous CSF venous fistulae have also been documented in at least 10 percent or more of patients. All are best treated initially by targeted occlusion with either autologous blood or fibrin glue, or a combination of both at the site of the fistula.[7–9] Surgical repair is reserved for those lesions that cannot be occluded percutaneously. So-called nontargeted blood patches, performed without knowledge of the precise location of the site of a fistula, can also be initially attempted and, if successful, can avoid the radiation and cost of more detailed localization examinations. Precise localization and targeted patching of a CSF leak, however, result in greater success rates and help guide subsequent surgical approaches, if required.[10] Thus, precisely locating a CSF leak is important in most cases of patients with SIH.

Conventional magnetic resonance (MR) scan sequences or CT myelography may detect SLEC in type 1 and 2 fistulas but often fail to detect the exact location of the leak, as CSF and/or extradural contrast often quickly extends in the epidural space, a distance from the site of a leak.[11,12] Type 3

CSF-venous fistulas are also not detected by conventional CT or MR techniques but rather require decubitus dynamic fluoroscopic-based myelography or dCTM for detection.[4,13,14] Therefore, all 3 types of CSF fistulas in the spine require a dynamic examination in order to precisely locate most fistulas.

ADVANTAGES OF DYNAMIC COMPUTED TOMOGRAPHY MYELOGRAPHY IN LOCALIZATION

dCTM offers several advantages in localizing spinal CSF leaks, providing valuable information for accurate diagnosis and appropriate management. The advantages of dCTM include the following:

1. Precise visualization of CSF contrast extravasation as well as venous fistulas.
2. High spatial and contrast resolution: CT imaging provides excellent spatial and contrast resolution of spinal structures, including discs, osteophytes, and surrounding osseous architecture and calcifications. This enables the identification of small transdural osteophytes (see **Figs. 1** and **2**). The use of submillimeter section CT imaging, even more so with newer photon-counting CT scanners, improves the spatial visualization of subtle leakage and CSF venous fistulas.[15]

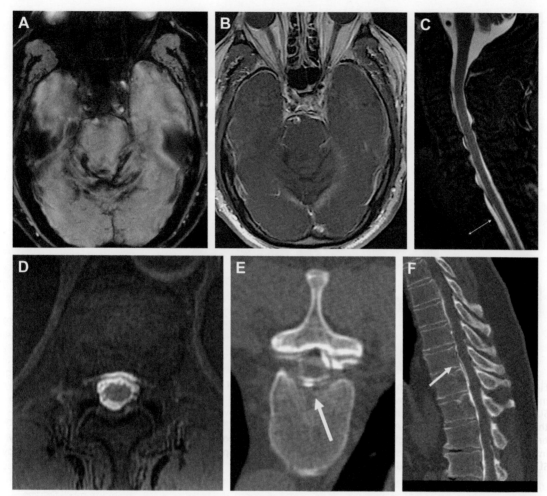

Fig. 2. SLEC. A 75-year-old with cognitive slowing.(*A*) Axial susceptibility-weighted images demonstrate pial siderosis indicative of chronic subarachnoid bleeding.(*B*) Axial post-gadolinium contrast T1-weighted image showing diffuse dural enhancement indicative of low CSF volume.(*C*) Sagittal T2-weighted MR image shows spinal extradural CSF collection (*arrow*).(*D*) Axial fat-saturated T2-weighted image shows spinal extradural CSF collection (*arrow*).(*E*) Axial prone CT scan following lumbar injection of iodinated contrast showing extradural contrast (*arrow*).(*F*) Sagittal reformation showing ventral extradural contrast (*arrow*) secondary to transdural osteophyte. CSF, cerebrospinal fluid; CT, computed tomography; MR, magnetic resonance; SLEC, spinal longitudinal extradural cerebrospinal fluid collection.

3. Multi-planar reconstructions: The generation of axial, sagittal, and coronal views provides a comprehensive assessment of the spinal canal, improving the ability to precisely identify the level and location of the leak.
4. Evaluation of associated abnormalities: In addition to CSF leak localization, dCTM enables the evaluation of associated spinal abnormalities, such as dural defects secondary to herniated discs or small osteophytes, meningeal diverticula, or spinal arachnoid cysts.
5. Integration with other imaging modalities: dCTM can be easily integrated with other imaging modalities, such as CT angiography or MRI, when necessary. For instance, MR myelography has been used with small injections of intrathecal gadolinium, which in rare cases can be helpful in detecting slow leaks or those around metal implants. Gadolinium can be injected along with the iodinated contrast at the time of CT myelography, and then subsequent MR is performed following CT.[16]
6. Availability and cost-effectiveness: CT scanners are fast and are a widely available and accessible diagnostic tool. General anesthesia is usually not required. Compared to other modalities such as MRI, dCTM is relatively more cost-effective and can be performed quickly,

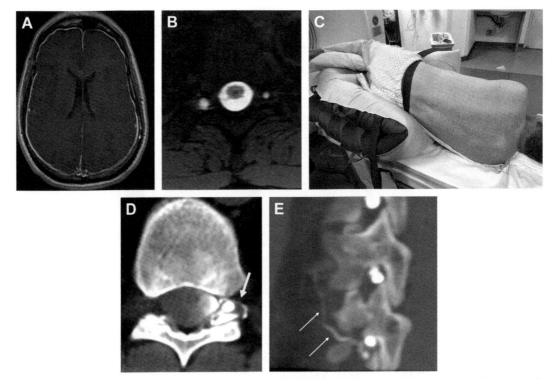

Fig. 3. CSF venous fistula.(*A*) Postcontrast MR scan showing typical dural enhancement related to low CSF volume.(*B*) Axial fat-saturated T2-weighted image showing enlarged perineural cysts and no extradural CSF (no SLEC).(*C*) Patient in lateral decubitus position after inflation of hover mat raises hips for 10 seconds after intrathecal injection of contrast.(*D*) Axial decubitus CT demonstrates a CSF venous fistula draining into internal vertebral vein (*arrow*).(*E*) Sagittal reformation demonstrates a CSF venous fistula draining superiorly and anteriorly into hemiazygos system (*arrows*). CSF, cerebrospinal fluid; CT, computed tomography; MR, magnetic resonance; SLEC, spinal longitudinal extradural cerebrospinal fluid collection.

leading to timely diagnosis and subsequent management decisions.

PRINCIPLES OF DYNAMIC COMPUTED TOMOGRAPHY MYELOGRAPHY

Dynamic myelography, whether performed fluoroscopically or with CT (dCTM), plays a crucial role in guiding the diagnosis and management of patients with spinal CSF leaks. dCTM combines the advantages of CT imaging with the rapid temporal resolution afforded by fast scanning immediately following the injection of contrast. The key points are proper preparation of the patient and attention to several technical nuances that increase the likelihood of detecting and then treating a CSF fistula.

TIPS AND TRICKS FOR OPTIMAL IMAGING

In the patient with suspected CSF leak, we perform an MR of the brain with contrast, as well as a T2-weighted MR of the spine with fat saturation. The presence or absence of SLEC in the

spine determines the positioning of the patient on the CT scanner during dCTM. If extradural CSF is present in the MR spine study, a prone dynamic CT is planned. In the absence of extradural contrast, a decubitus dCT myelogram is planned, which has been shown to increase the conspicuity of CSF venous fistula.[5,13,17] The patient lies prone or in the decubitus position on the CT table, either on a wedge pillow or a folded hover mat that can be inflated to allow transient Trendelenburg positioning (**Fig. 4**).[5,18]

An initial scout image in the anteroposterior (AP) and lateral planes is performed of the entire spine, which will be used for both the lumbar needle placement and subsequent dynamic total spine myelogram. A noncontrast CT is useful prior to myelography to identify small osteophytes and calcifications that can be obscured by contrast or confused with extradural contrast (see **Fig. 1**). Ideally the needle should be placed in the lateral decubitus position while the patient is positioned on a folded hover mat, positioned under their hips with the fold near the mid-thoracic region. The

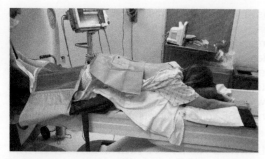

Fig. 4. Hover mat inflated for prone dynamic computed tomography myelography.

hover mat is transiently inflated after injection to raise the patient's hips and facilitate the cranial flow of contrast. The lateral decubitus position permits the measurement of an accurate opening pressure using a digital pressure gauge (Compass device, Centurion Medical Products, Williamston, MI, USA). Additionally, in this position it is easier to see CSF return in the needle hub and is more comfortable for the patient during scanning. While most patients with leaks have an opening pressure in the normal range, it serves as a baseline if the patient develops rebound intracranial hypertension after therapy and in the case of a patient who presents with headache secondary to other causes such as idiopathic intracranial hypertension.[19]

The prone position is used in patients with SLEC whose leak is suspected either ventrally or posterolaterally. If a prone scan is required, the patient can be carefully rolled while on a hover mat from the decubitus to the prone position, while carefully monitoring the needle in the back. This technique has also been used to perform both-sided decubitus myelography on the same day.[20] The hover mat is then inflated to raise the hips and facilitate contrast flow to the thoracic region. At times, however, especially in large patients, this may be difficult to achieve, and physical lifting may be required of the patient, transiently. If one chooses to perform the puncture on a wedge pillow in the prone position, careful attention to technique is necessary to prevent extradural injections of contrast, as the CSF pressure may be very low preventing CSF from appearing in the needle hub. In either case, one must try carefully not to inject contrast in the epidural or subdural space. We use intermittent low-dose (10–20 mA) targeted CT scans to monitor the placement of the needle into the thecal sac, verifying its final position by injecting a small amount (<1 cc) of contrast, which should sink to the bottom of the thecal sac if intrathecal. If contrast remains at the needle tip or is clearly extradural, one can try to manipulate the

needle into the thecal sac; however, the presence of extradural contrast will limit the precision of the study.

TIMING OF IMAGE ACQUISITION TO CAPTURE THE LEAK

Once the lumbar puncture has been performed and the needle is in the proper position, the radiologist and technologist plan the scan parameters using the whole-body scout images that were obtained for the placement of the needle. We use a high concentration (300%) of iodinated contrast material for dCTM when searching for a CSF leak. Dynamic CT is typically obtained back and forth from the sacrum to the cervical area, for a total of 2 to 3 passes using a diagnostic technique of 240 to 300 MA, 2.5 mm scan thickness, and 120 KVp. Thin 0.625-mm sections are reconstructed and sagittal and coronal reformations are saved for all passes (see **Figs. 1** and **2**). For those patients suspected of type 1 or 2 leaks, we inject contrast in the prone position and hover the mat up to raise the hips for a period of 6 to 10 seconds (see **Fig. 4**). We deflate the hover mat and begin the CT scanning immediately and will scan at least 2 passes of the spine. If using a wedge pillow, we inject contrast and immediately begin scanning inferior to superior and back, with the goal of visualizing the egress of the subarachnoid contrast column at the precise point of the fistula (see **Figs. 1** and **2**). One looks for a step-off of the contrast column ventrally or laterally, usually secondary to a ventral osteophyte or meningeal diverticula laterally at a thoracic level. If this is not seen in the prone position in a patient with suspected type 1 or 2 leaks, then repositioning the patient in the decubitus position and repeating a CT may identify a lateral leak. One pitfall in this technique is waiting too long to initiate the CT after injection as contrast may have leaked out quickly into the epidural space, above and below the site of the fistula, prohibiting its precise localization. A patient who has extensive extradural contrast on MR usually has such a fast leak and must be quickly scanned after injection when in Trendelenburg in order to catch the first egress of contrast out of the thecal sac.[21] Each of these techniques has advantages and disadvantages. Obese patients may find it difficult to position themselves on a wedge, but we may also have difficulty raising their hips on a hover mat sufficiently to position contrast over the thoracic kyphotic curve. Other techniques using motorized table accessories are in development (personal communication Andrew Callen, M.D.)

For those with suspected type 3 CSF venous fistula, scanning is performed in the decubitus position. Again, the lateral and AP scout CT localizer is obtained of the entire spine and the planned excursion of the dynamic scan is prescribed using diagnostic techniques. Once the needle is placed, a small amount (<1 cc) of contrast is injected to confirm the subarachnoid location of the needle. The CT technologist then sets up the scanning parameters, consisting of 3 passes of the entire spine using a diagnostic technique (equal or greater than 250 mA), from the sacrum to the cervical vertebrae (C1–C2), starting inferiorly and continually scanning inferior to superior, and back again. The patient is also instructed on the resistive inspiration technique of breathing slowly through the end of a 5-cc syringe with the plunger removed during scanning.[22] This technique decreases thoracic pressure and has been shown to increase the conspicuity of CSF venous fistulas.[23] Then 10 cc of contrast is injected and the needle is removed, and the folded hover mat, positioned under the hips and mid-thorax, is inflated for 10 to 15 seconds, raising the hips so contrast flows superiorly to the level of the foramen magnum. The hover mat is then quickly deflated, and the technologist immediately begins imaging while the patient begins restricted inspiration (the patient is instructed to breathe in slowly through the syringe, then at the peak inspiration, if still scanning, the patient may exhale and begin resisted inspiration again through the 5-cc syringe).

The acquired 2.5-mm CT images are reviewed, reconstructed into thin submillimeter sections, and reformatted into axial, sagittal, and coronal planes in order to provide a comprehensive evaluation of the spinal canal. A review of thin sections (0.625 mm) often helps confirm a CSF venous fistula. If no fistula is seen, the patient is carefully positioned on the opposite decubitus position and a repeat scan, of 1 pass, is performed. This may require a dynamic scan on this side on a different day if a fistula is highly suspected, as these can be elusive on delayed scans. As mentioned, a technique for bilateral dynamic decubitus CT myelograms at the same sitting has been reported by Carlton Jones and Goadsby,[20] requiring the needle to be kept in place while scanning after the injection of 6 to 8 cc of contrast, then turning the patient from one side to the other and reinjecting again.

In addition to resistive inspiration techniques, an injection of saline or mock CSF can be used to augment the pressure in those with low or low normal pressure. This involves saline aliquots that are infused to raise the CSF pressure to at least 20 cm of water before intrathecal contrast is injected. 5-cc aliquots of saline are injected until a rise in pressure is occurs, then 1 to 2-cc aliquots of saline and injected until 18 to 20 cm of pressure

is reached. The augmentation of CSF pressure using preservative-free saline or mock CSF has been reported to increase the visualization of CSF leaks.[24,25] This technique has been successfully employed in patients with very low pressures prior to injection of contrast intrathecally and in patients who are comatose secondary to several intracranial CSF volume depletion.[26]

LIMITING ARTIFACTS AND MOTION-RELATED ISSUES

The most common artifact during dCTM is motion from breathing during the scan, especially in the prone position as the patient's body moves with each breath. Patient movement secondary to leg or head pain is also an issue at times, especially when using a high concentration of contrast material, which can irritate lumbar nerve roots transiently or also cause headaches if it enters the intracranial compartment. For type 1 or 2 fistulas, it is best if the patient can suspend their breathing during CT in the prone position. In the decubitus position when looking for CSF venous fistula, the patient is instructed to slowly breathe in during restricted inspiration, as mentioned earlier. The patient is encouraged to lie as still as possible and not to cough or speak during the scanning. The use of several passes during dynamic CT often offsets these motion-related issues as 1 or more scans are typically motion-free.

INTERPRETATION AND LOCALIZATION OF SPINAL CEREBROSPINAL FLUID LEAKS

In the case of suspected type 1 or 2 leaks, one looks to detect the initial egress of contrast from the subarachnoid space into the epidural space. One carefully assesses the ventral epidural space, looking for subtle step-off of the contrast column, especially at locations of osteophytes, usually located at the upper thoracic levels. Small bony spicules that breach the ventral dura are easily obscured by the iodinated contrast and are often invisible on MR scans. Thus, it is useful to perform a noncontrast CT with a low-dose technique to detect these prior to injection of contrast media (see **Figs. 1** and **2**). If the egress of contrast is not seen on the prone dynamic myelogram, then the patient should be placed in the decubitus position and rescanned to assess the nerve root sleeves for type 2 meningeal diverticula.

Type 3 leaks are more difficult to detect and can be temporally elusive. The majority are found in the thoracic spine, and rarely in the cervical or sacral areas. They are usually solitary; however, multiple simultaneous fistulas have been reported, especially in patients with idiopathic intracranial hypertension. CSF venous fistulas are slightly more frequent on the right side and emanate most commonly from a perineural cyst or more centrally within the spinal canal, and drain into the paraspinous venous system, the internal and external vertebral veins and rarely into the basivertebral plexus. Normally a CSF venous fistula drains laterally into the azygos or hemiazygos veins. Careful assessment of the lateral paravertebral veins is important in localizing these type 3 fistulas; however, one must assess all the potential venous pathways of egress from the spinal canal so as not to miss a subtle fistula (see **Fig. 3**).[27]

The timing of the CSF venous fistula's appearance is critical to timing the CT scans following injection of contrast; however, a paucity of information is available regarding the dynamics of these lesions. Mark and colleagues, however, have reviewed digital dynamic myelographic data from Mayo Clinic and found that CSF venous fistulas appear a mean of 9 seconds after contrast infusion, with a range of 0 to 30 seconds.[28] A review of our own dynamic CT myelographic data shows that most are visualized on initial passes of the dCT; however, some appear on more delayed scans or are transient, appearing only on the second or third pass of the CT (ie, within 9–48 seconds after injection) and disappearing thereafter. Thus, we employ 3 passes with dCTM

to ensure we do not miss these somewhat slowly filling CSF venous fistulas (**Fig. 5**). It is also important to review thinner sections as CSF venous fistula may be poorly visualized on thicker sections.

On occasion, it has been difficult to precisely locate a leak on dynamic CT. In such cases, dynamic conventional myelography can be complementary, as the temporally dynamic nature of continuous fluoroscopic myelography is unsurpassed.[13] As the speed and resolution of CT improve, as with photon-counting CT scanners, more subtle fistulas may be visualized.[15] Nonetheless, in our own practice, we have at times performed conventional dynamic myelography especially when fast leaks cannot be precisely localized using CT. CSF venous fistulas may rarely occur from sacral root sleeves.[29] These must be examined in cases where no fistula is found in the typical thoracic locations. The patients are asked to either sit up briefly before rescanning, or one may use fluoroscopic dynamic myelography performed during reverse Trendelenberg positioning.

POTENTIAL COMPLICATIONS AND ADVERSE EFFECTS

Myelography is usually safe. The most common adverse effect is headache, which may occur due to intracranial spread of contrast or in a delayed postural fashion secondary to lumbar

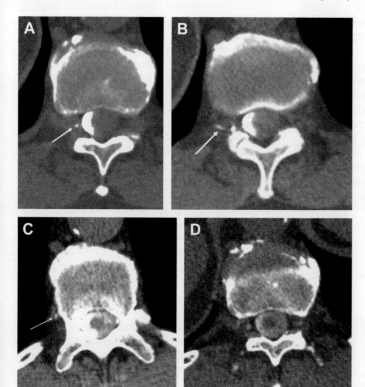

Fig. 5. Patient with long-standing symptoms of postural headache and brain fog. CSF opening pressure was 13 cm of water but then fell to 4 cm of water following removal of 4 cc of CSF for laboratory tests. 15 mL of preservative-free saline was then infused, and CSF pressure rises to 10 cm of water. CSF venous fistula was seen only on second pass of dynamic CTM. (A)Axial CT in decubitus position during the first pass. No fistula is seen. (B and C) Two CTs during the second CT pass a few seconds after A. Opacification of the CSF venous fistula is seen (arrows).(D) The third pass of CT shows CSF venous fistula no longer is visible. The transient opacification makes the diagnosis difficult in some cases. CSF, cerebrospinal fluid; CT, computed tomography; CTM, computed tomography myelography.

puncture (LP)–related CSF leakage. Postural puncture headaches can be minimized with the use of smaller gauge, noncutting lumbar puncture needles, such as a 25-gauge pencil point Whitacre, Sprott, or 24-gauge Gerty Marx needles. However, it must be noted that viscous 300% iodine concentration may take longer to inject through these smaller gauge needles. Several interventions such as bed rest, hydration, caffeine administration, as well as epidural blood patching can minimize or treat post-LP headaches.

Headache can also occur secondary to raised intracranial pressure during injection of saline along with intrathecal contrast. This is typically transient but can be severe for a short while and exacerbated by the spread of intracranial contrast. Rebound headaches may also develop following successful treatment of these lesions and usually respond to acetazolamide.

Radiation exposure remains one of the largest drawbacks to dCTM, especially in younger patients. In order to detect these small lesions, a high radiation dose is required, and several CT passes are typically performed. This can be minimized with the use of modern CT modulation techniques. Nonetheless, especially in younger patients, we may choose to start with nontargeted blood patches prior to performing CT myelography in order to minimize radiation dose, particularly in those with extradural CSF on the MR spine. This is sometimes curative and can spare a patient the discomfort and radiation dose of dynamic CT or myelography. Mamlouk and colleagues have also reported on radiation-reduced techniques for dCTM.[5] In summary, dCTM plays a crucial role in localizing spinal CSF leaks, providing valuable information for diagnosis and treatment planning. By understanding the technique's nuances and pitfalls, radiologists can optimize image acquisition, interpretation, and localization for subsequent attempts at percutaneous or surgical therapy. Careful attention to tips, tricks, and potential pitfalls helps minimize errors and improve patient care in the realm of spinal CSF leak diagnosis.

DISCLOSURE

The author has no financial or commercial conflict of interest.

REFERENCES

1. Hoxworth JM, Patel AC, Bosch EP, et al. Localization of a rapid CSF leak with digital subtraction myelography. AJNR Am J Neuroradiol 2009;30(3):516–9.

2. Schievink WI, Moser FG, Maya MM, et al. Digital subtraction myelography for the identification of spontaneous spinal CSF-venous fistulas. J Neurosurg Spine 2016;24(6):960–4.

3. Dobrocky T, Mosimann PJ, Zibold F, et al. Cryptogenic Cerebrospinal Fluid Leaks in Spontaneous Intracranial Hypotension: Role of Dynamic CT Myelography. Radiology 2018;289(3):766–72.

4. Luetmer PH, Mokri B. Dynamic CT myelography: a technique for localizing high-flow spinal cerebrospinal fluid leaks. AJNR Am J Neuroradiol 2003;24(8):1711–4.

5. Mamlouk MD, Ochi RP, Jun P, et al. Decubitus CT Myelography for CSF-Venous Fistulas: A Procedural Approach. AJNR Am J Neuroradiol 2021;42(1):32–6.

6. Madhavan AA, Benson JC, Cutsforth-Gregory JK, et al. Co-existing fast CSF leaks and CSF-venous fistulas on dynamic CT myelography. Radiol Case Rep 2022;17(9):2968–71.

7. Mokri B. Spontaneous low pressure, low CSF volume headaches: spontaneous CSF leaks. Headache 2013;53(7):1034–53.

8. Elwood JJ, Dewan M, Smith JM, et al. Efficacy of epidural blood patch with fibrin glue additive in refractory headache due to intracranial hypotension: preliminary report. SpringerPlus 2016;5:317.

9. Mamlouk MD, Shen PY, Sedrak MF, et al. CT-guided Fibrin Glue Occlusion of Cerebrospinal Fluid–Venous Fistulas. Radiology 2021;299(2):409–18.

10. Cho KI, Moon HS, Jeon HJ, et al. Spontaneous intracranial hypotension: efficacy of radiologic targeting vs blind blood patch. Neurology 2011;76(13):1139–44.

11. Dillon WP, Fishman RA. Some lessons learned about the diagnosis and treatment of spontaneous intracranial hypotension. AJNR Am J Neuroradiol 1998;19(6):1001–2.

12. Dillon WP. Spinal manifestations of intracranial hypotension. AJNR Am J Neuroradiol 2001;22(7):1233–4.

13. Schievink WI, Marcel Maya M, Moser FG, et al. Lateral decubitus digital subtraction myelography to identify spinal CSF–venous fistulas in spontaneous intracranial hypotension. J Neurosurg Spine 2019;31(6):902–5.

14. Kranz PG, Gray L, Amrhein TJ. Decubitus CT Myelography for Detecting Subtle CSF Leaks in Spontaneous Intracranial Hypotension. AJNR Am J Neuroradiol 2019;40(4):754–6.

15. Schwartz FR, Malinzak MD, Amrhein TJ. Photon-Counting Computed Tomography Scan of a Cerebrospinal Fluid Venous Fistula. JAMA Neurol 2022;79(6):628–9.

16. Chazen JL, Talbott JF, Lantos JE, et al. MR myelography for identification of spinal CSF leak in spontaneous intracranial hypotension. AJNR Am J Neuroradiol 2014. Published online. http://www.ajnr.org/content/early/2014/05/22/ajnr.A3975.abstract.

17. Farb RI, Nicholson PJ, Peng PW, et al. Spontaneous Intracranial Hypotension: A Systematic Imaging Approach for CSF Leak Localization and Management Based on MRI and Digital Subtraction Myelography. AJNR Am J Neuroradiol 2019;40(4):745–53.

18. Callen AL, Timpone VM, Schwertner A, et al. Algorithmic Multimodality Approach to Diagnosis and Treatment of Spinal CSF Leak and Venous Fistula in Patients With Spontaneous Intracranial Hypotension. AJR Am J Roentgenol 2022;219(2):292–301.

19. Kranz PG, Tanpitukpongse TP, Choudhury KR, et al. How common is normal cerebrospinal fluid pressure in spontaneous intracranial hypotension? Cephalalgia 2016;36(13):1209–17.

20. Carlton Jones L, Goadsby PJ. Same-Day Bilateral Decubitus CT Myelography for Detecting CSF-Venous Fistulas in Spontaneous Intracranial Hypotension. AJNR Am J Neuroradiol 2022;43(4):645–8.

21. Mamlouk MD, Shen PY, Dahlin BC. Modified dynamic CT myelography for type 1 and 2 CSF leaks: A procedural approach. AJNR Am J Neuroradiol 2023;44(3):341–6.

22. Mark IT, Amans MR, Shah VN, et al. Resisted Inspiration: A New Technique to Aid in the Detection of CSF-Venous Fistulas. AJNR Am J Neuroradiol 2022;43(10):1544–7.

23. Kranz PG, Malinzak MD, Gray L, et al. Resisted Inspiration Improves Visualization of CSF-Venous Fistulas in Spontaneous Intracranial Hypotension. AJNR Am J Neuroradiol 2023. https://doi.org/10.3174/ajnr.A7927.

24. Kootar S, Walavalkar A, Kumar A, et al. Modification in MRI contrast myelogram by instillation of intrathecal preservative-free normal saline to demonstrate CSF spinal leaks. Neurol India 2018;66(4):1187–9.

25. Griauzde J, Gemmete JJ, Pandey AS, et al. Intrathecal preservative-free normal saline challenge magnetic resonance myelography for the identification of cerebrospinal fluid leaks in spontaneous intracranial hypotension. J Neurosurg 2015;123(3):732–6.

26. Binder DK, Dillon WP, Fishman RA, et al. Intrathecal saline infusion in the treatment of obtundation associated with spontaneous intracranial hypotension: technical case report. Neurosurgery 2002;51(3):830–6. discussion 836-837.

27. Kranz PG, Amrhein TJ, Gray L. CSF Venous Fistulas in Spontaneous Intracranial Hypotension: Imaging Characteristics on Dynamic and CT Myelography. AJR Am J Roentgenol 2017;209(6):1360–6.

28. Mark I, Madhavan A, Oien M, et al. Temporal Characteristics of CSF-Venous Fistulas on Digital Subtraction Myelography. AJNR Am J Neuroradiol 2023;44(4):492–5.

29. Mark IT, Morris PP, Brinjikji W, et al. Sacral CSF-Venous Fistulas and Potential Imaging Techniques. AJNR Am J Neuroradiol 2022;43(12):1824–6.

Spinal Cerebrospinal Fluid Leak Localization with Digital Subtraction Myelography: Tips, Tricks, and Pitfalls

Javier Galvan, MD, MPH[a,b], Marcel Maya, MD[a,b,*], Ravi S. Prasad, MD[b],
Vikram S. Wadhwa, MD[b], Wouter Schievink, MD[b,c]

KEYWORDS

- Cerebrospinal fluid leak • Spontaneous intracranial hypotension • Digital subtraction myelography
- MR myelography • CT myelography • Cerebrospinal fluid-venous fistula

KEY POINTS

- Digital subtraction myelography has high sensitivity for identifying leak site.
- A hyperdense paraspinal vein sign may be a false localizing sign of CSF-venous fistulas.
- Paraspinal fluid in the C1-2 region does not correspond to site of CSF leak and is known as the false localizing sign of C1-2.
- CSF leaks in the cervicothoracic region seen on spinal imaging are rarely the site of leak and targeted treatment in this region is not likely to result in lasting symptom relief.
- While rare, skull-based CSF leaks can cause SIH.

 Video content accompanies this article at http://www.radiologic.theclinics.com

INTRODUCTION

Cerebrospinal fluid (CSF) leak is a condition in which there is a loss of CSF which leads to spontaneous intracranial hypotension (SIH). SIH can cause a variety of neurologic symptoms, but orthostatic headache due to intracranial hypotension is the most characteristic (Table 1).[1,2] On brain magnetic resonance imaging (MRI), there are characteristic imaging findings associated with intracranial hypotension. These findings encompass subdural fluid collections, pachymeningeal enhancement, engorged venous structures, a hyperemic pituitary gland, and sagging of the brain which can be remembered with the mnemonic SEEPS.[3] These findings along with the appropriate clinical context can be used to clinically diagnose a CSF leak and proceed with conservative treatment or epidural blood patching.[3] In the event that first line treatment with conservative management or epidural patching is not helpful, further diagnostic imaging to localize a CSF leak can be performed.

There are 4 types of CSF leaks (Table 2), CSF leaks that are a result of dural tears are classified as type 1 (Figs. 1 and 2), a CSF leak resulting from a meningeal diverticulum is a type 2 CSF leak (Fig. 3), a type 3 CSF leak is due to a CSF-venous fistula (Figs. 4 and 5), and indeterminate CSF leaks are classified as type 4.[1] Brain and spine imaging play a critical role in the diagnosis of SIH. Historically, computed tomography (CT) myelogram has been the gold standard for detecting and localizing spinal CSF leaks.[4] At our institution our approach is

[a] Department of Imaging, Cedars-Sinai Medical Center; [b] Department of Imaging, Cedars Sinai Medical Center, 8700 Beverly Boulevard Taper Mezzanine M-335, Los Angeles, CA 90048; [c] Department of Neurosurgery, Cedars-Sinai Medical Center
* Corresponding author. Cedars Sinai Medical Center, 8700 Beverly Boulevard Taper Mezzanine M-335, Los Angeles, CA 90048.
E-mail address: Marcel.Maya@cshs.org

Radiol Clin N Am 62 (2024) 321–332
https://doi.org/10.1016/j.rcl.2023.10.004
0033-8389/24/© 2023 Elsevier Inc. All rights reserved.

Table 1 Modified ICHD-3 diagnostic criteria for headache caused by spontaneous intracranial hypotension	
Criterion	Description
A	Any headache attributed to low CSF pressure or CSF leakage that meets criterion C, below
B	Either or both of the following: • Low CSF pressure (<60 mm CSF) • Evidence of CSF leakage on imaging
C	Headache that developed in temporal relation to the low CSF pressure or CSF leakage or that led to its discovery
D	Headache not better accounted for by another ICHD-III diagnosis.

Abbreviation: CSF, cerebrospinal fluid; ICHD, International Classification of Headache Disorders

to first obtain MR brain with contrast and MR spine using heavily weighted T2 sequences (MR myelogram) as these studies have been shown to have similar sensitivity for identifying the presence of CSF leak.[3–5] A flow diagram demonstrating our approach is shown in **Fig. 6**. MR brain and spine are favored for diagnostic purposes because of its noninvasive nature and the absence of radiation exposure. It is important to remember that up to 20% of patients with SIH have a normal brain MRI.[3] In cases where patients who exhibit severe and disabling symptoms digital subtraction myelography (DSM) can be performed as it offers the highest sensitivity for identifying the leak site.[6]

In this article, we will discuss our experience and technique using DSM for the detection of CSF leaks with a focus on a 5-step mnemonic called the "5 P's to success," and potential diagnostic pitfalls to avoid.

Table 2 Classification of spontaneous spinal CSF leaks	
Type 1	Dural tear a. Ventral b. (Postero-)lateral
Type 2	Meningeal Diverticulum a. Simple b. Complex/dural ectasia
Type 3	CSF-venous fistula
Type 4	Indeterminate

Abbreviation: CSF, cerebrospinal fluid

NORMAL ANATOMY AND IMAGING TECHNIQUE

CSF is a vital component of the central nervous system, distributed within the cerebral ventricles, and subarachnoid spaces of the brain and spinal cord. CSF production begins in the arachnoid plexus and is secreted into the cerebral ventricles. From there, CSF courses craniocaudally through the ventricular system in a unidirectional manner where it reaches the subarachnoid spaces, which is multidirectional, via the medial foramen of Magendie and the lateral foramina of Luschka. The mean volume of CSF is approximately 150 cc and regulated through production and absorption. Insufficient CSF volume can lead to intracranial hypotension, whereas excessive CSF volume can cause hydrocephalus. CSF is absorbed within the subarachnoid villi within the dural sinuses where it enters the systemic circulation. One of the primary functions of CSF is to "provide a hydromechanical protective role for the brain and spinal cord."[3,7]

The most common first line study ordered in the emergency setting for headaches is a noncontrast head CT.[3] Although cranial CT has limited sensitivity, it is widely accessible and can potentially show signs of SIH such as basal cistern effacement, downward displacement of the cerebellar tonsils or subdural fluid collections. Effacement of the basal cisterns causes increased attenuation which is occasionally seen and can potentially be mistaken for a subarachnoid hemorrhage.

Initial imaging evaluation involves brain MRI and spinal MRI for the initial detection of CSF leaks.[6] Traditionally, CT myelogram has been the gold standard for detecting CSF leaks; however, this has been supplanted by newer techniques such as dynamic CT myelogram and DSM for the accurate localization of CSF leaks.[6,8] CT myelography involves the administration of intrathecal iodinated contrast after a lumbar puncture, followed by obtaining thin-cut CT images of the spine. However, 1 limitation of CT myelography is that in cases of high-flow CSF leaks, the extravasation of CSF can occur rapidly, leading to widespread distribution of the extradural CSF collection at the time of image acquisition that makes identifying a specific leak site challenging.[9,10]

Brain MRI with intravenous contrast is an excellent initial test for the evaluation of SIH. It offers several advantages, including wide availability, absence of radiation exposure, and high sensitivity for detecting signs indicative of SIH. Specifically, it detects diffuse pachymeningeal enhancement in 73% of SIH patients.[6] Brain MRI however does have its limitations, and it is important to remember that it can be normal in up to 20% of patients with SIH.[3,6]

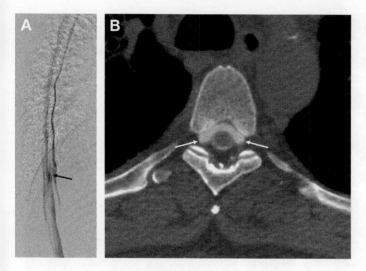

Fig. 1. 48-year-old male with bibrachial amyotrophy due to cerebrospinal fluid (CSF) leak. Prone digital subtraction myelography shows a ventral leak at the level of T9-10 (*A*, lateral projection). CT post myelogram of the thoracic spine shows large ventral extradural collection throughout the thoracic spine (*B*). Lateral projection DSM cine of ventral leak in another patient is provided in Video 1.

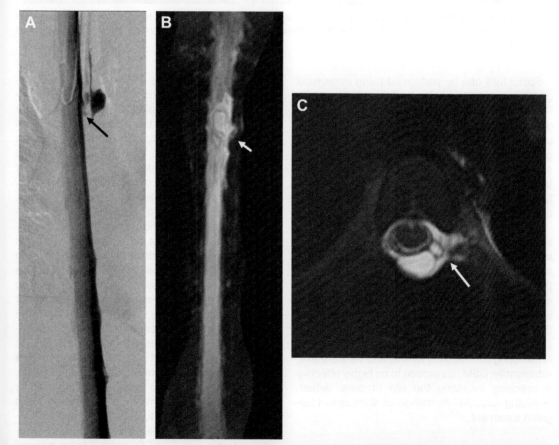

Fig. 2. 23-year-old patient with a history of orthostatic headaches secondary to spontaneous intracranial hypotension (SIH). Digital subtraction myelography (DSM) in the left lateral decubitus positions shows a lateral leak at T4-5 (*A*). Corresponding MR myelography shows an extradural cerebrospinal fluid (CSF) collection at T4-5 (*B*). MRI of the thoracic spine shows circumferential CSF leak at this site (*C*). Frontal projection DSM cine is provided in Video 2.

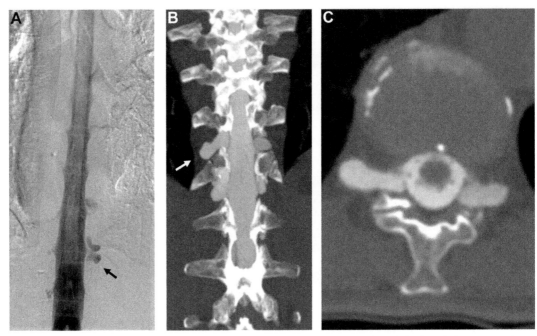

Fig. 3. 64-year-old patient with a history of SIH. Prone digital subtraction myelography (DSM) shows a meningeal diverticulum at T12-L1 (*A, arrow*). Post DSM CT myelography shows large thoracic nerve root cysts (*B* – coronal MIP, *C* – axial).

Spinal MRI can be performed using intrathecal gadolinium or with heavily weighted T2 sequences (**Table 3**). Heavily weighted T2 spinal MRI has demonstrated similar sensitivity to CT myelography, as reported in previous studies.[11] Intrathecal gadolinium spinal MR has not been shown to be superior to heavily weighted T2 spinal MR. Therefore, it is preferable to utilize spinal MRI with heavily weighted T2 sequences in conjunction with brain MR as part of the initial workup of SIH.[6,12]

Digital subtraction myelogram is more invasive but has the highest sensitivity for localizing CSF leaks with comparable radiation dosing to CT myelogram.[6,10] At our institution we now use DSM to identify and locate CSF leaks in a wider range of cases, including those with low-flow leaks which are typically reserved for CT myelogram. Based on our experience, DSM has demonstrated superior sensitivity compared to other imaging test in detecting CSF-venous fistulas and ventral leaks. Additionally, DSM has proven to be highly effective in precisely localizing the site of dural defect, providing valuable information for subsequent targeted treatment.[3,13–15]

HISTORY

It is important to remember that spinal neuroimaging, although used for the initial diagnosis of CSF leak, has been found to yield negative results "in

48% to 76% of patients."[6] One potential explanation for the negative findings on spinal CT or MR imaging, particularly in cases where there are larger dural tears leading to extensive extrathecal contrast spanning multiple levels, is the limitation of temporal resolution. This limitation can make precise localization challenging. In 2003, Luetmer and Mokri introduced dynamic CT myelography to overcome this challenge.[9] Although dynamic CT myelography offered improved temporal resolution, it still had limitations attributed "to the volume of tissue that must be imaged" as this leads to a higher radiation dose to the patient.[8,16] In 2002, Philips, and colleagues,[17] presented a case in which, despite utilizing conventional imaging techniques such as myelogram, CT myelogram or MRI, the authors were unable to identify a CSF leak. Since no leak was seen on imaging, a neurosurgical procedure was conducted, but it also failed to identify a leak. It was only when the authors performed a DSM, a novel technique at the time, that they were able to successfully diagnose a postoperative pseudomeningocele. Seven years after DSM was used to localize a pseudomeningocele, Hoxworth and colleagues used DSM to accurately identify high-flow CSF leaks.[16] In the authors' experience, conventional imaging techniques could detect the presence of a CSF leak, but due to the high-flow of the leaks, they were unable to precisely determine the location of CSF leak

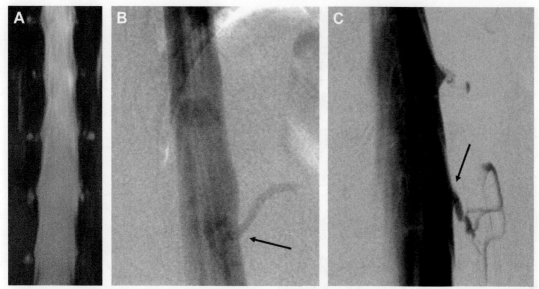

Fig. 4. 46-year-old patient with orthostatic headaches. MRI of the spine shows only small cyst without a cerebrospinal fluid (CSF) leak (*A*, MR myelography). The patient then underwent a left lateral decubitus digital subtraction myelogram which shows a CSF-venous fistula at T11 -12 (*B*, lateral projection, *C*, frontal projection).

without the higher temporal resolution provided by DSM. In 2012, Luetmer and colleagues[8] proposed a new algorithm to determine which patients should undergo dynamic CT myelography. In their paper, the authors recommend that patients proceed directly to dynamic CT myelography if the initial spinal MR demonstrates an extradural CSF collection.[8] At our institution, we adopted a comparable algorithm based on the presence or absence of spinal longitudinal extradural collections to determine the patient's positioning at DSM (**Fig. 6**).

In 2013, Schievink, and colleagues, showcased the utilization of DSM for the identification of a CSF-venous fistula in patients with SIH.[14] At the time of the publication, this radiographic finding had not been previously reported. Beyond increased temporal resolution, DSM provides a diagnostic tool that offers about the same radiation dose as conventional CT myelography and about a third of the dose of dynamic CT myelography.[18] In 2018 Farb and colleagues introduced the lateral decubitus position for DSM to increase the sensitivity of visualization of CSF venous fistulas.[19] In their article, they categorized patients into the prone position if spinal MR showed an extradural CSF collection and the left lateral decubitus position if no extradural CSF collection was seen on spinal imaging. If the initial left lateral decubitus DSM was negative, the patient would return in a couple of weeks for a DSM on the contralateral side. This distinction between the presence of extradural CSF collection or not highlights the importance of pre-DSM planning.

APPROACH ("5 P'S TO SUCCESS")
Planning

At our institution, we have performed 2588 DSMs since 2009. Pre-DSM planning is imperative in the diagnosis and management of CSF leaks. The diagnostic process begins with MR brain to look for signs of intracranial hypotension and MR spine to determine for the presence of extradural fluid collections, as this will guide the patient's positioning during the subsequent DSM. Heavily T2 weighted myelographic sequences are important to determine positioning as the presence of large and/or irregular cysts will guide management to that specific spinal segment.[20] Based on the type of leak identified, the patient can be placed in various positions: prone for ventral leaks, lateral decubitus for lateral leaks, supine for posterior leaks, or lateral decubitus for CSF-venous fistulas.

Patient Preparation

Although DSM can be conducted with or without moderate sedation or general anesthesia, we prefer general endotracheal anesthesia with the patient in deep paralysis.[21] In our experience this approach is well tolerated by patients while minimizing nondiagnostic examinations due to patient motion, but also ensures optimal detail and temporal resolution by facilitating controlled suspended respiration throughout the procedure. Three to 5 minutes prior to contrast bolus we ask the anesthesiologist to administer additional rocuronium to ensure full paralysis and avoid breathing attempts and

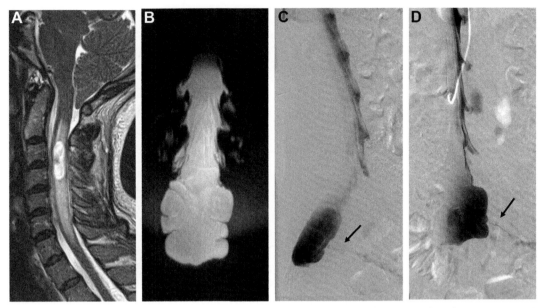

Fig. 5. 39-year-old patient with spontaneous intracranial hypotension (SIH) presented with upper extremity myelopathy and was found to have a spinal cord syrinx at C3-5 on MR C-Spine (*A*). Initial workup revealed a large sacral Tarlov cyst on MR myelography (*B*) which was the focus of interrogation on subsequent digital subtraction myelography. Lateral projection (*C*) and ventral projection (*D*) Digital subtraction myelography (DSM) in the left lateral decubitus position show a cerebrospinal fluid (CSF)-venous fistula arising from the very large sacral Tarlov cyst at approximately the S2-3 level. Frontal and lateral projection DSM cine is provided in Videos 3 and 4.

diaphragm spasms that may contribute to respiratory motion during image acquisition.

Positioning

Using a biplane angiography suite equipped with a tilt table, the patient can then be positioned in either the prone or lateral decubitus position. The table can then be adjusted to overcome lumbar lordosis and thoracic kyphosis. If the patient is in the prone position, this is done by tilting the table to greater than 15°. The lateral decubitus position requires less tilt than the prone position (**Fig. 7**). In the absence of tilt table, the patient can be

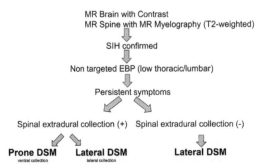

Fig. 6. Cedars-Sinai diagnostic approach for patients with suspected spontaneous intracranial hypotension (SIH).

further positioned using pillows and custom wedges to help overcome lumbar lordosis.[21] To enhance the diagnostic yield of DSM for the diagnosis CSF-venous fistulas, patients are positioned in the lateral decubitus position. In our institutional experience, we have demonstrated that this position increased our diagnostic yield from 15% to 75%.[15]

Puncture

Under fluoroscopic guidance, a Gertie-Marx 22-gauge needle is placed midline at the L2-3 level taking caution to avoid tenting and prevent a subdural injection. Opening pressure is then obtained and 0.5 cc of iohexol 240 mg/mL or 300 mg/mL contrast (Omnipaque; GE Healthcare, Marlborough, Massachusetts) is injected to determine needle position. Once the intradural position of the needle is confirmed during the procedure, the patient can then be repositioned to optimize the diagnostic yield and concentrate on a specific region of greatest interest. This repositioning allows for a more targeted approach, enhancing the accuracy and effectiveness of the procedure.

Procedure Imaging

Images are acquired at a frame rate of 1 frame per second using a 75 second breath hold with manual

Table 3
Imaging protocols

CT brain without contrast	Helical scan at 0.5 s tube rotation with 0.625 thickness 2 mm reformats in the sagittal and coronal plane
CT myelogram	Helical scan at 1 s tube rotation with 0.625 thickness for cervical spine Helical scan at 0.6 s tube rotation with 0.625 thickness for thoracic and lumbar spine 2 mm reformats in the sagittal and coronal plane
Dynamic CT myelogram	Dynamic CT myelogram can be performed in various positions and with rapid repositioning to elucidate otherwise difficult to detect leaks Helical scans at 0.6 s tube rotation with 2.5 mm thickness Five scan acquisitions in the prone (arms up), left lateral decubitus, right lateral decubitus, prone (arms up), supine (arms up)
MR brain with and without contrast	Sagittal Tl, axial diffusion weighted imaging, axial FLAIR, axial T2, coronal T2 FS, axial susceptibility-weighted imaging, sagittal T2, axial Tl MPRAGE post, sagittal MPR post, Coronal MPR post
MR spine with myelogram	Sagittal Tl, sagittal T2, sagittal STIR, axial T2, and coronal T2 haste with 3D, sagittal Tl post FS, and 3D maximum intensity projection reconstructions
Digital subtraction myelogram	Digital subtraction fluoroscopy during intrathecal contrast injection Performed with general endotracheal anesthesia

injection of 12 cc of iohexol 240 mg/mL or 300 mg/mL at a rate of 1 cc per second. This is followed by a 20 cc saline flush. It is our standard practice that all patients undergo a CT myelogram 1-hour post-DSM. This additional imaging procedure is essential and complements the diagnostic process. A recent article by Lutzen, and colleagues, demonstrated a novel use of ultrahigh-resolution cone-beam CT (UHR-CBT) following DSM to identify a CSF venous fistula in a patient with negative MR spine and CT myelogram.[22] While it is unclear if the CSF venous

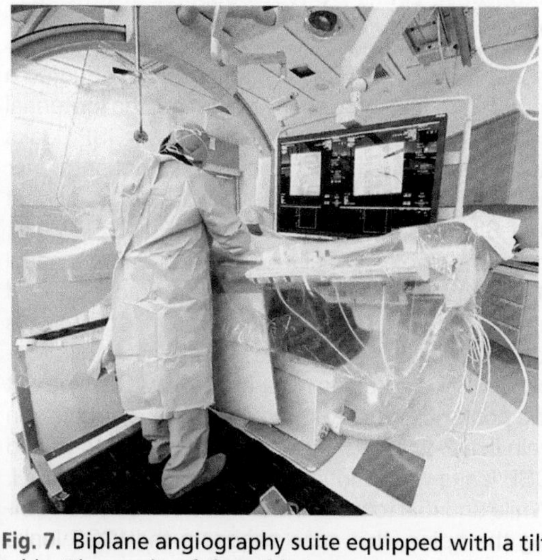

Fig. 7. Biplane angiography suite equipped with a tilt table. The angle of the table is greater than 15°.

fistula was diagnosed during the preceding DSM, the increased spatial resolution achieved with UHR-CBT provides an additional tool to add to the growing arsenal of techniques being developed and advancing the field of spinal CSF leak localization.

PITFALLS AND LIMITATIONS
False Localizing Signs

During the pre-DSM planning phase, fluid collections in the upper cervical spine at the C1-2 level are occasionally observed on spinal imaging (Fig. 8). It has been commonly believed that these fluid collections correspond to the site of CSF leak and treatment has been directed at the C1-2 level.[23–25] Yousry and colleagues[26] were the first to propose that these retrospinal fluid collections did not accurately represent the site of CSF leak but rather represented fluid collections caused by paraspinal venous transudate or exudate. Schievink and colleagues[27] found that these retrospinal fluid collections did indeed originate from CSF leakage from the epidural space that then extend cranially where they ultimately extravasate into the surrounding C1-2 soft tissues.[28] It is important to recognize this distinction to avoid inadvertently directing therapy at the wrong level. A paraspinal fluid collection at the high cervical region has been termed the "false localizing sign of C1-2."[27]

Another false localizing sign that has been previously described is contrast extravasation in the

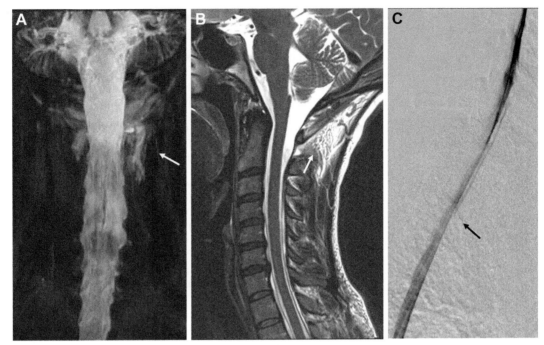

Fig. 8. 40-year-old patient with spontaneous intracranial hypotension (SIH). MR myelography (*A*) and sagittal T2 MR of the cervical spine (*B*) show extensive extradural cerebrospinal fluid (CSF) collection in the posterior soft tissues of the upper cervical spine consistent with false localizing sign of C1-2. Subsequent digital subtraction myelography (DSM) in the prone position (lateral projection) shows the site of ventral CSF leak to be at T2-3 (*C*).

cervicothoracic region. A study at our institution looking at 11 patients with preplanning imaging showing fluid collections at the cervicothoracic region demonstrated that these fluid collections were not indicative of the site of leak.[29] As a result, treatment targeted at the region of fluid collection in the cervicothoracic region is not likely to result in prolonged symptom improvements for patients. This finding has been termed the false localizing sign of cervicothoracic CSF leak (**Fig. 9**).

Although MR myelography is the preferred initial imaging of choice, up to 50% of SIH cases have negative spinal imaging.[6] Patients with CSF-venous fistulas are more likely to have no CSF leak identified on conventional imaging. Not all patients undergo DSM, therefore, it is important to recognize secondary findings that suggest the presence of CSF-venous fistula on CT myelography. One of those signs is the presence of a hyper-attenuating paraspinal vein which has been appropriately named the "hyperdense paraspinal vein sign."[30] While initially thought to correspond to the level of CSF-venous fistula localization, Schievink, and colleagues,[31] demonstrated a case of 2 patients with hyperdense paraspinal veins who underwent treatment with surgery or glue injection whose CSF-venous fistula was not at the same level or laterality as the draining veins. The authors

concluded that while the hyperdense paraspinal vein sign was indicative of a CSF-venous fistula, consideration should be given to DSM or dynamic myelography prior to treatment to avoid the potential pitfall of directing treatment at the incorrect site. This potential pitfall is known as the false localizing sign of CSF-venous fistulas.[31]

Skull Base Leaks Do Not Cause Spontaneous Intracranial Hypotension

In 2012, Schievink, and colleagues,[32] conducted a study with the aim of investigating the potential causal association between cranial CSF leaks and SIH. The authors identified 315 patients over a 9-year period and found no evidence to suggest that SIH was caused by base of skull CSF leaks. Instead, they concluded that "clear nasal discharge in patients with SIH can be considered a false localizing sign."[32] It took almost 10 years for Schievink and colleagues to utilize lateral decubitus DSM and discover a rapid-flow CSF leak at the posterior fossa that drained into the subclavian vein in a 2-year old boy.[33] Historically, skull-based CSF leaks were thought not to be a cause of SIH. While unusual to have a CSF leak not located within the spine, this case suggests that CSF leaks from the posterior fossa can cause SIH, albeit

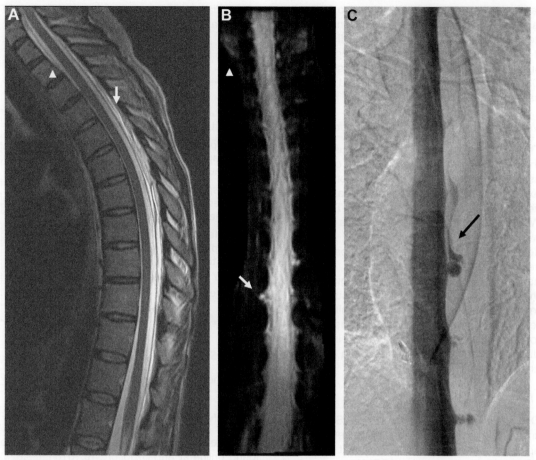

Fig. 9. 43-year-old patient with orthostatic headaches. MR T-spine (*A*) shows dorsal (*arrow*) and ventral (*arrow-head*) epidural fluid collections. Heavily T2-weighted spinal MRI MIP images (*B*) show a complex meningeal diverticulum at T10 to 11 (*arrow*) and false localizing sign of the cervicothoracic spine (*arrowhead*). Digital subtraction myelography in the left lateral decubitus position (frontal projection) show epidural cerebrospinal fluid (CSF) leak associated with a lateral tear at T9-10 meningeal diverticulum.

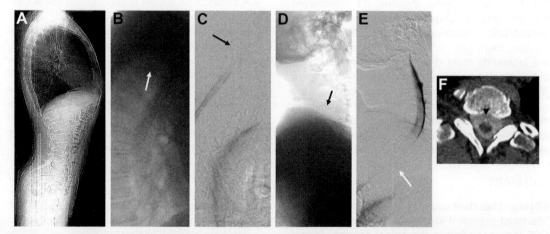

Fig. 10. Scout image demonstrates thoracic kyphosis and lumbar lordosis (*A*). Digital subtraction myelography (DSM) without bone suppression (*B, D*) and with bone suppression (*C, E*) show under penetration of the spine at the cervicothoracic region with poor visualization of the contrast column at this level. Post DSM CT myelogram shows calcification at the site of the dural tear (*F*).

rarely. Another potential pitfall related to CSF leaks is a subset of patients who in addition to having headaches and SIH, have clear nasal discharge.[32] It is important for clinicals to have a high index of suspicion for SIH in patients with skull-based CSF leaks, as delayed diagnosis and treatment can have debilitating consequences.[33,34]

Venolymphatic Vascular Malformations

Thus far we have discussed CSF-venous fistulas in the context of high-flow leaks, but they can also be associated with slow-flow vascular anomalies. For example, in 2014, Mokri reported 2 cases of patients with CSF leaks and Klippel-Trenaunay-Weber syndrome.[35] Since then, 5 cases of patients with venous/venolymphatic vascular malformations and SIH have been identified; 3 patients had venous/venolymphatic malformations, 1 patient had a venous malformation (hemangioma), and the last patient had a pelvic/sacral vascular malformation.[36–38] Although there is no definitive causal relationship between venolymphatic vascular malformations and SIH, it is important to include the diagnosis in the differential when both conditions are observed simultaneously.

Limitations

One of the limitations inherent to DSMs is the limited field of view which may not cover the entire spinal column. In this instance, a repeat procedure may be necessary. Additional DSM is also required to assess CSF venous fistulas in lateral decubitus positions on different days.[21] While most CSF venous fistulas are apparent within 60 seconds of DSM run,[20] some ventral leaks are too slow to visualize during the 60 to 80 seconds DSM run. For these slower leaks, dynamic CT myelogram with imaging at longer intervals may be more appropriate.[9,10] Additionally, given different body habitus, there are certain anatomic areas which are inherently more difficult to evaluate such as the cervicothoracic region overlying the shoulders (**Fig. 10**). Future refinements in technique may overcome some of the limitations which include newer equipment with increased detector size and cone beam CT which has been used to detect slow flow leaks not detected on DSM.[39]

SUMMARY

SIH is an important cause of orthostatic headache. The most prevalent identifiable cause of SIH is a CSF leak occurring in the spinal column. Digital subtraction myelography is the most sensitive imaging technique for pinpointing the precise location of the CSF leak. Moreover, DSM is well tolerated with radiation doses comparable to those of CT myelography.

CLINICS CARE POINTS

- Digital subtraction myelography has high sensitivity for identifying leak site.
- A hyperdense paraspinal vein sign on CT myelography may be a false localizing sign of CSF-venous fistulas.
- Paraspinal fluid in the C1-2 region does not correspond to site of CSF leak and is known as the false localizing sign of C1-2.
- CSF leaks in the cervicothoracic region seen on spinal imaging are rarely the site of leak and targeted treatment in this region is not likely to result in lasting symptom relief.
- While rare, skull-based CSF leaks can cause SIH.

DISCLOSURE

The authors have nothing to disclose.

SUPPLEMENTARY DATA

Supplementary data related to this article can be found online at https://doi.org/10.1016/j.rcl.2023.10.004

REFERENCES

1. Schievink WI, Maya MM, Jean-Pierre S, et al. A classification system of spontaneous spinal CSF leaks. Neurology 2016;87(7):673–9.
2. Schievink WI, Maya MM, Moser FG, et al. Incidence of spontaneous intracranial hypotension in a community: Beverly hills, California, 2006–2020. Cephalalgia 2022;42(4–5):312–6.
3. Chan SM, Chodakiewitz YG, et al. Intracranial hypotension and cerebrospinal fluid leak. Neuroimaging Clin 2019;29(2):213–26.
4. Schievink WI. Novel neuroimaging modalities in the evaluation of spontaneous cerebrospinal fluid leaks. Curr Neurol Neurosci Rep 2013;13(7):358.
5. Tay ASS, Maya M, Moser FG, et al. Computed tomography vs heavily T2-weighted magnetic resonance myelography for the initial evaluation of patients with spontaneous intracranial hypotension. JAMA Neurol 2021;78(10):1275–6.
6. D'Antona L, Merchan MAJ, Vassiliou A, et al. Clinical presentation, investigation findings, and treatment outcomes of spontaneous intracranial hypotension

syndrome. JAMA Neurol 2021;78(3). https://doi.org/
10.1001/jamaneurol.2020.4799.

7. Sakka L, Coll G, Chazal J. Anatomy and physiology of cerebrospinal fluid. European Annals of Otorhinolaryngology, Head and Neck Diseases 2011;128(6): 309–16.

8. Luetmer PH, Schwartz KM, Eckel LJ, et al. When should I do dynamic CT myelography? predicting fast spinal CSF leaks in patients with spontaneous intracranial hypotension. Am J Neuroradiol 2012; 33(4):690–4.

9. Luetmer PH, Mokri B. Dynamic CT myelography: A technique for localizing high-flow spinal cerebrospinal fluid leaks. Am J Neuroradiol 2003;24(8):1711–4.

10. Kranz PG, Luetmer PH, Diehn FE, et al. Myelographic techniques for the detection of spinal CSF leaks in spontaneous intracranial hypotension. Am J Roentgenol 2016;206(1):8–19.

11. Wang Y-, Lirng J-, Fuh J-, et al. Heavily T2-weighted MR myelography vs CT myelography in spontaneous intracranial hypotension. Neurology 2009; 73(22):1892–8.

12. Dobrocky T, Winklehner A, Breiding PS, et al. Spine MRI in spontaneous intracranial hypotension for CSF leak detection: Nonsuperiority of intrathecal gadolinium to heavily T2-weighted fat-saturated sequences. Am J Neuroradiol 2020;41(7):1309–15.

13. Schievink WI, Moser FG, Maya MM, et al. Digital subtraction myelography for the identification of spontaneous spinal CSF-venous fistulas. J Neurosurg Spine 2016;24(6):960–4.

14. Schievink WI, Moser FG, Maya MM. CSF–venous fistula in spontaneous intracranial hypotension. Neurology 2014;83(5):472–3.

15. Schievink WI, Maya MM, Moser FG, et al. Lateral decubitus digital subtraction myelography to identify spinal CSF–venous fistulas in spontaneous intracranial hypotension. J Neurosurg Spine 2019;31(6):1–905.

16. Hoxworth JM, Patel AC, Bosch EP, et al. Localization of a rapid CSF leak with digital subtraction myelography. Am J Neuroradiol 2009;30(3):516–9.

17. Phillips CD, Kaptain GJ, Razack N. Depiction of a postoperative pseudomeningocele with digital subtraction myelography. Am J Neuroradiol 2002;23(2): 337–8.

18. Nicholson PJ, Guest WC, van Prooijen M, et al. Digital subtraction myelography is associated with less radiation dose than CT-based techniques. Clin Neuroradiol 2021;31(3):627–31.

19. Farb RI, Nicholson PJ, Peng PW, et al. Spontaneous intracranial hypotension: A systematic imaging approach for CSF leak localization and management based on MRI and digital subtraction myelography. Am J Neuroradiol 2019;40(4):745–53.

20. Mark I, Madhavan A, Oien M, et al. Temporal characteristics of CSF-venous fistulas on digital subtraction myelography. Am J Neuroradiol 2023;44(4):492–5.

21. Kim DK, Brinjikji W, Morris PP, et al. Lateral decubitus digital subtraction myelography: Tips, tricks, and pitfalls. Am J Neuroradiol 2020;41(1):21–8.

22. Lützen N, Beck J, Urbach H. Cerebrospinal fluid venous fistula imaging with ultrahigh-resolution cone-beam computed tomography. JAMA Neurol 2023. https://doi.org/10.1001/jamaneurol.2023.1640.

23. Beck J, Raabe A, Seifert V, et al. Intracranial hypotension after chiropractic manipulation of the cervical spine. J Neurol Neurosurg Psychiatr 2003; 74(6):821–2.

24. Kamada M, Fujita Y, Ishii R, et al. Spontaneous intracranial hypotension successfully treated by epidural patching with fibrin glue. Headache 2000;40(10): 844–7.

25. Kasner SE, Rosenfeld J, Farber RE. Spontaneous intracranial hypotension: Headache with a reversible Arnold-Chiari malformation. Headache 1995;35(9): 557–9.

26. Yousry I, Forderreuther S, Moriggl B, et al. Cervical MR imaging in postural headache: MR signs and pathophysiological implications. Am J Neuroradiol 2001;22(7):1239–50.

27. Schievink WI, Maya MM, Tourje J. False localizing sign of C1–2 cerebrospinal fluid leak in spontaneous intracranial hypotension. J Neurosurg 2004;100(4): 639–44.

28. Schievink WI, Maya MM, Moser F, et al. Multiple spinal CSF leaks in spontaneous intracranial hypotension: Do they exist? Neurology. Clin Pract 2021;11(5): e691–7.

29. Schievink WI, Maya MM, Chu RM, et al. False localizing sign of cervico-thoracic CSF leak in spontaneous intracranial hypotension. Neurology 2015; 84(24):2445–8.

30. Kranz PG, Amrhein TJ, Schievink WI, et al. The hyperdense paraspinal vein sign: A marker of CSF-venous fistula. Am J Neuroradiol 2016;37(7):1379–81.

31. Schievink WI, Maya MM, Moser FG. False localizing signs of spinal CSF–venous fistulas in spontaneous intracranial hypotension: Report of 2 cases. J Neurosurg Spine 2019;31(5):1–767.

32. Schievink WI, Schwartz MS, Maya M, et al. Lack of causal association between spontaneous intracranial hypotension and cranial cerebrospinal fluid leaks: Clinical article. J Neurosurg 2012;116(4):749–54.

33. Schievink WI, Michael LM, Maya M, et al. Spontaneous intracranial hypotension due to Skull-Base cerebrospinal fluid leak. Ann Neurol 2021;90(3): 514–6.

34. Schievink WI. Spontaneous intracranial hypotension. N Engl J Med 2021;385(23):2173–8.

35. Mokri B. Klippel-trenaunay-weber syndrome (KTWS) and spontaneous spinal CSF leak: Coincidence or link. Headache 2014;54(4):726–31.

36. Schievink WI, Maya MM, Moser FG, et al. Spontaneous spinal CSF–venous fistulas associated with venous/

venolymphatic vascular malformations: Report of 3 cases. J Neurosurg Spine 2019;32(2):305–10.

37. Chan JL, Maya MM, Schievink WI. Open repair of Hemangioma-Associated cerebrospinal Fluid-Venous fistula. Ann Neurol 2021;89(3):621–2.

38. Schievink WI, Maya MM, Borst AJ. Adolescent headache due to congenital pelvic/sacral vascular malformation. Ann Neurol 2023. https://doi.org/10.1002/ana.26651.

39. Lützen N, Demerath T, Volz F, et al. Conebeam CT as an additional tool in digital subtraction myelography for the detection of spinal lateral dural tears. Am J Neuroradiol 2023;44(6):745–7.

Percutaneous Treatment and Post-treatment Management of CSF Leaks and CSF-Venous Fistulas in Spontaneous Intracranial Hypotension

Jessica L. Houk, MD*, Peter G. Kranz, MD, Timothy J. Amrhein, MD

KEYWORDS

- Spontaneous intracranial hypotension • Cerebrospinal fluid leak • CSF-Venous fistula
- Epidural blood patching • Rebound intracranial hypertension

KEY POINTS

- SIH is a treatable cause of orthostatic headaches secondary to pathologic cerebrospinal fluid (CSF) leak from the subarachnoid space.
- CSF leaks can be caused by dural tears from disc osteophytes, leaks arising from nerve root sleeve diverticula, or CSF-venous fistulas.
- Epidural blood patching (EBP) remains first-line therapy for SIH. Surgery or transvenous embolization are alternative methods for treatment if EBP is unsuccessful.
- Percutaneous treatment of CSF leaks requires an in-depth knowledge of preprocedural work up, procedure technique, and post-procedural management.

INTRODUCTION

Spontaneous intracranial hypotension (SIH) is a treatable cause of orthostatic headaches secondary to pathologic loss of cerebrospinal fluid (CSF) from the subarachnoid space. Patients present with a variety of symptoms which, in addition to headache, can include disequilibrium, sensorineural hearing loss, cranial neuropathies, and cognitive dysfunction. The reported incidence of SIH has been estimated at 5 in 100,000 but is likely greater given high rates of misdiagnosis.[1,2]

SIH has several known pathologic causes, nearly always arising from the spine including dural tears from disc osteophytes, leaks emanating from nerve root sleeve diverticula, and CSF-venous fistulas (CVFs).[3,4] Each of these distinct etiologies of CSF volume depletion has specific approaches to treatment. Depending on the type of leak, surgical repair or endovascular techniques may be options for definite treatment. However, epidural blood patching (EBP) with or without fibrin glue remains the first-line therapy due to its long track record, broad availability, and relatively lower risk profile.

With the growing recognition of SIH and a resultant increased number of cases requiring treatment, physicians should familiarize themselves with available treatment options and post-treatment management. The purpose of this article is to review the indications and techniques for the percutaneous treatment of SIH and to provide an

Department of Radiology, Duke University Medical Center, 2301 Erwin Road, Box 3808, Durham, NC 27710, USA
* Corresponding author.
E-mail address: jessica.houk@duke.edu

Radiol Clin N Am 62 (2024) 333–343
https://doi.org/10.1016/j.rcl.2023.09.003
0033-8389/24/© 2023 Elsevier Inc. All rights reserved.

overview of post-procedural considerations and management of these patients.

TYPES OF CSF LEAKS

Deciding on the appropriate treatment for an SIH patient depends on the accurate localization and identification of the type of CSF leak. A commonly employed CSF leak classification system defines 3 types of leaks. Type 1 leaks consist of dural tears caused by an osteophyte spur, which are usually associated with extradural fluid collections. These are divided further based on the location of the tear with 1a leaks being ventral due to disc degenerative changes, and 1b leaks posterolateral, often secondary to facet hypertrophic changes. Type 2 leaks are those arising from nerve root diverticula, usually at the level of the nerve root axilla. These occur due to denuding of dura mater and extension of more friable arachnoid matter through the defect and can be associated with epidural fluid collections. Finally, Type 3 leaks, or CVFs, are abnormal fistulous connections between the subarachnoid space and epidural venous structures, which do not result in extradural fluid collections.[3]

A variety of different imaging modalities can be used to identify and localize the causative spinal CSF leak including heavily T2-weighted MRI, computed tomography (CT) myelography, ultrafast CT myelography, and digital subtraction myelography.[5–8] Each of these modalities offers particular advantages and disadvantages. However, a detailed review of their individual utility is outside the scope of this review and has been covered extensively elsewhere.[9–11]

PREPROCEDURAL ASSESSMENT

Potential treatment options for SIH include conservative management (ie, caffeine, hydration, and recumbency), EBP with or without fibrin glue, transvenous embolization (TVE), or surgery. Fibrin glue is a biological pharmaceutical agent that emulates the final stages of the normal coagulation cascade and is often used as an adjunct to EBP. Conservative management is generally unsuccessful or provides only transient relief and consequently will not be discussed further.[12] This review will focus on percutaneous treatment techniques, primarily EBP (with or without the use of fibrin glue).

Prior to treatment, a thorough preprocedural assessment must be completed that should include screening for coagulopathic states, infection, malignancy, medication allergies, and general assessment of sedation requirements. At the authors' institution, the authors do not routinely check labs prior to EBP or TVE in the absence of known coagulopathic states. If labs are available, a platelet count greater than 50,000 and international normalized ratio (INR) less than 1.5 is generally considered acceptable prior to any percutaneous procedure, though there are guidelines to suggest more liberal cutoff values may be reasonable.[13] Anticoagulants are discontinued according to the most up-to-date recommendations.[14,15] If the patient currently is bacteremic or septic, the procedure is delayed until health is optimized. Similarly, if there is a superficial infection (eg, abscess or cellulitis) in the area of planned intervention, the procedure is delayed until resolution or a different approach/trajectory is taken to avoid the region of concern.

Rarely, hematologic or solid organ malignancy is encountered in a patient requiring EBP. EBP is considered safe in this population as the limited retrospective published data on this scenario do not support the theory that epidural placement of autologous blood will result in malignant seeding of the neuraxis.[16,17]

A diagnosis of SIH in pregnancy is rare. However, no evidence exists to suggest that pregnancy itself should be considered a strict contraindication to proceeding with percutaneous treatment of CSF leaks.[18] Certainly, radiation dose to the fetus is an important consideration and therefore treatment is often delayed until after delivery, if possible.

Patient allergies are thoroughly reviewed prior to beginning the procedure. Allergic reactions to fibrin glue, including severe reactions and anaphylaxis, have been documented in patients previously exposed to fibrin glue (either during a prior EBP or during other open surgical procedures).[19] Thus, the patient should be screened for prior exposure and the authors' group recommends that any patient undergoing repeat EBP with fibrin glue be treated preprocedurally with 50 mg of intravenous diphenhydramine approximately 1 hour prior to the procedure. Moreover, true allergies to local anesthetic are encountered rarely and require switching to a different family of anesthetics (ie, amide for an esther allergy and vice versa).[20] Finally, if patient is allergic to iodinated contrast, a small volume of gadolinium contrast material can be used as an alternative for the epidurogram prior to administration of patching material. While gadolinium has a sufficient density to provide an analogous epidurogram, use in this manner is off label and physicians should be aware of the potential risks of inadvertent intrathecal administration, specifically neurotoxicity at higher doses.[21]

Most patients who undergo percutaneous procedures EBP will do so under moderate sedation with nursing staff present and standard doses of analgesic and benzodiazepines (usually fentanyl and versed), safely titrated up as necessary. The level of sedation is ultimately up to the discretion of the treating physician, taking into account specific patient considerations including anxiety, tolerance, and risk factors. Occasionally, EBP can be performed via a single agent or solely using local anesthetic (eg, lidocaine). Basic moderate sedation protocols are followed prior to the procedure, including instruction to fast >6 hours before the procedure start time. A driver must be present prior to beginning the procedure.

TREATMENT PROCEDURES
Epidural Blood Patch

General EBP principles
The purpose of an EBP is to place autologous blood within the epidural space. The exact mechanism by which this results in symptom relief is uncertain, but the 2 main theories are (1) direct sealing of the CSF leak, and (2) displacement of CSF cranially by pressure exerted on the thecal sac. While the term "EBP" is often used to broadly reference the percutaneous placement of patching material within the epidural space, technical variations exist. EBP can be performed with imaging guidance (ie, using computed tomography [CT] or fluoroscopic guidance) or without imaging guidance ("blind" patching). The procedure can also be performed using a targeted approach (ie, targeting the exact site of CSF leak) or can be non-targeted. The administration of patching material without the use of imaging guidance does not allow for direct visualization of critical structures, creating the potential for false loss of resistance (false identification of the epidural space).[22] The use of CT provides some advantages as it allows for visualization of the soft tissues and direct visualization of the needle tip within the epidural space, but is dependent on institutional availability. Radiation doses for CT fluoroscopic-guided procedures are comparable to those of traditional fluoroscopy.[23,24] Finally, one must decide whether to perform the patch with autologous blood only, fibrin glue only, or a combination of autologous blood and fibrin glue. No conclusive data exist yet regarding which of these patching methods is superior.

EBP technique
For any percutaneous EBP, standard procedural technique involves sterilizing the patient's skin and subcutaneous administration of local anesthetic. A spinal needle (our group uses a 22-gauge Quincke point tip needle) is then placed into the epidural space under imaging guidance. Correct needle tip placement is confirmed with an epidurogram by injecting approximately 0.2 mL of contrast material prior to the injection of blood and/or fibrin glue. The reason for this is 3-fold: to assess the potential spread and distribution of patching material, to exclude intravascular placement, and to thereby minimize the risk of allergic reaction to fibrin glue.[25,26] Extravascular positioning of the needle tip is also important since intravenous injection has the potential to be less efficacious given the resultant systemic administration of patching material, rather than localized placement within the epidural space or at the site of leak. Assessing the epidurogram for inadvertent intravascular needle tip positioning is well covered elsewhere.[26]

Once the epidural space is confidently accessed, sterile autologous blood and/or fibrin glue is injected at the intended location. Clotting of blood prior to injection can be a significant problem. In order to mitigate this, our group draws the blood as the last step prior to beginning the procedure. A small volume of contrast (1–2 mL) is added to each syringe in order to promote visualization of patching material. **Fig. 1** demonstrates a standard tray used for EBP at our institution.

The amount of blood used is generally determined by the type of patch (eg, targeted vs nontargeted), the needle approach, and the patient's ability to tolerate the associated mass effect. Three distinct needle approaches can be used with selection dependent on the type of leak and on the physician preference. Interlaminar and transforaminal epidural approaches are analogous to those for epidural steroid injections performed for pain procedures.[27–29] Ventral epidural needle placement in patients with ventral dural defects (type 1a CSF leaks) has been shown to have greater rates of spread across the ventral dural surface.[30] A range of 3 to 20 mL is used for interlaminar approaches and 1 to 5 mL for both transforaminal and ventral epidural approaches. An important consideration here is that CT fluoroscopic guidance enables cross-sectional visualization, allowing one to determine the extent of mass effect on critical structures (eg, the spinal cord and nerves) in real time.

There is a wide range of reported efficacy of EBP (36%–90%), leading to some uncertainty about the true rate of response to this treatment, whether targeted or non-targeted in approach.[31–38] Further, the literature guiding decision making is limited by a lack of level 1 evidence and very few comparative studies.[39] In some cases, more than 1 EBP (either targeted or non-targeted) is necessary for symptomatic relief.

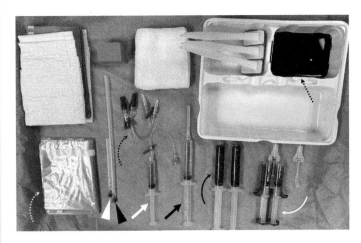

Fig. 1. Epidural blood patching (EBP) Tray Components. Sterile draping (*white curved dotted arrow*), 3 ½ inch 22-gauge spinal needle (*white arrowhead*), 5 inch 22-gauge spinal needle (*black arrowhead*), connector tubing (*black curved dotted arrow*), contrast within a 5 mL syringe (*white arrowhead*), lidocaine (*black arrow*), autologous blood (*curved black arrow*), betadine (*dotted black arrow*), fibrin glue (*curved thin white arrow*).

While the efficacy of non-targeted EBP in treating CVFs has not yet been specifically studied, some investigators believe that targeted patching at the location of the underlying pathologic connection can result in symptom resolution.[40] To our knowledge, no studies have directly addressed comparative efficacy of EBP, TVE, or surgical ligation in treating CVFs.

Use of fibrin glue

Fibrin glue is a pharmaceutical product composed of both thrombin and fibrinogen, designed to mimic the end of the clotting cascade. It can be used alone or in combination with sterile autologous blood. Notably, percutaneous injection of fibrin sealant for EBP is considered an off-label use by the Food and Drug Administration (FDA). The primary safety concerns with fibrin glue are the possibility of thromboembolic events as a result of intravascular coagulation and hypersensitivity reactions to aprotinin, a proteinase inhibitor and component of the glue used to prevent lysis of the created clot.[25,41,42]

Non-targeted EBP

A non-targeted approach to EBP involves injecting patching material into the epidural space without knowledge of the exact location of the CSF leak. This technique is often performed prior to myelography for CSF leak localization and therefore allows one to forego invasive diagnostic imaging procedures that would require an SIH specialist. Some authors advocate for performing non-targeted EBP as first-line therapy in those patients presenting with imaging findings definitive for SIH (ie, positive brain MRI or extradural collection on heavily T2-weighted MRI) with subsequent targeted EBP if there is no response.[43]

Since the exact CSF leak site is unknown with non-targeted EBP, ample spread of patching material throughout the epidural space is important in an attempt to cover the affected site. Several modifications to the procedure can be considered with this goal in mind: an interlaminar approach is often employed with the use of larger volumes of blood (>20 mL), injecting at the thoracolumbar junction (as most leaks arise cranial to this level), or performing multi-level injections throughout the spine to maximize craniocaudal coverage (**Fig. 2**).[1]

Targeted epidural blood patch

Targeted EBP is performed when the exact location of the spinal CSF leak is known and therefore autologous blood and/or fibrin glue can be placed directly at the site of the abnormality. Thus, targeted patching requires the precise identification and localization of the site of the CSF leak or CVF, usually requiring imaging experts and invasive procedures (eg, CT myelography). Many investigators believe that targeted patching is superior to non-targeted approaches, but the literature is not conclusive and further research is needed on this topic, including comparative studies.

The location of each subtype of leak ultimately dictates procedural approach and needle tip placement. For nerve root sleeve diverticulum leaks and CVFs, a transforaminal needle approach is preferred with or without a simultaneous interlaminar approach given the relatively lateral location of the abnormality (**Fig. 3**). Ventral dural tears often require a transforaminal approach; optimal positioning of the needle tip in these cases is within the ventral epidural space (**Fig. 4**).[30] Some authors report definitive treatment with targeted EBP using fibrin glue in the case of CVFs.[40]

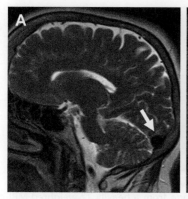
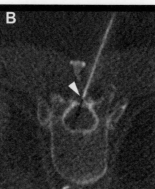

Fig. 2. Interlaminar Approach for Needle Placement. A 67-year-old female presented with brain MRI demonstrating venous distension sign (*white arrow*) consistent with spontaneous intracranial hypotension (SIH). She underwent non-targeted EBP using autologous blood at the T12-L1 interspace via an interlaminar approach to epidural needle placement (*white arrowhead*).

However, caution is advised given the previously discussed potentially increased risks of hypersensitivity reactions and thromboembolic events with intravenous injection of fibrin glue.

TRANSVENOUS EMBOLIZATION OF CEREBROSPINAL FLUID-VENOUS FISTULAS

Given the overall greater risk profile for open surgery, minimally invasive approaches to treatment of CVFs (eg, transvenous embolization [TVE] or EBP) are generally considered first-line for SIH. However, patients who are refractory to EBP may elect for open surgical procedures as these may provide more definitive and durable treatments.

TVE is a relatively novel treatment for CVFs with the initial publication describing this technique by Brinjikji et el. in 2021.[44] This procedure involves directing a catheter through the venous system and gaining access to the azygos, hemiazygos, or superior intercostal veins in order to select the paraspinal vein associated with the CVF. The proceduralist then directly embolizes the abnormal fistulous connection using Onyx (Medtronic, Minnesota, USA) (Fig. 5).[44] Early studies on transvenous embolization demonstrate promising results, though it remains uncertain whether EBP or TVE is superior.[44,45] TVE will not be discussed in detail in this review but can be found in other excellent contemporaneous reviews.[46,47]

Decisions about the techniques employed for an open surgical approach to repair a dural tear or ligate a CVF are generally driven by on the location of the spinal pathology and by the surgeon preference and expertise. These have been thoroughly discussed elsewhere in the literature.[48–50]

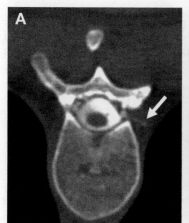
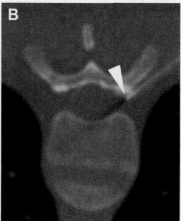
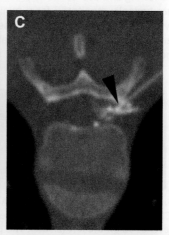

Fig. 3. Transforaminal Needle Placement. A 26-year-old-male presented with orthostatic headache and positive brain MRI for SIH (not shown). (*A*) Subsequent computed tomography (CT) myelography demonstrated a cerebrospinal fuid (CSF)-venous fistula on the right at T10 with opacification of the radicular and segmental veins (*white arrow*). (*B*) Transforaminal approach needle placement (*white arrowhead*) is demonstrated at the time of epidural blood patch (EBP). (*C*) Successful EBP with use of autologous blood and fibrin glue at the site of the fistula (*black arrowhead*).

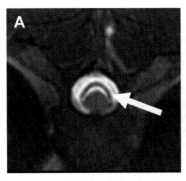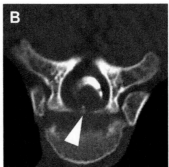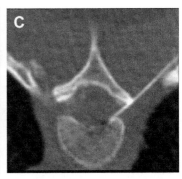

Fig. 4. Ventral Epidural Needle Placement. A 25-year-old female presented with abrupt onset of positional head-ache and brain MRI positive for findings of SIH (not shown). (*A*) Axial image from a heavily T2-weighted MRI sequence of the spine demonstrated a longitudinally extensive, circumferential epidural fluid collection (*white arrow*), and small central disc protrusion at the level of T2-3. (*B*) Subsequent prone CT myelography demonstrated a small, calcified disc protrusion at this level at the site of the confirmed CSF leak (*white arrowhead*). (*C*) Ventral epidural placement of the needle is demonstrated during EBP.

POST-TREATMENT MANAGEMENT

Extensive literature exists on the diagnosis and treatment of CSF leaks and CVFs; however, rela-tively little is published on the post procedural management of these patients. Treating physi-cians should be knowledgeable about potential complications, indications for further imaging, and the long-term sequelae of untreated SIH. There are no consensus guidelines on the appro-priate post-procedural care of SIH patients after treatment with EBP or TVE. Herein, the authors provide their recommendations.

Immediate Post-Treatment Management

Recovery room

Following the use of moderate sedation, patients are typically monitored for a minimum of 2 hours with standard recovery room observation protocol and monitoring of vital signs. Patients should be positioned recumbent such that they are parallel to the floor to decrease hydrostatic pressure on the nascent patch. Anti-emetics are given as needed for nausea.

Post-procedure activity restrictions

It is worth emphasizing that no evidence exists regarding post-procedural restrictions and the guidelines provided here reflect the authors' opin-ions. The authors encourage bed rest for the initial 24 hours post EBP. Patients are advised to lift no more than 10 lbs and to avoid any strenuous bending or twisting. Patients should restart any held anticoagulation 24 hours after the procedure according to available guidelines. Showering is permitted; however, patients are instructed not to bathe or swim within the first 72 hours following the procedure to reduce the risk of infection at the injection sites.

Restrictions gradually become more lenient over the first 3 months following EBP. During the first month, the authors recommend resuming light

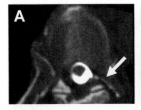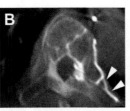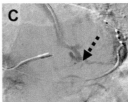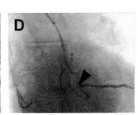

Fig. 5. Transvenous Embolization. A 71-year-old male presented with brain MRI positive for SIH (not shown). (*A*) CT myelography performed in the left lateral decubitus position demonstrated a CSF-venous fistula arising at the level of T8 on the left (*arrow*). The patient was referred for transvenous embolization (TVE). (*B*) Intraprocedural cone-beam CT) confirmed correct distribution of contrast material (*white arrowheads*) prior to administration of embolic material. (*C*) The azygos system was accessed and the left T8 segmental vein was selected to delineate anatomy prior to embolization. This demonstrated the left T8 segmental vein communicating with the radicular veins and epidural venous plexus (*dashed arrow*). (*D*) Given satisfactory catheter positioning, embolization at the level of the distal segmental vein (*black arrowhead*) was performed using Onyx liquid embolic system with a balloon inflated proximally to the level of administration.

activity as tolerated but no intentional exercise. Patients are instructed not to lift anything greater than 10 lbs. During the second and third months post treatment, patients may gradually return to light and low-impact exercises and are permitted to lift items up to 20 lbs. Beyond 3 months, the authors recommend to continue to avoid strenuous bending, twisting, or lifting exercises.

Potential complications

Minor/expected Patients may experience localized back pain at the site of the procedure in the immediate post-procedural period (within the first 7 days). Usually, the pain is localized to the procedure site and is self-limited, typically resolving within 48 hours. Use of local heat or ice is suggested along with the use of acetaminophen.

Major/unexpected Prior to discharge, patients should be counseled about potential signs and symptoms that may require them to seek emergency medical treatment and be provided clinic contact information as well as instructions for emergent management. Fortunately, these major complications are rare, but when they occur they are typically secondary to mass effect on the spinal cord/nerves (due to postoperative epidural hematoma or patching material) or infection. Symptoms therefore include the development of severe back pain, lower extremity weakness, fecal incontinence, urinary retention, severe nausea/vomiting, or fever.

Rebound intracranial hypertension Some patients may experience a change in headache phenotype following treatment with EBP or TVE. Most commonly this change occurs due to rebound intracranial hypertension (RIH) (ie, the development of elevated CSF pressures after treatment).[51] Several unproven theories exist as to the underlying physiology causing the development of RIH. One potential contributing factor is the mass effect within the epidural space from the injected patching material, which then causes direct pressure on the thecal sac resulting in increased CSF pressures. Other proposed mechanisms include the persistence of pre-treatment compensatory physiologic changes that were in place to manage low CSF volumes (eg, continued increased CSF production or engorgement of the venous plexus despite a sealed CSF leak).[51]

Given that the primary symptom of RIH is headache, some patients may erroneously attribute this new headache to persistent SIH. Thus, recognition of this condition is critical in order to further direct care and to avoid further invasive diagnostic procedures or treatment in a patient who has been adequately treated for SIH. Diagnosis of RIH can be challenging; however, several features can be used to distinguish RIH from persistent/refractory SIH including symptom profile, responsiveness to CSF pressure-lowering medications (eg, acetazolamide), and, if necessary, remeasuring the opening CSF pressure.

Initial evaluation of a patient with new headaches in the post-treatment period should be focused on determining if there are any changes in phenotype from the pretreatment headache. RIH headaches typically manifest as frontal/periorbital in location and classically worsen with recumbency. This is in contradistinction to SIH in which the headache is usually occipital and worsens upon standing upright.[51] Other symptoms suggestive of RIH include significant nausea, vomiting, and blurred vision. While nausea and vomiting can also occur with SIH, blurred vision is highly specific for RIH (mirroring the well-established symptoms of blurred vision in patients with idiopathic intracranial hypertension).[52] The onset of RIH headache following treatment can vary substantially, with 1 study reporting that most patients present within the first 48 hours (range 2 hours to 1 year).[51] Finally, definitive diagnosis of RIH can be established with measuring of opening pressure as some of these patients will demonstrate a marked interval increase in pressure.[51]

First-line management for patients presenting with symptoms of RIH is a trial of acetazolamide. No studies providing evidence-based guidelines on a starting dose exist; however, at the authors' institution, a total of 500 to 1000 mg divided throughout the day is generally the initial regimen. This dosing can be increased or decreased based on the severity of RIH symptoms. Acetazolamide is a potent carbonic anhydrase inhibitor and known diuretic with the potential to cause severe metabolic acidosis if used over the long term or at higher doses. In most patients, RIH resolves within the first several days after onset. If a longer period of treatment is necessary, hydration is encouraged and labs are obtained to assess for hypokalemia, with potassium supplements prescribed as needed. Finally, referral to other specialists (neurology or ophthalmology) may be needed if remaining on the medication long term or if visual symptoms are present. Patients should also be informed of potential benign side effects of acetazolamide, to include paresthesias of the mouth/face and extremities.

Rarely, severe RIH requires treatment via therapeutic removal of CSF with serial lumbar punctures. Treatment of long-term persistent RIH may include CSF diversion with surgically implanted shunts, but is not without the risk for complications and should be reserved for severe/medically refractory patients and preceded by multidisciplinary discussion.

Arachnoiditis Arachnoiditis has been reported as a delayed complication most often following "blind" EBP (ie, without the use of imaging guidance).[53] This complication may arise secondary to inadvertent placement of blood and/or fibrin glue into the subarachnoid space. The use of imaging guidance should ensure proper needle placement in the epidural space and markedly reduce the probability of this rare complication.

Post-treatment Follow-up

The importance of continued communication with patients following treatment cannot be overstated. While monitoring for the previously discussed post-treatment complications is important, confirmation of resolution of symptoms is equally important. Persistent symptoms of SIH will necessitate that the patient returns for additional imaging or treatment.

Following treatment, a brain MRI may be ordered within 1 to 2 months in order to document resolution of brain MRI findings of SIH (eg, dural enhancement, brain sagging, venous distension). One should also consider obtaining a follow-up MRI of the spine to document resolution of extradural collections in the case of type 1 or 2 CSF leaks, as persistent extradural collections have been cited as the cause for developing superficial siderosis.[54] While some institutions may advocate for repeat myelograms to confirm resolution of causative spinal pathology, in asymptomatic patients the authors avoid invasive tests requiring dural puncture as there is a small risk of causing an iatrogenic leak.

Patients with persistent symptoms of SIH following percutaneous treatment may require repeat treatment (additional EBP) and/or repeat spinal imaging if the leak was not definitively localized initially (perhaps using specialized secondary imaging with decubitus positioning, photon counting CT, digital subtraction myelography, etc).[7,11,55] If the leak was already definitively localized, treated with a targeted EBP, and the patient remains symptomatic, then options include either repeat targeted EBP or referral for an alternative treatment (eg, surgery or TVE).

Some patients will have an asymptomatic period after treatment suggestive of cure followed by the development of new symptoms that cannot be definitively classified as recurrent SIH, RIH, or a new cause of headaches. Given the uncertainty in this scenario, a new diagnostic work up may be necessary. In these instances, repeat brain MRI with contrast or spinal imaging can be helpful with subsequent treatment as necessary.

Risks associated with untreated chronic SIH

A minority of SIH patients may have a CSF leak on imaging but remain asymptomatic or minimally symptomatic. Management of these patients can be particularly challenging as one needs to weigh the risks of treatment in the absence of significant symptoms against the risks of continued conservative management. During the management discussion, the patient should be made aware that opting to forgo all treatment is not entirely without risk. Debilitating consequences of untreated SIH have been well-documented in the literature including superficial siderosis and bibrachial amyotrophy, with the probability of developing these complications ranging from 0% at 48 months to 58% at 16 years.[54]

Superficial siderosis

Superficial siderosis is defined as hemosiderin deposition along the surfaces of the brain, usually in the setting of recurrent subarachnoid hemorrhage. While this finding is often encountered on brain MRI, it is most commonly diffuse or supratentorial predominant. Superficial siderosis confined to the infratentorial compartment has a known association with untreated SIH and is usually associated with a dural defect (ie, type 1 or 2 leak).

Patients with superficial siderosis can develop cranial nerve palsies, ataxia, and sensorineural hearing loss causing a substantial impact on quality of life. While there have been reports of radiographic reversal following chelation therapy or surgical treatment, these findings are generally thought of as irreversible. Thus, patients should be counseled about the possibility of developing these complications when discussing the risks and benefits of pursuing treatment.[4,56]

Bibrachial Amyotrophy

Bibrachial amyotrophy is another potentially devastating consequence of delayed treatment, particularly in patients with large extradural collections. This condition manifests as progressive weakness and atrophy of the upper extremities, and its clinical presentation can overlap with that of amyotrophic lateral sclerosis. While the mechanism is unknown, it is hypothesized that injury to the cervical nerves occurs as a result of mass effect from the extradural collection.[54]

SUMMARY

SIH is increasingly recognized resulting in larger numbers of patients presenting for treatment.

Decisions regarding the appropriate treatment approach depend, in part, on the underlying CSF leak subtype. Percutaneous treatments, such as EBP, remain the first-line treatment for SIH. Effective percutaneous treatment requires an in-depth knowledge of preprocedural planning, technical approach, and postprocedural complications as well as the ability to recognize signs of unsuccessful treatment and indications to reimage the patient.

CLINICS CARE POINTS

- Selection of a therapeutic approach for the treatment of SIH is dependent upon the underlying spinal pathology. Non-targeted EBP does not require identifying and localizing the spinal CSF leak or CVF obviating the need for invasive diagnostic imaging (eg, myelography). However, such imaging is required for more advanced treatment approaches that are thought to impart improved therapeutic efficacy including targeted EBP, transvenous embolization, and open surgery.

- Treating physicians should be aware of the potential complications after treatment of SIH, including rebound intracranial hypertension (RIH). RIH is the development of elevated CSF pressures after successful treatment of a CSF leak or CVF and manifests as a headache with a new phenotype from the pretreatment presentation, most commonly frontal/periorbital and one that worsens with recumbency.

- Providers should continue to follow SIH patients after treatment until confirmation of resolution of the patient's symptoms of SIH and brain MRI findings. Continued symptoms after an EBP could represent persistent SIH requiring further treatment with TVE or open surgery, or RIH that may require CSF pressure-lowering medications or therapeutic removal of CSF via lumbar puncture.

DISCLOSURE

None.

REFERENCES

1. D'Antona L, Jaime Merchan MA, Vassiliou A, et al. Clinical Presentation, Investigation Findings, and Treatment Outcomes of Spontaneous Intracranial Hypotension Syndrome: A Systematic Review and Meta-analysis. JAMA Neurol 2021;78(3):329–37.
2. Schievink WI. Misdiagnosis of spontaneous intracranial hypotension. Arch Neurol 2003;60(12):1713–8.
3. Schievink WI, Maya MM, Jean-Pierre S, et al. A classification system of spontaneous spinal CSF leaks. Neurology 2016;87(7):673–9.
4. Beck J, Ulrich CT, Fung C, et al. Diskogenic microspurs as a major cause of intractable spontaneous intracranial hypotension. Neurology 2016;87(12):1220–6.
5. Dobrocky T, Mosimann PJ, Zibold F, et al. Cryptogenic Cerebrospinal Fluid Leaks in Spontaneous Intracranial Hypotension: Role of Dynamic CT Myelography. Radiology 2018;289(3):766–72.
6. Hoxworth JM, Trentman TL, Kotsenas AL, et al. The role of digital subtraction myelography in the diagnosis and localization of spontaneous spinal CSF leaks. AJR Am J Roentgenol 2012;199(3):649–53.
7. Schievink WI, Moser FG, Maya MM, et al. Digital subtraction myelography for the identification of spontaneous spinal CSF-venous fistulas. J Neurosurg Spine 2016;24(6):960–4.
8. Thielen KR, Sillery JC, Morris JM, et al. Ultrafast dynamic computed tomography myelography for the precise identification of high-flow cerebrospinal fluid leaks caused by spiculated spinal osteophytes. J Neurosurg Spine 2015;22(3):324–31.
9. Amrhein TJ, Kranz PG. Spontaneous Intracranial Hypotension: Imaging in Diagnosis and Treatment. Radiol Clin North Am 2019;57(2):439–51.
10. Callen AL, Timpone VM, Schwertner A, et al. Algorithmic Multimodality Approach to Diagnosis and Treatment of Spinal CSF Leak and Venous Fistula in Patients With Spontaneous Intracranial Hypotension. AJR Am J Roentgenol 2022;219(2):292–301.
11. Kranz PG, Gray L, Malinzak MD, et al. CSF-Venous Fistulas: Anatomy and Diagnostic Imaging. AJR Am J Roentgenol 2021;217(6):1418–29.
12. Kong DS, Park K, Nam DH, et al. Clinical features and long-term results of spontaneous intracranial hypotension. Neurosurgery 2005;57(1):91–6. discussion 91-6.
13. Patel IJ, Rahim S, Davidson JC, et al. Society of Interventional Radiology Consensus Guidelines for the Periprocedural Management of Thrombotic and Bleeding Risk in Patients Undergoing Percutaneous Image-Guided Interventions-Part II: Recommendations: Endorsed by the Canadian Association for Interventional Radiology and the Cardiovascular and Interventional Radiological Society of Europe. J Vasc Interv Radiol 2019;30(8):1168–1184 e1.
14. Jaffe TA, Raiff D, Ho LM, et al. Management of Anticoagulant and Antiplatelet Medications in Adults Undergoing Percutaneous Interventions. AJR Am J Roentgenol 2015;205(2):421–8.

15. Patel IJ, Davidson JC, Nikolic B, et al. Consensus guidelines for periprocedural management of coagulation status and hemostasis risk in percutaneous image-guided interventions. J Vasc Interv Radiol 2012;23(6):727–36.

16. Demaree CJ, Soliz JM, Gebhardt R. Cancer Seeding Risk from an Epidural Blood Patch in Patients with Leukemia or Lymphoma. Pain Med 2017;18(4):786–90.

17. Uppal V, Russell R, Sondekoppam RV, et al. Evidence-based clinical practice guidelines on postdural puncture headache: a consensus report from a multisociety international working group. Reg Anesth Pain Med 2023. https://doi.org/10.1136/rapm-2023-104817.

18. Ferrante E, Trimboli M, Petrecca G, et al. Management of Spontaneous Intracranial Hypotension During Pregnancy: A Case Series. Headache 2020;60(8):1777–87.

19. Schievink WI, Georganos SA, Maya MM, et al. Anaphylactic reactions to fibrin sealant injection for spontaneous spinal CSF leaks. Neurology 2008;70(11):885–7.

20. Becker DE, Reed KL. Essentials of local anesthetic pharmacology. Anesth Prog. Fall 2006;53(3):98–108. quiz 109-10.

21. Provenzano DA, Pellis Z, DeRiggi L. Fatal gadolinium-induced encephalopathy following accidental intrathecal administration: a case report and a comprehensive evidence-based review. Reg Anesth Pain Med 2019. https://doi.org/10.1136/rapm-2019-100422.

22. Bartynski WS, Grahovac SZ, Rothfus WE. Incorrect needle position during lumbar epidural steroid administration: inaccuracy of loss of air pressure resistance and requirement of fluoroscopy and epidurography during needle insertion. AJNR Am J Neuroradiol 2005;26(3):502–5.

23. Amrhein TJ, Schauberger JS, Kranz PG, et al. Reducing Patient Radiation Exposure From CT Fluoroscopy-Guided Lumbar Spine Pain Injections by Targeting the Planning CT. AJR Am J Roentgenol 2016;206(2):390–4.

24. Hoang JK, Yoshizumi TT, Toncheva G, et al. Radiation dose exposure for lumbar spine epidural steroid injections: a comparison of conventional fluoroscopy data and CT fluoroscopy techniques. AJR Am J Roentgenol 2011;197(4):778–82.

25. Beierlein W, Scheule AM, Dietrich W, et al. Forty years of clinical aprotinin use: a review of 124 hypersensitivity reactions. Ann Thorac Surg 2005;79(2):741–8.

26. Kranz PG, Amrhein TJ, Gray L. Incidence of Inadvertent Intravascular Injection during CT Fluoroscopy-Guided Epidural Steroid Injections. AJNR Am J Neuroradiol 2015;36(5):1000–7.

27. Kranz PG, Raduazo PA. Technique for CT fluoroscopy-guided cervical interlaminar steroid injections. AJR Am J Roentgenol 2012;198(3):675–7.

28. Wagner AL. Selective lumbar nerve root blocks with CT fluoroscopic guidance: technique, results, procedure time, and radiation dose. AJNR Am J Neuroradiol 2004;25(9):1592–4.

29. Wagner AL, Murtagh FR. Selective nerve root blocks. Tech Vasc Interv Radiol 2002;5(4):194–200.

30. Amrhein TJ, Befera NT, Gray L, et al. CT Fluoroscopy-Guided Blood Patching of Ventral CSF Leaks by Direct Needle Placement in the Ventral Epidural Space Using a Transforaminal Approach. AJNR Am J Neuroradiol 2016;37(10):1951–6.

31. Ahn C, Lee E, Lee JW, et al. Two-site blind epidural blood patch versus targeted epidural blood patch in spontaneous intracranial hypotension. J Clin Neurosci 2019;62:147–54.

32. Berroir S, Loisel B, Ducros A, et al. Early epidural blood patch in spontaneous intracranial hypotension. Neurology 2004;63(10):1950–1.

33. Cho KI, Moon HS, Jeon HJ, et al. Spontaneous intracranial hypotension: efficacy of radiologic targeting vs blind blood patch. Neurology 2011;76(13):1139–44.

34. Chung SJ, Lee JH, Im JH, et al. Short- and long-term outcomes of spontaneous CSF hypovolemia. Eur Neurol 2005;54(2):63–7.

35. He FF, Li L, Liu MJ, et al. Targeted Epidural Blood Patch Treatment for Refractory Spontaneous Intracranial Hypotension in China. J Neurol Surg B Skull Base 2018;79(3):217–23.

36. Sencakova D, Mokri B, McClelland RL. The efficacy of epidural blood patch in spontaneous CSF leaks. Neurology 2001;57(10):1921–3.

37. Wu JW, Hseu SS, Fuh JL, et al. Factors predicting response to the first epidural blood patch in spontaneous intracranial hypotension. Brain 2017;140(2):344–52.

38. Piechowiak EI, Aeschimann B, Hani L, et al. Epidural Blood Patching in Spontaneous Intracranial Hypotension-Do we Really Seal the Leak? Clin Neuroradiol 2023;33(1):211–8.

39. Amrhein TJ, Williams JW Jr, Gray L, et al. Efficacy of Epidural Blood Patching or Surgery in Spontaneous Intracranial Hypotension: A Systematic Review and Evidence Map. AJNR Am J Neuroradiol 2023;44(6):730–9.

40. Mamlouk MD, Shen PY, Sedrak MF, et al. CT-guided Fibrin Glue Occlusion of Cerebrospinal Fluid-Venous Fistulas. Radiology 2021;299(2):409–18.

41. Beierlein W, Scheule AM, Antoniadis G, et al. An immediate, allergic skin reaction to aprotinin after reexposure to fibrin sealant. Transfusion 2000;40(3):302–5.

42. Dietrich W, Spath P, Zuhlsdorf M, et al. Anaphylactic reactions to aprotinin reexposure in cardiac surgery: relation to antiaprotinin immunoglobulin G and E antibodies. Anesthesiology 2001;95(1):64–71. discussion 5A-6A.

43. Cheema S, Anderson J, Angus-Leppan H, et al. Multidisciplinary consensus guideline for the diagnosis and management of spontaneous intracranial hypotension. J Neurol Neurosurg Psychiatry 2023. https://doi.org/10.1136/jnnp-2023-331166.

44. Brinjikji W, Savastano LE, Atkinson JLD, et al. A Novel Endovascular Therapy for CSF Hypotension Secondary to CSF-Venous Fistulas. AJNR Am J Neuroradiol 2021;42(5):882–7.

45. Brinjikji W, Garza I, Whealy M, et al. Clinical and imaging outcomes of cerebrospinal fluid-venous fistula embolization. J Neurointerv Surg 2022;14(10):953–6.

46. Borg N, Oushy S, Savastano L, et al. Transvenous embolization of a cerebrospinal fluid-venous fistula for the treatment of spontaneous intracranial hypotension. J Neurointerv Surg 2022;14(9):948.

47. Borg N, Cutsforth-Gregory J, Oushy S, et al. Anatomy of Spinal Venous Drainage for the Neurointerventionalist: From Puncture Site to Intervertebral Foramen. AJNR Am J Neuroradiol 2022;43(4):517–25.

48. Beck J, Raabe A, Schievink WI, et al. Posterior Approach and Spinal Cord Release for 360 degrees Repair of Dural Defects in Spontaneous Intracranial Hypotension. Neurosurgery 2019;84(6):E345–51.

49. Kamenova M, Schaeren S, Wasner MG. Intradural extraarachnoid sutureless technique combined with laminoplasty for indirect repair of ventral dural defects in spontaneous intracranial hypotension: technical note and case series. Acta Neurochir 2021;163(9):2551–6.

50. Wang TY, Karikari IO, Amrhein TJ, et al. Clinical Outcomes Following Surgical Ligation of Cerebrospinal Fluid-Venous Fistula in Patients With Spontaneous Intracranial Hypotension: A Prospective Case Series. Oper Neurosurg (Hagerstown) 2020;18(3):239–45.

51. Kranz PG, Amrhein TJ, Gray L. Rebound intracranial hypertension: a complication of epidural blood patching for intracranial hypotension. AJNR Am J Neuroradiol 2014;35(6):1237–40.

52. Wall M. Update on Idiopathic Intracranial Hypertension. Neurol Clin 2017;35(1):45–57.

53. Chazen JL, Amrhein TJ. Arachnoiditis following epidural blood patch-An avoidable rare complication due to blind technique. Headache 2021;61(6):972–3.

54. Schievink WI, Maya M, Moser F, et al. Long-term Risks of Persistent Ventral Spinal CSF Leaks in SIH: Superficial Siderosis and Bibrachial Amyotrophy. Neurology 2021;97(19):e1964–70.

55. Madhavan AA, Yu L, Brinjikji W, et al. Utility of Photon-Counting Detector CT Myelography for the Detection of CSF-Venous Fistulas. AJNR Am J Neuroradiol 2023;44(6):740–4.

56. Kessler RA, Li X, Schwartz K, et al. Two-year observational study of deferiprone in superficial siderosis. CNS Neurosci Ther 2018;24(3):187–92.

Endovascular Embolization Techniques for Cerebrospinal Fluid-Venous Fistula in the Treatment of Spontaneous Intracranial Hypotension

Atakan Orscelik, MD[a,*], Jeremy K. Cutsforth-Gregory, MD[b],
Ajay Madhavan, MD[a], Yigit Can Senol, MD[a,c], Hassan Kobeissi, MD[a],
Gokce Belge Bilgin, MD[a], Cem Bilgin, MD[a], David F. Kallmes, MD[a],
Waleed Brinjikji, MD[a,c]

KEYWORDS

- Spontaneous intracranial hypotension • Cerebrospinal fluid-venous fistula
- Endovascular embolization

KEY POINTS

- Endovascular embolization is a effective and minimally invasive treatment for cerebrospinal fluid-venous fistula (CVF), which is abnormal communication between the cerebrospinal fluid and venous systems.
- Transvenous embolization techniques involve selective catheterization of the paraspinal vein and deployment of embolic agents, and have demonstrated high rates of symptom resolution in patients.
- The pressure cooker embolization technique, using balloons and coils, enhances embolic agent penetration into the foraminal venous plexus and minimizes reflux risk.
- Accurate diagnosis and localization of CVFs using advanced imaging technique such as lateral decubitus digital subtraction myelography are essential for effective treatment planning.

INTRODUCTION

Spontaneous intracranial hypotension (SIH) is a relatively rare but increasingly recognized cause of headache and is often associated with disabling symptoms that can significantly reduce patients' quality of life.[1] This condition is caused by low cerebrospinal fluid (CSF) volume due to spontaneous CSF leakage at any level of the spine.[2] Orthostatic headache is a characteristic feature, and most patients experience other postural symptoms such as nausea, vomiting, neck pain, tinnitus, and cognitive impairment.[1,2] It is estimated to affect 4 to 5 per 100,000 individuals per year; however, it is likely underdiagnosed.[3] Several types of spontaneous spinal CSF leak have been described, although why they occur in a given patient is unknown. Some patients have connective tissue disorders or a history of intracranial hypertension before the onset of CSF leak.[2,4,5] The diagnosis of SIH requires a comprehensive workup of patients, including clinical examination, imaging

[a] Department of Radiology, Mayo Clinic, Rochester, MN, USA; [b] Department of Neurology, Mayo Clinic, Rochester, MN, USA; [c] Department of Neurologic Surgery, Mayo Clinic, Rochester, MN, USA
* Corresponding author. Mayo Clinic Department of Radiology, 200 First Street, SW Rochester, MN 55905.
E-mail address: atakanorscelik@gmail.com

Radiol Clin N Am 62 (2024) 345–354
https://doi.org/10.1016/j.rcl.2023.10.006
0033-8389/24/© 2023 Elsevier Inc. All rights reserved.

studies, and invasive procedures such as radionuclide cisternography or myelography.[3,6,7]

CSF-venous fistula (CVF) is a type of spinal CSF leak caused by abnormal communication between the spinal subarachnoid space and adjacent spinal epidural veins.[8] Diagnosis and localization of CVF are crucial to treating SIH. The most effective techniques for precisely localizing CVFs include decubitus digital subtraction myelography (DSM) and decubitus CT myelography.[9,10] Embolization of the CVF has emerged as a minimally invasive and effective treatment option.[2] The embolization technique involves the injection of embolic agents such as Onyx (Medtronic, Minnesota, USA) and coils into the affected veins to occlude the site of CSF leakage and block the abnormal communication between the CSF and venous systems.[2,6,8] Apart from embolization, other treatment options for CVF include conservative management, epidural blood patching, targeted epidural saline injection, and surgical repair.[9]

In this review article, we provide a comprehensive overview of the embolization procedure technique and other treatment options for the management of CVF in SIH. We aim to describe in detail the technical aspects of embolization for CVF, including patient demographics, procedure equipment, embolic agents, and clinical improvement.

METHODS

We searched Pubmed to identify articles in English focusing the pathogenesis, diagnosis, endovascular techniques and alternative treatment options of CVF from inception through April 2023. We used combinations of search terms including "spontaneous intracranial hypotension," "cerebrospinal fluid-venous fistula," "endovascular," "embolization," "imaging," "pathogenesis," "surgical," "conservative," and "percutaneous." We found 7 studies that reported endovascular embolization techniques in the treatment of CVF as case reports, case series, and retrospective studies. These techniques and their outcomes are discussed comprehensively in this article.

ANATOMY AND PATHOGENESIS OF CEREBROSPINAL FLUID-VENOUS FISTULA FORMATION

CVFs are aberrant connections between spinal dura and the venous system, leading to unregulated leakage of CSF into the venous circulation and causing decreased intracranial CSF volume and associated symptoms.[8] The typical presentation of patients with spontaneous spinal CSF leak secondary to CVF includes orthostatic headache (worsens with standing and improves with recumbency), Valsalva headache, neck pain, tinnitus, hearing loss, visual disturbances, and other neurologic symptoms.[10] Understanding the anatomy and pathogenesis of CVFs is crucial for diagnosis and management. Although the exact pathogenesis of CVFs remains incompletely understood, several structural abnormalities such as dural defects and meningeal diverticula have been associated with the development of CVFs.[8,11] The aberrant connections that constitute CVFs can occur via dysfunction of arachnoid granulations, due to factors such as trauma, inflammation, or anatomic variation. When arachnoid granulations are compromised, they can lose their ability to maintain the one-way flow of CSF into the venous sinuses, potentially leading to a CVF (Fig. 1).

Spinal veins drain into the azygos and hemiazygos systems, then the inferior or superior vena cava.[12] In contrast to the cranial venous system, the spinal venous system lacks valves, making it more susceptible to reflux of CSF than its cranial counterpart.[11] CVFs can occur anywhere along the spinal venous drainage system, with the most common location being the thoracic spine.[11,12] The anatomy of the spinal venous drainage system in these areas is particularly complex, with multiple veins draining into a single vein and veins changing course abruptly.[11] These complex venous structures likely contribute to the development of the fistula and can make them difficult to diagnose. Once the fistula develops, pulsations of CSF during normal physiologic movements may cause it to enlarge.[11] The spinal venous drainage system consists of the internal vertebral venous plexus (IVVP), also referred to as the epidural venous plexus, the external vertebral venous plexus (EVVP), and radicular veins.[12] The IVVP is a network of veins that runs along the spinal cord and vertebral column and communicates with the intracranial venous system through the foramen magnum. The EVVP is a network of veins that runs outside the dura mater and vertebral column within the paravertebral soft tissues and communicates with the paraspinal veins and systemic venous system. The radicular veins drain the spinal cord and nerve roots and empty into the vertebral venous plexuses. Both the IVVP and EVVP have connections with the CSF-filled spaces around the spinal cord and communicate with each other through the intervertebral foramina, which are the most common site of CVF.[12]

IMAGING TECHNIQUES IN THE DIAGNOSIS OF CEREBROSPINAL FLUID-VENOUS FISTULAS

Intracranial imaging findings of SIH include pachymeningeal enhancement, pituitary engorgement,

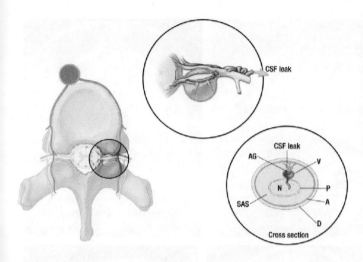

Fig. 1. The role of arachnoid granulations in the pathogenesis of CVF formation. Under normal conditions, arachnoid granulations facilitate one-way flow of CSF into the venous sinuses. However, they can become disrupted or damaged due to various factors, leading to the abnormal connection between the subarachnoid space and the venous system. This disruption results in a CVF, causing the leakage of CSF into the venous sinuses and associated clinical symptoms. A, arachnoid matter; AG, arachnoid granulations; CSF, cerebrospinal fluid; D, dua mater; P, pia mater; SAS, subarachnoid space; V, vein.

hygromas, and dural venous sinus engorgement (**Fig. 2**). However, the diagnosis of CVFs can be challenging due to nonspecific symptoms and insensitive imaging markers. Timely and accurate diagnosis is crucial for effective treatment planning, and early diagnosis and treatment may prevent irreversible neurologic deficits and chronic disability and improve patient outcomes. In recent years, various advanced imaging modalities have been used to localize CVFs, each with relative advantages and limitations. Roytman and colleagues emphasize a multimodality approach to identifying the site of leak.[8] Callen and colleagues suggested an algorithmic approach to the diagnosis and treatment of spinal CSF leak and venous fistula in patients with SIH that considers the relative diagnostic yields of the various imaging modalities available.[13] Computed tomography (CT) myelography is a well-established imaging technique that combines myelography and CT imaging to provide a detailed delineation of pathologic spine conditions, especially those involving the thecal sac and its contents.[14] Caton Jr and colleagues described the use of spinal compliance curves,[15] a technique that involves measuring the CSF pressure at different spinal levels using a manometer during dynamic CT myelography. The authors found that this tool helped localize the fistula in 8 of 22 patients (36%). Decubitus CT myelography is another procedural approach that involves the injection of contrast dye into the spinal canal while the patient is in the right or left lateral decubitus position. Mamlouk and colleagues reported that this technique has a diagnostic yield of 50% and concluded that it is a safe and effective imaging modality with a higher diagnostic yield than standard CT myelography.[16,17] Recently, decubitus photon counting detector CT myelography was described as a potentially beneficial technique,

with early data showing that it may detect CVFs missed on standard decubitus CT myelography.[18]

Intrathecal gadolinium magnetic resonance myelography (ITG-MRM) is an off-label modification of MR myelography that uses gadolinium-based contrast agents to enhance the signal intensity of CSF and visualize spinal fluid leaks and fistulas. In a study by Madhavan and colleagues, ITG-MRM was found to have a diagnostic yield of 14% (14 out of 97) for localizing CSF leaks, with CVFs in 9 patients and distal nerve root sleeve tears in 5 patients.[19] The authors concluded that other imaging techniques should be attempted before performing ITG-MRM.

DSM is a technique that uses computer software to subtract the precontrast images from the postcontrast images, providing a more precise visualization of contrast-filled structures. Schievink and colleagues conducted a study on 53 patients with suspected spontaneous spinal CVFs and found that DSM had a diagnostic yield of 19%.[20] Lateral decubitus DSM (LDDSM) is a modified technique that increases the sensitivity of DSM for CVFs; yield was 53% in a cohort of 62 patients reported by Kim and colleagues.[21] A practical guide to performing LDDSM, including common pitfalls, was published by Kim and colleagues in 2020.[22]

EMBOLIZATION TREATMENT OF CEREBROSPINAL FLUID-VENOUS FISTULAS

Traditional treatment options for CVFs mirror those historically used for the classic spinal CSF leak types of dural rent or nerve root sleeve tear, namely bedrest, epidural blood or fibrin patching, and surgical repair. Endovascular embolization has recently emerged, however, as a minimally invasive approach for the management of CVFs (**Table 1**).

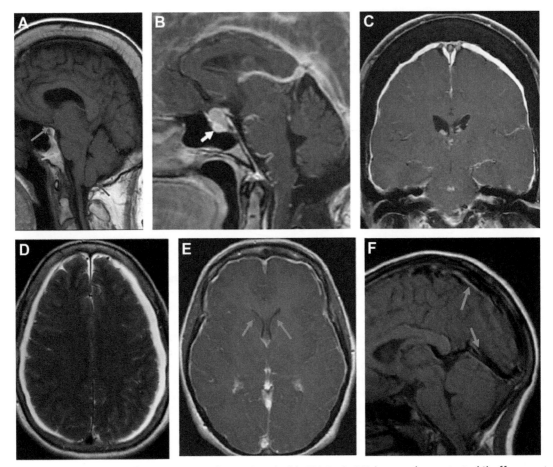

Fig. 2. Intracranial image findings commonly associated with SIH. Brain MR images demonstrate (*A*) effacement of the suprasellar cistern (*orange arrow*), flattening of the ventral pons (green *arrow*), low-lying tonsils (*purple arrow*), (*B*) pituitary engorgement (*white arrow*), (*C*) bilateral hygromas, (*D*) pachymeningeal enhancement, (*E*) ventricular collapse (*orange arrow*), and (*F*) dural venous sinus engorgement (*orange arrow*).

Brinjikji and colleagues proposed a novel embolization technique for the venous component of the fistula for the first time in 5 patients.[23] This technique involves selective catheterization of the paraspinal vein using the 5 Fr Vertebral catheter (Merit Medical, Utah, USA) and Headway Duo microcatheter (Microvention, California, USA) through the common femoral or internal jugular vein and Azygos vein, and subsequent embolization using Onyx 34 to create a plug and Onyx 18 to fill the network surrounding the nerve root sleeve (**Figs. 3** and **4**). The authors reported complete resolution of symptoms in 4 patients and 50% improvement in 1 patient using this technique, with no significant complications. Borg and colleagues then published a technical video explaining this transvenous embolization technique using a 5 Fr intermediate catheter and balloon microcatheter.[24] Following their promising results, Brinjikji and colleagues also reported the largest case series to date on

endovascular treatment of CVF.[25] The study included 40 patients and showed that transvenous embolization is highly effective for CVFs, with much or very much improvement in 33 patients (82.5%) and at least minimal improvement in 36 patients (90%) on the Patient Global Impression of Change (PGIC) scales. The authors also reported 7 patients (17.5%) who may have developed rebound intracranial hypertension that required medical treatment and 12 patients (30%) who experienced persistent local pain at the embolization site for 3 months after embolization. Furthermore, Noufal and colleagues performed transvenous embolization of the radicular vein and its anastomoses with the intercostal vein and other veins using Onyx 18 and the help of Scepter XC balloon microcatheter (Microvention, California, USA).[26] The technique was successful in all cases, and there were no major complications. Four of 5 (80%) patients experienced complete or near-complete resolution of

Table 1
Main studies included endovascular embolization of cerebrospinal fluid-venous fistula in patients with spontaneous intracranial hypotension

Study	Type of Study	Number of Patients	Imaging Technique Used for Diagnosis	CVF Level (Number of CVFs Treated)	Venous Access Route	Procedural Equipment	Clinical Improvement at the Last Follow-Up (Number of patients)
Brinjikji et al,[23] 2021	Case series	5	LDDSM	Right/Bilateral T4-T9 (5)	CFV/IJV → azygos vein → paraspinal vein	5 Fr Vertebral, Headway Duo, Onyx 18/34	Complete resolution of symptoms (4), 50% improvement (1)
Borg et al,[24] 2022	Case report	1	LDDSM	Right T10	CFV → azygos vein → foraminal and paraspinal veins	5 Fr intermediate, balloon microcatheter, Onyx	Significant improvement in symptoms
Brinjikji et al,[25] 2022	Retrospective single-center	40	LDDSM	Cervical spine (3), right/left T1-T12 (46), left lumbar spine (1)	N/A → azygos vein/ ascending lumbar vein/vertebral vein → paraspinal ± foraminal veins	6 Fr Benchmark, 5 Fr Vertebral, Headway Duo ± Scepter XC, Onyx 18/34	At least minimal improvement (36) and much or very much improvement (33) on PGIC scale
Parizadeh et al,[27] 2022	Case report	1	Lateral decubitus CT myelogram	Left L1	Basilic vein → azygos vein/hemiazygos vein → ascending lumbar vein → lateral epidural venous plexus, foraminal venous plexus, and dorsal muscular vein	6 Fr Benchmark, Headway Duo, Scepter XC, Onyx 18 + 34, Coils	Resolution of symptoms and return to work
Noufal et al,[26] 2022	Case series	5	Decubitus DSM ± decubitus CT myelogram	Right/Left T6-T11 (9)	CFV → azygos vein/hemiazygos vein → spinal segmental vein → radicular vein	6 Fr Benchmark, 5 Fr Vert, Phenom 045, Scepter XC, Onyx 18	Complete or near-complete resolution of symptoms (4), remitting relapses (1)

(continued on next page)

Table 1
(continued)

Study	Type of Study	Number of Patients	Imaging Technique Used for Diagnosis	CVF Level (Number of CVFs Treated)	Venous Access Route	Procedural Equipment	Clinical Improvement at the Last Follow-Up (Number of patients)
Parizadeh et al,[28] 2023	Retrospective single-center	18	LDDSM or lateral decubitus CT myelogram	Right C7 (1), left L1 (1), right/left T1-T10 (16)	Antecubital vein, basilic vein or CFV → azygos vein/hemiazygos vein/vertebral vein/ superior intercostal vein → foraminal venous plexus and adjacent venous tributaries (segmental/ intercostal veins, lateral epidural venous plexus, dorsal muscular/ laminar veins)	6 Fr Benchmark, 5 Fr Vertebral, 5 Fr Cobra, 7 Fr Rist, Headway Duo ± Scepter XC/ Eclipse, Onyx 18/ 34 ± Coils	At least minimal improvement (17) and much or very much improvement (16) on PGIC scale

Abbreviations: CFV, common femoral vein; CT, computed tomography; CVF, cerebrospinal fluid-venous fistula; DSM, digital subtraction myelogram; IJV, internal jugular vein; MR, magnetic resonance; N/A, not available; PGIC, Patient Global Impression of Change.

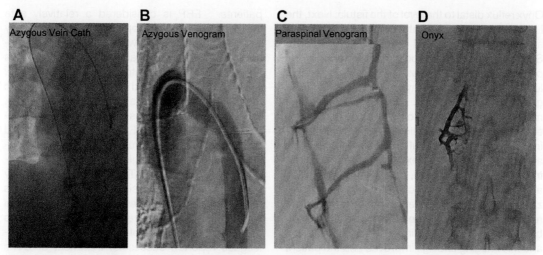

Fig. 3. Venogram images of transvenous embolization technique of CVF. (*A*) Venogram of azygos vein catheter placement. The catheter is navigated through the common femoral or internal jugular vein and advanced into the azygos vein to gain access to the paraspinal venous system. (*B*) Venogram of the azygos vein, highlighting the roadmap for the procedure. This step illustrates the contrast injection to delineate the paraspinal venous anatomy. (*C*) Venogram of the paraspinal vein showing selective catheterization and the microcatheter positioned within the paraspinal venous network. (*D*) Venogram of Onyx injection postembolization, demonstrating the formation of an embolic plug within the paraspinal vein. Onyx is used to create a plug and to fill the network surrounding the nerve root sleeve, effectively occluding the fistula.

symptoms and were able to resume their baseline function and work.

In a recent technical video, Parizadeh and colleagues described a modified embolization technique using Onyx and a double microcatheter for occlusion of the fistula that involves a pressure cooker technique including a balloon and coil.[27] This technique aimed to maximize the penetration of Onyx into the foraminal venous plexus, where

CVFs are usually located, and to reduce reflux of Onyx to the systemic circulation. The initial step involves accessing the basilic vein in the upper extremity, followed by the advance of a 6 Fr Benchmark guide catheter and a 5 Fr Berenstein diagnostic catheter into the Azygos and hemiazygos veins. Helical coils are then deployed into the exiting venous tributaries, including the lumbar vein and distal ascending lumbar vein, to prevent

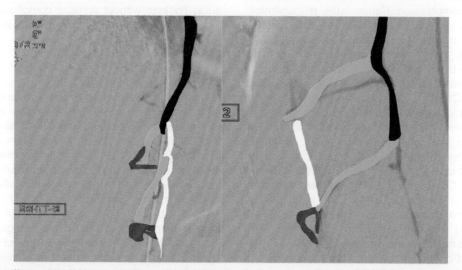

Fig. 4. An illustration drawn over the venogram image to show more clearly the veins undergoing embolization. The dark blue color line was drawn for the azygos vein, green lines for the paraspinal vein, white line for intersegmental anastomosis, and purple lines for the intercostal vein.

Onyx reflux distal to the level of the fistula. Next, the Headway Duo microcatheter is placed immediately adjacent to the foraminal venous plexus, and the Scepter XC balloon microcatheter is placed in the proximal foraminal venous plexus and ascending lumbar vein to prevent Onyx reflux to the hemiazygos vein when inflated. Once the appropriate microcatheter position is confirmed by microcatheter venogram, embolization is first performed using Onyx 34 for the lateral epidural venous plexus and then Onyx 18 for all exiting venous tributaries, including the lumbar vein, ascending lumbar vein, and dorsal muscular branch. Following the embolization procedure, the patient experienced transient rebound intracranial hypertension and local pain but SIH symptoms including orthostatic headache and MR imaging findings improved and the patient returned to work. Parizadeh and colleagues later published a retrospective study of 18 patients treated by the pressure cooker embolization technique.[28] Significant clinical and radiographic improvement was observed in 16 patients (89%). Fifteen patients experienced transient back pain at the embolization site, and 9 patients developed rebound intracranial pressure that required medical treatment.

OTHER TREATMENT OPTIONS FOR CEREBROSPINAL FLUID-VENOUS FISTULAS

Several alternative treatment options can be effective in certain cases, even though endovascular treatment has become the preferred method for managing CVFs. These alternatives include conservative management, percutaneous techniques, and surgical options such as ligation, dural repair, and decompression. Conservative management, such as bed rest, oral caffeine, and fluid intake, may be beneficial for some patients with SIH,[29] whereas more invasive procedures, such as epidural blood patching or surgical ligation, may be necessary for patients with symptomatic or significant CVFs.[30]

When conservative treatment fails, the first-choice treatment option for patients with SIH is often an epidural blood patch (EBP), which involves the injection of autologous blood into the epidural space of the spine to form a clot and seal the CVFs. Berroir and colleagues conducted a study on the use of EBP for CVFs in 40 patients and demonstrated that only 1 patient (1 out of 40) achieved long-term resolution of symptoms and required no further intervention.[31] Similarly, Schievink and colleagues reported that 6 patients with CVFs who underwent EBP for fistulas responded positively but the symptoms resolved temporarily and surgical ligation was performed for all

patients.[32] EBP is considered a relatively safe and effective treatment option for CVF, especially when the leak site is known and localized. However, its efficacy is significantly limited and patients often require further treatment. In our experience, EBP has only provided transient symptomatic improvement in patients with CVFs. Therefore, we generally prefer transvenous Onyx embolization when the site of CVF is clearly demonstrated on imaging. Another percutaneous treatment option is CT-guided fibrin glue occlusion. This technique involves using CT guidance to precisely inject fibrin glue at the site of the CVFs and has the advantage of being less invasive than surgical ligation. The fibrin glue creates a sealant and helps prevent further leakage of CSF. Mamlouk and colleagues reported successful treatment of CVFs using this technique in their case series, which resulted in complete resolution of symptoms and improvement in posttreatment cranial imaging in all patients after 1 to 3 sessions of fibrin injection.[33]

Surgical ligation of the CVF allows direct obliteration of the fistulous connection through open or minimally invasive techniques, although not at the levels of appendicular roots or the artery of Adamkiewicz. Wang and colleagues conducted a prospective case series of 20 patients to evaluate the clinical outcomes of surgical ligation of the fistula.[34] They reported that surgical ligation provided clinically significant treatment satisfaction in all patients and a major improvement in headache severity in 83% of patients. Lohkamp and colleagues also reported the use of minimally invasive surgery for CVF ligation.[35] The authors reported successful outcomes in their patient with improvement of symptoms and brain MR imaging findings without surgical complications or requiring conversion to an open procedure.

SUMMARY

CVFs are a major cause of CSF leak and of SIH. Although the underlying pathogenesis is not fully understood, the advent of advanced imaging techniques such as decubitus CT myelography and LDDSM has made successful diagnosis and treatment possible. Endovascular treatment has emerged as a promising approach to the management of CVFs and has been shown to effectively resolve the clinical symptoms and imaging abnormalities with low complication rates. Alternative treatment options, such as EBP and surgical ligation, may also be considered in select cases. Careful patient selection and multidisciplinary collaboration among neurologists, neuroradiologists, and neurosurgeons can provide successful management of SIH associated with CVF, achieving impressive clinical outcomes and increasing quality of life for patients. Endovascular treatment is a growing tool for managing this challenging condition, and further prospective and multicenter investigations are needed to confirm its safety and efficacy.

CLINICS CARE POINTS

- Endovascular treatment of CVFs has shown a high success rate in improving SIH symptoms. Studies have reported significant clinical improvement in the majority of patients, with some experiencing complete resolution of symptoms.

- Following embolization, a small percentage of patients may develop transient complications, including rebound intracranial hypertension and local pain at the embolization site. Prompt management of these complications is important for optimal patient care.

- Timely and accurate diagnosis of CVF in SIH is crucial for preventing irreversible neurologic deficits and chronic disability. A multimodality approach to identifying the site of the leak is emphasized because CVF diagnosis can be challenging, especially due to nonspecific symptoms. Clinicians should consider advanced imaging modalities to improve diagnostic accuracy and plan for prompt intervention.

- The management of patients with CVFs and SIH often requires a multidisciplinary approach involving neurologists, interventional neuroradiologists, and neurosurgeons. Collaboration among specialists is crucial to accurately diagnose, plan the treatment, and provide comprehensive care to improve patient outcomes.

DISCLOSURE

W. Brinjikji holds equity in Nested Knowledge, Superior Medical Editors, Piraeus Medical, Sonoris Medical, and MIVI Neurovascular. He receives royalties from Medtronic and Balloon Guide Catheter Technology. He receives consulting fees from Medtronic, Stryker, Imperative Care, Microvention, MIVI Neurovascular, Cerenovus, Asahi, and Balt. He serves in a leadership or fiduciary role for MIVI Neurovascular, Marblehead Medical LLC, Interventional Neuroradiology (Editor in Chief), Piraeus Medical, and WFITN. D. F. Kallmes holds equity in Nested Knowledge, Superior Medical Editors, and Conway Medical, Marblehead Medical, and Piraeus Medical. He receives grant support from MicroVention, Medtronic, Balt, and Insera Therapeutics; has served on the Data Safety Monitoring Board for Vesalio; and received royalties from Medtronic.

REFERENCES

1. Urbach H, Fung C, Dovi-Akue P, et al. Spontaneous intracranial hypotension. Dtsch Arzteblatt Int 2020; 117(27–28):480–7.
2. Carlton Jones L, Butteriss D, Scoffings D. Spontaneous intracranial hypotension: the role of radiology in diagnosis and management. Clin Radiol 2022; 77(3):e181–94.
3. Luetzen N, Dovi-Akue P, Fung C, et al. Spontaneous intracranial hypotension: diagnostic and therapeutic workup. Neuroradiology 2021;63(11):1765–72.
4. Kranz PG, Malinzak MD, Amrhein TJ, et al. Update on the diagnosis and treatment of spontaneous intracranial hypotension. Curr Pain Headache Rep 2017;21(8):37.
5. Mokri B, Maher CO, Sencakova D. Spontaneous CSF leaks: underlying disorder of connective tissue. Neurology 2002;58(5):814–6.
6. Amrhein TJ, Kranz PG. Spontaneous intracranial hypotension: imaging in diagnosis and treatment. Radiol Clin North Am 2019;57(2):439–51.
7. Mehta D, Cheema S, Davagnanam I, et al. Diagnosis and treatment evaluation in patients with spontaneous intracranial hypotension. Front Neurol 2023; 14:1145949.
8. Roytman M, Salama G, Robbins MS, et al. CSF-venous fistula. Curr Pain Headache Rep 2021; 25(1):5.
9. Shlobin NA, Shah VN, Chin CT, et al. Cerebrospinal fluid-venous fistulas: a systematic review and examination of individual patient data. Neurosurgery 2021;88(5):931–41.
10. Duvall JR, Robertson CE, Cutsforth-Gregory JK, et al. Headache due to spontaneous spinal cerebrospinal fluid leak secondary to cerebrospinal fluid-venous fistula: case series. Cephalalgia Int J Headache 2019;39(14):1847–54.
11. Kranz PG, Gray L, Malinzak MD, et al. CSF-venous fistulas: anatomy and diagnostic imaging. AJR Am J Roentgenol 2021;217(6):1418–29.
12. Borg N, Cutsforth-Gregory J, Oushy S, et al. Anatomy of spinal venous drainage for the neurointerventionalist: from puncture site to intervertebral foramen. AJNR Am J Neuroradiol 2022;43(4):517–25.
13. Callen AL, Timpone VM, Schwertner A, et al. Algorithmic multimodality approach to diagnosis and treatment of spinal CSF leak and venous fistula in patients with spontaneous intracranial hypotension. AJR Am J Roentgenol 2022;219(2):292–301.

14. Patel DM, Weinberg BD, Hoch MJ. CT myelography: clinical indications and imaging findings. Radiogr Rev Publ Radiol Soc N Am Inc 2020;40(2):470–84.

15. Caton MT, Laguna B, Soderlund KA, et al. Spinal compliance curves: preliminary experience with a new tool for evaluating suspected CSF venous fistulas on CT myelography in patients with spontaneous intracranial hypotension. AJNR Am J Neuroradiol 2021;42(5):986–92.

16. Mamlouk MD, Ochi RP, Jun P, et al. Decubitus CT myelography for CSF-venous fistulas: a procedural approach. AJNR Am J Neuroradiol 2021;42(1):32–6.

17. Madhavan AA, Verdoorn JT, Shlapak DP, et al. Lateral decubitus dynamic CT myelography for fast cerebrospinal fluid leak localization. Neuroradiology 2022;64(9):1897–903.

18. Schwartz FR, Malinzak MD, Amrhein TJ. Photon-counting computed tomography scan of a cerebrospinal fluid venous fistula. JAMA Neurol 2022;79(6):628–9.

19. Madhavan AA, Carr CM, Benson JC, et al. Diagnostic yield of intrathecal gadolinium mr myelography for CSF leak localization. Clin Neuroradiol 2022;32(2):537–45.

20. Schievink WI, Moser FG, Maya MM, et al. Digital subtraction myelography for the identification of spontaneous spinal CSF-venous fistulas. J Neurosurg Spine 2016;24(6):960–4.

21. Kim DK, Carr CM, Benson JC, et al. Diagnostic yield of lateral decubitus digital subtraction myelogram stratified by brain MRI findings. Neurology 2021;96(9):e1312–8.

22. Kim DK, Brinjikji W, Morris PP, et al. Lateral decubitus digital subtraction myelography: tips, tricks, and pitfalls. AJNR Am J Neuroradiol 2020;41(1):21–8.

23. Brinjikji W, Savastano LE, Atkinson JLD, et al. A novel endovascular therapy for CSF hypotension secondary to CSF-venous fistulas. AJNR Am J Neuroradiol 2021;42(5):882–7.

24. Borg N, Oushy S, Savastano L, et al. Transvenous embolization of a cerebrospinal fluid-venous fistula for the treatment of spontaneous intracranial hypotension. J Neurointerventional Surg 2022;14(9):948.

25. Brinjikji W, Garza I, Whealy M, et al. Clinical and imaging outcomes of cerebrospinal fluid-venous fistula embolization. J Neurointerventional Surg 2022;14(10):953–6.

26. Noufal M, Liang CW, Negus J. Transvenous embolization for cerebrospinal fluid-venous fistula. a case series from a single community-academic center. World Neurosurg 2022;168:e613–20.

27. Parizadeh D, Vasconcelos AHC, Miller DA, et al. Dual microcatheter and coil/balloon pressure cooker technique for transvenous embolization of cerebrospinal fluid-venous fistulas. J Neurointerventional Surg 2022;neurintsurg-2022:019005.

28. Parizadeh D, Fermo O, Vibhute P, et al. Transvenous embolization of cerebrospinal fluid-venous fistulas: Independent validation and feasibility of upper-extremity approach and using dual-microcatheter and balloon pressure cooker technique. J Neurointerventional Surg 2023;jnis-2022:019946.

29. Kong DS, Park K, Nam DH, et al. Clinical features and long-term results of spontaneous intracranial hypotension. Neurosurgery 2005;57:91–6 [discussion: 91–6].

30. Montenegro MM, Kissoon NR, Atkinson JLD, et al. Clinical and imaging outcomes of surgically repaired cerebrospinal fluid-venous fistulas identified by lateral decubitus digital subtraction myelography. World Neurosurg 2023;S1878-8750(23):00831–8.

31. Berroir S, Loisel B, Ducros A, et al. Early epidural blood patch in spontaneous intracranial hypotension. Neurology 2004;63(10):1950–1.

32. Schievink WI, Maya M, Prasad RS, et al. Spontaneous spinal cerebrospinal fluid-venous fistulas in patients with orthostatic headaches and normal conventional brain and spine imaging. Headache 2021 Feb;61(2):387–91.

33. Mamlouk MD, Shen PY, Sedrak MF, et al. CT-guided fibrin glue occlusion of cerebrospinal fluid-venous fistulas. Radiology 2021;299(2):409–18.

34. Wang TY, Karikari IO, Amrhein TJ, et al. Clinical outcomes following surgical ligation of cerebrospinal fluid-venous fistula in patients with spontaneous intracranial hypotension: a prospective case series. Oper Neurosurg Hagerstown Md 2020;18(3):239–45.

35. Lohkamp LN, Marathe N, Nicholson P, et al. Minimally invasive surgery for spinal cerebrospinal fluid-venous fistula ligation: patient series. J Neurosurg Case Lessons 2022;3(18):CASE21730.

Practical Applications of Artificial Intelligence in Spine Imaging: A Review

Upasana Upadhyay Bharadwaj, MD[a,1], Cynthia T. Chin, MD[b,1,*], Sharmila Majumdar, PhD[a]

KEYWORDS

- Artificial intelligence • Machine learning • Deep learning • Spine

KEY POINTS

- Artificial intelligence (AI) tools enable automated vertebral, disc, neuroforamen, canal, and facet segmentation.
- AI may enhance spine imaging reconstruction improving image quality, acquisition time, and reduced radiation dose.
- AI may assist characterizing common spine conditions: degeneration; infection; inflammation; trauma; metastatic disease; and deformity.
- AI clinical deployment may assist semiautomated reporting under radiologist supervision to provide more consistent, objective, and efficient reporting.

INTRODUCTION

Recent artificial intelligence (AI) advances may potentially transform all aspects of radiology including acquisition, interpretation, and radiology report generation, enhancing accuracy, efficiency, and clinical utility.[1–6]

AI enables automated vertebral, disc, and canal segmentation even with noise, artifacts, and anatomic variations.[7,8] Models for training large data sets can identify complex features, enhancing diagnosis and classification of fractures, tumors, or degeneration.[9] Specialized algorithms and variational autoencoders may reconstruct images from undersampled/noisy data, resulting in faster acquisition times while preserving diagnostic accuracy.[10,11]

AI capabilities present opportunities for clinical applications in spine imaging: early detection improving patient outcomes, enhanced diagnosis and surgical planning, improved patient experience with faster acquisition times, and assisting radiologists' efficiency with end-to-end tools for automation.[12]

With exponential increased publications on novel imaging AI, assessing a particular approach's practical utility and clinical relevance is challenging. This review presents an AI overview for practical spine imaging and potential clinical adoption.

OVERVIEW OF ARTIFICIAL INTELLIGENCE

AI broadly encompasses techniques enabling computer systems to perform tasks typically requiring human intelligence.[13] AI algorithms enable computers to learn and perceive, through problem-solving, pattern recognition, decision-making, and natural language understanding.

AI can be classified into two main categories: narrow AI and general AI. Narrow AI systems perform specific tasks: image recognition, language translation, or playing chess and cannot

[a] Department of Radiology and Biomedical Imaging, University of California San Francisco, 1700 4th Street, Byers Hall, Suite 203, Room 203D, San Francisco, CA 94158, USA; [b] Department of Radiology and Biomedical Imaging, University of California San Francisco, 505 Parnassus Avenue, Box 0628, San Francisco, CA 94143, USA
[1] CT Chin and UU Bharadwaj contributed equally to the manuscript.
* Corresponding author.
E-mail address: cynthia.t.chin@ucsf.edu

Radiol Clin N Am 62 (2024) 355–370
https://doi.org/10.1016/j.rcl.2023.10.005

generalize beyond their specific expertise.[14] General AI represents autonomous systems that learn and apply knowledge across various domains. General AI, while a goal for future research and development, is largely a theoretic discipline.

Although AI, "machine learning" (ML), and "deep learning" (DL) are sometimes used interchangeably, there are major differences between each of these related terms (**Fig. 1**).

Machine Learning

ML, the foundation of AI, is a subset focusing on algorithms and statistical models enabling computers to automatically learn and make predictions or decisions based on data. ML can be broadly categorized into supervised, unsupervised, and reinforcement learning.[15]

Supervised learning involves training a model on labeled data, the input data and corresponding output or target labels are provided. The model learns to generalize from the training data and make predictions or decisions on new, unseen data. This approach is commonly used for classification, regression, and object detection tasks in medical imaging applications.[16]

Unsupervised learning trains models on unlabeled data, discovering hidden patterns, structures, or relationships. Clustering, dimensionality reduction, and anomaly detection are some common applications of unsupervised learning. In medical imaging, unsupervised learning techniques can aid in tasks such as data exploration, grouping similar images, or identifying outliers.[17,18]

In reinforcement learning, an agent interacts with an environment and improves its performance by receiving feedback (rewards or penalties). This approach, used in robotics and control systems, learns optimal actions through trial and error. It has limited practical use in medical imaging but has potential for future applications such as optimizing imaging protocols or designing personalized treatment plans.[19]

Deep Learning

DL, a subset of ML, has recently gained tremendous success.[1,20] It involves training artificial neural networks with multiple layers, allowing the model to learn complex hierarchical representations directly from raw data. Neural networks, mathematical or computer models mimicking the structure and function of biological neural networks (the central nervous system—the brain), consist of a large number of artificial neurons made using a variety of connection techniques: convolutional neural network (CNN), generative adversarial networks (GANs), and recurrent neural networks are examples.[21]

CNN, a widely used DL medical imaging architecture, excels in image reconstruction, segmentation, and classification.[22–25] AI's success in medical imaging is driven by the availability of large, labeled data sets, advancements in computational power, and development of DL models.[26]

APPLICATIONS IN SPINE IMAGING
Image Reconstruction and Acquisition

AI may enhance spine imaging reconstruction, improve image quality, acquisition time, and reduce radiation dose.

AI can reduce MR imaging (MRI) and CT image noise, using DL techniques learning noise patterns in data. DL noise reduction algorithm improved signal-to-noise ratio (SNR) of lumbar spine (LS) MRI scans up to 30%.[27] DL reconstruction algorithms can enhance MR image resolution by learning relationships between different coordinates in the image, significantly improving LS MR image quality.[28,29]

LS CT studies show DL-enhanced images have significantly lower noise compared with the original scan.[30] Reducing radiation dose in LS CT scans is an important direction in image reconstruction from fewer data points with high-quality images acquired at doses up to 72% lower than standard of care (SOC).[31]

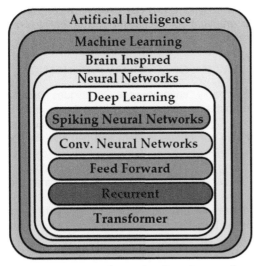

Fig. 1. AI taxonomy with associated learning paradigms. (https://www.researchgate.net/figure/Taxonomy-of-AI-and-its-sub-fields_fig1_352189762.) Khan, F.H.; Pasha, M.A.; Masud, S. Advancements in Microprocessor Architecture for Ubiquitous AI—An Overview on History, Evolution, and Upcoming Challenges in AI Implementation. Micromachines 2021, 12, 665. https://doi.org/10.3390/mi12060665.

Fast MR Acquisition

Reconstruction and noise reduction techniques can also reduce LS MR imaging acquisition times. A rapid LS MR imaging protocol, 3D imaging with DL reconstruction, yielded 54% acquisition time reduction.[32]

Fast MR acquisitions modify conventional imaging protocol parameters, decreasing scan times while maintaining resolution at the cost of increased image noise (reduced SNR). Common strategies shortening acquisition times exploit k-space data redundancy or spatial correlation. Modifications include reducing excitations, raising bandwidth, and increasing parallel imaging factors. These acceleration approaches inherently suffer from reduced SNR, blurring, resulting in insufficient imaging quality. DL-based image denoising methods applied to compromised fast scan data can restore SNR, maintaining image sharpness and SOC quality.[33]

Using a DL reconstruction method to improve SNR and reduce artifacts (commercially available AIR Recon DL, GE Healthcare) on LS MR images, Han and colleagues demonstrated DL reconstruction combined with fast acquisitions has potential for diagnostic image quality noninferior to SOC LS MRIs. The LS MR imaging protocol was 52% faster and able to provide scores noninferior to the standard protocol for apparent SNR, anatomic structure visualization, and diagnostic confidence as evaluated in a blinded fashion by one junior and two senior subspecialty radiologists[34] **(Fig. 2)**.

A prospective, randomized, multicenter study assessed DL enhancement to preserve perceived spine MR imaging quality despite 40% scan time reduction. Three experienced neuroradiologists rated perceived superiority of 61 spine MR images for SNR; spatial resolution; imaging artifacts; cord delineation; cord/cerebrospinal fluid (CSF) contrast; disc pathology; bone lesions; and facet/ligamentous pathology. The readers assessed image consistency for anatomy and pathology and found overall diagnostic quality of DL-enhanced MR images statistically equivalent or subjectively better (perceived benefits in SNR and artifact reduction) than SOC across all assessed features, suggesting potential for clinical practice utility.[35]

Synthetic Artificial Intelligence

Synthesizing new images from available images is an active MR imaging research area. DL reconstruction can create synthetic images from existing data sets. Virtually generated MR imaging may make the physical acquisition of particular sequences no longer necessary. GANs can generate synthetic images from different MR contrasts as input. A GAN (generator network and discriminator network) learns to synthesize realistic images (generator) and distinguish real from fake (synthesized) images (discriminator). During the learning process, these networks compete against each other, resulting in the generator network progressively learning to synthesize images with more and more realistic appearances.[36]

T2-weighted (T2W) fat sat (FS) spine sequences are important, requiring significant scan time. Using GAN-generated T2WFS images from conventional T1W and non-FS T2W images, Schlaeger and colleagues compared synthetic T2WFS images to their true counterparts for image quality, FS quality, and diagnostic agreement.

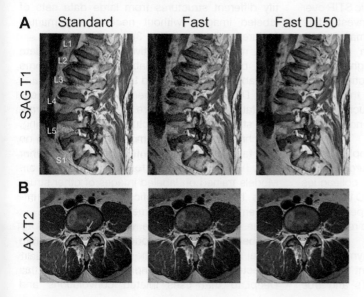

A Standard   Fast   Fast DL50

SAG T1

B

AX T2

Fig. 2. Comparison of standard versus fast versus fast DL50 imaging on sag T1 axial T2 sequences. (*A*) L5–S1 transitional anatomy, moderate NF stenosis (solid *arrow*), severe L4–L5 facet arthropathy (dashed *arrows*). (*B*) Central annular fissure (solid *arrow*). These features are well delineated on fast DL50 images.[34]

Apparent signal- and contrast-to-noise ratios measured in true and synthetic T2WFS sequences by two neuroradiologists were not significantly different. Subjective image quality was graded higher for synthetic T2WFS (*P*=.023). In a Turing test, synthetic and true T2WFS could not be distinguished from each other. The inter-method agreement between synthetic and original protocol ranged from substantial to almost perfect agreement for six evaluated spine pathologies. Overall scan time was reduced approximately 40% compared with conventional spine examinations.[37]

A multicenter, multireader study evaluated synthetically created short tau inversion recovery (STIR) spine MR images compared with acquired STIR. A digital imaging and communications in medicine (DICOM)-based DL application generated a synthetically created STIR series from sagittal T1 and T2 images. Three neuroradiologists, one musculoskeletal (MSK) radiologist, and one general radiologist rated STIR quality and classified disease pathology; assessed presence/absence of findings typically evaluated with STIR in trauma. The radiologists evaluated either acquired STIR or synthetically created STIR in a blinded and randomized fashion with a 1-month washout period. The interchangeability of acquired and synthetically created STIR was assessed using a noninferiority threshold of 10%.

For classification, there was a decrease in inter-reader agreement expected by randomly introducing synthetically created STIR of 3.23%. For trauma, there was an overall increase in inter-reader agreement by 11.9%. The lower bound of confidence for both exceeded the noninferiority threshold, indicating interchangeability of synthetically created with acquired STIR. Results showed higher image quality scores for synthetic STIR over acquired STIR (*P*<.0001). The investigators concluded synthetic STIR spine MR images were diagnostically interchangeable with acquired STIR while providing significantly higher image quality, suggesting routine clinical practice potential. The investigators also avoided the use of GANs, which can be prone to introducing structures in synthesized images that are not present in the source images.[38]

CT and MR imaging are complimentary, routinely obtained for evaluation and surgical planning in spine patients. Roberts and colleagues developed a DL algorithm producing 3D LS CT images from MR imaging data using a supervised 3D cycle-GAN model, thus the potential to reduce patient radiation.[36]

They evaluated the accuracy of synthetic LS CTs by comparing 24 clinically relevant measurements on 20 matched synthetic CTs and true CTs by four clinical evaluators (neurosurgeons and radiologists). The outcome measured was the mean difference in measurements performed by the group of evaluators between real CT and synthetic CTs. Measurements in the sagittal plane had a10% relative error and pedicle measurements in the axial plane were considerably less accurate (relative error up to 34%). The investigators concluded that computer-generated synthetic CTs demonstrated a high level of accuracy when performed in-plane to original MR images used for synthesis. Measurements performed on axial reconstructed images were less accurate, attributable to the images being synthesized from nonvolumetric sagittal T1W MR images.[36]

LOCALIZATION OF SPINAL STRUCTURES

Localization of spinal structures on imaging is essential for accurate diagnosis and treatment.[7,8,39,40] They are used to enhance the performance of end-to-end DL systems and also as intermediate visualization tools that can assist diagnosis. The finest form of localization is segmentation, structural delineation from images. Similarity of various vertebrae, curvature, hardware artifacts, and transitional vertebrae are some challenges developing and implementing AI solutions for automatic labeling.[41,42]

Before DL, segmented structures were traditionally processed with thresholding (classifying pixels as foreground or background based on intensity, texture features). More sophisticated techniques such as contour modeling and watershed transform group pixels iteratively based on image gradients improved performance.[43]

DL, a powerful tool for segmentation, can identify different structures from large data sets of labeled images, without necessitating manual feature engineering[8] (**Fig. 3**).

DL models require relatively large, labeled data sets, because as more labeled images become available, the models tend to be more accurate.[44] New DL architectures specifically for spine segmentation tend to be more efficient and accurate than standard DL architectures. Transfer learning, a technique allowing DL models to be trained on one task and subsequently applied to another task, has been effective for spine segmentation. Models trained on labeled images of other structures have shown significant performance improvements to spine segmentation.[45]

The U-Net architecture with skip connections has been the de facto model to precisely localize spinal structures using the encoder–decoder architecture.[46] Several improvements, such as DeepLab that uses dilated convolutions and

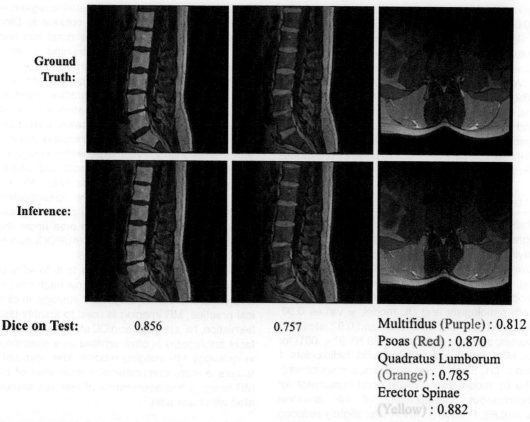

Ground Truth:

Inference:

Dice on Test: 0.856   0.757   Multifidus (Purple) : 0.812
Psoas (Red) : 0.870
Quadratus Lumborum
(Orange) : 0.785
Erector Spinae
(Yellow) : 0.882

Fig. 3. Vertebral, disc, and paraspinal muscle segmentation results (first, second, and third columns, respectively).[8]

atrous spatial pyramid pooling, have become popular given their overall performance and ability to capture multiscale contextual information for accurate spine segmentation.[47] A recent study using U-Net achieved a dice score of 0.85 for segmenting discs on spine MR images.[7,8,48,49] Using Deep-Lab achieved a Jaccard index of 0.82 for vertebral CT segmentation. Three-dimensional (3D) CNNs have shown superior performance in segmenting complex spine structures, achieving dice scores over 0.90 for various structures.[7,8]

CLASSIFYING AND DIAGNOSING SPINE PATHOLOGIES
Degenerative Spine

Given the increasing prevalence of spinal degenerative disease, there is great potential for AI-assisted ML MR imaging interpretation to streamline care for these patients. In providing rapid automated analysis of MR imaging scans, ML technology may also assist in reducing radiologist workloads. ML models can generate quantitative parameters

from imaging data, which are time-consuming for a radiologist to produce.

Spinal Stenosis

Clinically, spinal stenosis (SS) diagnosis relies on subjective evaluation, and spine MRIs are essential for accurate evaluation. DL is promising in automatically learning representative imaging features to perform classifications. Initially focused on automating vertebral numbering and disk classification, DL more recently has assessed automated SS grading. Studies have looked at individual ordinal/multiclass (normal, mild, moderate, severe) and binary/dichotomous stenosis grading (stenosis vs no stenosis; normal–mild vs moderate–severe; normal-mild-moderate vs severe).

Lu and colleagues developed a DL model (Deep Spine) to grade central canal (CC) and neural foramen (NF) stenosis using axial and sagittal T2W images. A large data set of LS MRIs was used but relied on natural language processing labels from existing radiology reports. Average class accuracy (normal, mild, moderate, or severe stenoses) was 70.6% CC and 67.1% NF stenosis.[49]

SpineNet,[42] a multitask architecture, developed automated classification of several spinal conditions, including CC stenosis on sagittal and axial T2W images.[50] SpineNet achieved agreement of 65.7% for ordinal gradings (normal, mild, moderate, or severe) compared with an expert radiologist and 94% (κ = 0.75) for binary/dichotomous grading of normal-mild-moderate versus severe stenosis compared with an experienced orthopedic surgeon.[51]

Lateral Recess Stenosis

Hallinan and colleagues showed comparable agreement with subspecialist radiologists for classifying CC and lateral recess stenosis, with slightly lower agreement for NF stenosis on LS MR imaging. Dichotomous classification (normal/mild vs moderate/severe) showed good agreement for both radiologists and DL model: κ values 0.98, 0.98, and 0.96 CC; 0.92, 0.95, and 0.92 lateral recesses; and 0.94, 0.95, and 0.89 NF (P < .001) for an MSK radiologist, subspecialist radiologists 1 and 2, (31, 5 and 9 year experience, respectively). The DL model also showed good agreement for dichotomous classification of NF stenosis (κ = 0.89; P < .001), which was slightly reduced compared with subspecialist radiologists (κ = 0.94, 0.95; P < .001). These results compare favorably with the average DL model from the SpineNet study, which had κ values 0.82, 0.96 for ordinal and dichotomous classification of CC stenosis, respectively (P < .001).[40]

Facet Arthropathy

Bharadwaj and colleagues proposed a two-staged learning system that automatically evaluated T2W axial LS MR images classifying CC and NF stenosis and for the first time facet arthropathy (Fig. 4).

The first stage—localization of anatomic regions—was performant with excellent volumetric Dice scores (well above 0.90) for the dural sac and disk, and with no additional training or fine-tuning, localization of the foramen and facet was also favorable. In the second stage, the interpretable approach to multiclass grading (normal, mild, moderate, severe) of CC stenosis was in line with pairwise agreements between three radiologists (two senior subspecialty radiologists each with greater than 20 year experience; one junior radiologist with 3 year experience) and significantly outperformed a black-box CNN. Models also showed accurate binary classification (normal/mild vs moderate/severe) of both NF stenosis and facet arthropathy with area under the receiver operating characteristic (AUROC) curves 0.92 and 0.93, respectively (Fig. 5).

Facet arthropathy, prevalent in 15% to 45% of patients presenting with chronic low back pain, is a very important underdiagnosed etiology. In clinical practice, MR imaging is used to identify disc herniation, NF stenosis, and CC stenosis, whereas facet arthropathy is often omitted as a descriptor in radiology MR imaging reports. This approach targets a more comprehensive evaluation of LS MR imaging and assessment of features associated with back pain.[7]

Modic Changes

Modic changes (MCs), endplate–adjacent marrow signal abnormalities representing sequela of structural and inflammatory changes, are hypothesized to be potentially associated with pain. MC type 1: edema or fibrovascular changes (hypointense T1W, hyperintense T2W images); MC type 2: fatty marrow (hyperintense T1W, iso-hyperintense T2WFS, and non-FS T2W sequences, respectively); MC type 3: sclerotic (hypointense on both sequences). The semiquantitative nature of MC classification is highly susceptible to variability in

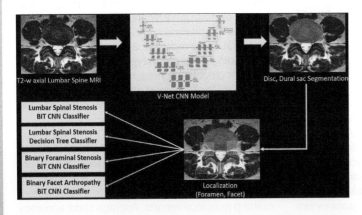

Fig. 4. Overview of DL-pipeline. Axial T2-weighted slices passed into V-Net segmentation models obtain masks for disc and dural sac (DDS). Geometric rules based on DDS localize foramen and facet bounding boxes and passes into its corresponding classifier: Big Transfer (BiT) CNN classifies lumbar SS, foraminal stenosis, and facet arthropathy. Lumbar SS interpretable classification (decision tree) relies on additional quantitative metrics extracted from the DDS segmentations.[7]

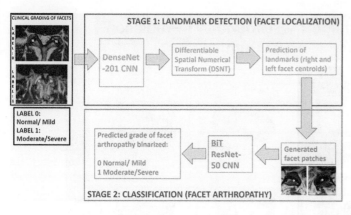

Fig. 5. Second stage: landmark detection (facet localization) and binary classification (facet arthropathy). Landmark coordinate regression system uses a DSNT (differentiable spatial-to-numerical transform) layer on the top of a DenseNet–CNN backbone architecture to predict two coordinates per slice, corresponding to right and left facet. Crop patches of facets (36 mm × 36 mm bounding boxes) center around predicted facet landmarks. Green, ground truth; Red, model prediction. Binary classification model (BiT) with a ResNet-50 backbone architecture classifies the patches from first stage as normal/mild versus moderate/severe arthropathy.[7].

non-standardized imaging.[52] Wang and colleagues extracted morphologic and signal intensity-based metrics from contours of MCs, reporting improved inter- and intra-rater agreement compared with unassisted MC classification.[53] The need for labor-intensive manual demarcation of MCs is a significant limitation.

Gao and colleagues used DL-based models to automatically map MCs. Overall, these results demonstrate substantial agreement of the detection model with radiologist-annotated grading and a novel Modic mapping technique providing grading assistance. MCs are often transitional (27.2% regarded as mixed, comprising characteristics of multiple Modic types).[54] Capturing this granularity of mixed MCs is challenging for the human eye. A voxel-wise MC segmentation method was therefore implemented due to its key capability of visualizing the heterogeneity of mixed MCs. In addition, the segmentation methodology offers higher degree of supervision, retaining context of the neighboring tissue and improving label specificity. Further works using this approach can unravel attributes of progressive or transitional MCs that may interact with pain, as heterogeneous tissues are often correlated with degeneration[9] (Fig. 6).

In the MC detection component, the distribution of predicted MCs across the LS was predominantly in the L4–S1 range (74.4%), matching well with the radiologist annotations (78.8%) and past work (75.5%).[54] MC voxel-wise classification yielded high predictive value of MC types 1 and 2, the groups most important to classify due to their prevalence and strong association of MC 1 with nonspecific low back pain (LBP).[55] The additional utility of the model predictions improved agreement of the junior radiologist (3 year experience) grading the MCs with the two senior (each >25 year experience) subspecialty radiologists ($\Delta\kappa = +0.06$ and $\Delta\kappa = +0.03$ reader 1 and reader 2, respectively).[9]

Spine Infection and Inflammation

Modic changes versus pyogenic spondylitis

Spinal infection diagnosis is difficult due to nonspecific clinical and laboratory findings. Noninfectious conditions can mimic the imaging findings of spondylodiscitis and it can be difficult to distinguish between degenerative and infectious endplate abnormalities.

MC type 1 can mimic infection on MR imaging. Differences between inflammatory, degenerative, and infectious pathologies have a significant impact on prognosis. Many imaging techniques, including conventional plain radiography, CT, MR imaging, and radionuclide studies, have been used to diagnose spinal infections.

A retrospective study evaluated the performance of a CNN to differentiate pyogenic spondylitis from MC on MR imaging. Fifty MRIs, each from pyogenic spondylitis and MC patients, were reviewed, comparing the performance of the CNN to four clinicians: a radiologist, spine surgeon, and two orthopedic surgeons (17, 20, 5–6 year experience, respectively).

The CNN-based AUROC curve from the T1 weighted image (T1W), T2W, and STIR images was 0.95, 0.94, and 0.95, respectively. The accuracy of the CNN was significantly greater than that of the four clinicians on T1W and STIR ($P < .05$), and better than a radiologist and one orthopedic surgeon on the T2W ($P < .05$). The sensitivity was significantly better than the four clinicians on T1W and STIR ($P < .05$) and better than a radiologist and one orthopedic surgeon on the T2W ($P < .05$). The specificity was significantly better than one orthopedic surgeon on T1W and T2W ($P < .05$) and better than both orthopedic

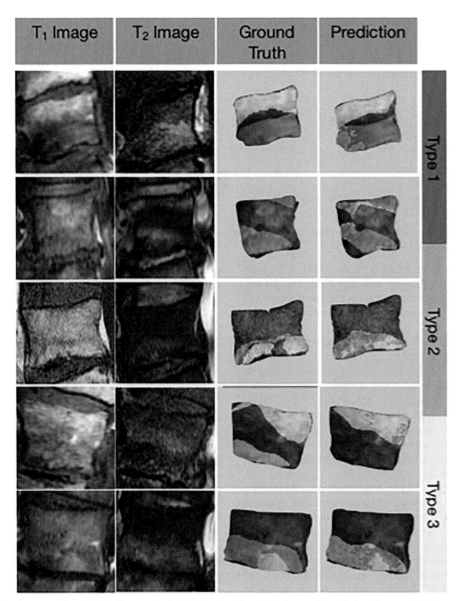

Fig. 6. Modic maps. Representative examples of inputs (T$_1$ and T$_2$ images), radiologist-annotated ground truth segmentations, predicted Modic maps. Model is advantageous for visualizing heterogeneity and transitional pathology: top row: model detects MC type 3 in anterior inferior endplate; second row: small MC type1 region in anterior superior endplate, unmarked by the radiologist and annotated by the model.[9]

surgeons on STIR (P < .05). The investigators concluded that the CNN model was able to differentiate between MCs and pyogenic spondylitis and the model performance was comparable to, or better than, that of the radiologist, spine surgeon, and two orthopedic surgeons.[56]

Multiple sclerosis

The spinal cord (SC) is frequently affected by demyelinating lesions and atrophy in multiple sclerosis (MS) patients. Spinal cord and lesion segmentation may provide diagnosis, prognosis, and longitudinal monitoring in MS. Automating segmentation may assist in decreasing inter-rater variability and increase efficiency of large-throughput analysis pipelines. Precise outlining of lesions is challenging due to their heterogeneity, and reliable segmentation across multisite SC data is difficult due to variability related to acquisition parameters and image artifacts.

Gros and colleagues created an original automated SC and MS lesion segmentation method based on two CNNs (Spinal Cord Toolbox [SCT], open-source readily available). When compared against manual segmentation, the investigators demonstrated this CNN-based approach showed a median Dice of 95% versus 88% compared with PropSeg (P < .05), a state-of-the-art SC segmentation method. On MS data, the framework provided a Dice of 60%, a relative volume difference of 15%, and a lesion-wise detection sensitivity and precision of 83% and 77%, respectively. Their SC segmentation results outperformed a state-of-the-art method on a multisite and highly heterogeneous clinical data set. Lesion segmentation results were generally within range of manual segmentations, although the false-positive rate (FP) warrants further investigations.[57]

Spine Trauma

Fracture

AI has been studied for detecting both osteoporotic and traumatic spinal fractures. The clinical management of these patients requires timely and accurate interpretation of volumetric imaging. Automated image analysis has the potential to streamline care of patient with spinal fractures.

Osteoporotic Tomita and colleagues compared a CNN model detecting osteoporotic vertebral fractures (VFs) to the radiologists' diagnoses from 1432 CT scan radiology reports. The CNN achieved an accuracy of 89.2% and F1 score of 90.8% on the test/validation data set (F1 score: ML metric measuring model accuracy). Although the F1 score for the model matched the performance of practicing radiologists on the test set, the radiologists' diagnoses were more precise and had higher specificity relative to the model. The investigators proposed the model could be used to assist and improve the diagnosis of osteoporotic VFs in clinical settings by pre-screening routine CT examinations and flagging suspicious cases before review by radiologists.[58]

Bush and colleagues created an automated ML system to detect and classify osteoporotic VFs according to Genant standards and to measure bone density of thoracic and lumbar vertebral bodies on CT using 3D CT images. They retrospectively analyzed 210 thoracic and lumbar vertebrae with VFs that were electronically marked and classified by a radiologist.

The sensitivity for detection/localization was 95.7% with a FP of 0.29 per patient. Sensitivity was 98.7% and specificity was 77.3% at case-based ROC curve analysis. Accuracy for classification by Genant type (anterior, middle, or posterior height loss) was 0.95 with weighted κ = 0.90. Accuracy for categorization by Genant height loss grade was 0.68, with a weighted κ = 0.59. The average bone attenuation for

T12–L4 vertebrae was 146 HU±29 (standard deviation) in patients versus 173 HU±42 in controls (P < .001).[59]

Traumatic thoracic lumbar Murata and colleagues used a CNN on anteroposterior and lateral thoracolumbar radiographs of 300 patients to detect VFs with accuracy 86% and sensitivity 84.7%. They compared model performance with orthopedic surgeons and residents and determined it was non-inferior to orthopedic surgeons and had superior sensitivity compared with orthopedic residents. The model did not reveal which vertebra was fractured.[60]

Burns and colleagues also designed an automated system for retrospective detection/localization of traumatic thoracic and lumbar VFs on CT in 104 patients compared with the localizations and classifications marked by a radiologist according to Denis column involvement.

Testing set sensitivity for the detection and localization of fractures within each vertebra was 0.81, with an FP of 2.7. The most common cause of FPs was nutrient foramina (39%).

Origins of false-negative (FN) findings (misses) and FP fracture line detections were decided in a consensus review by two board-certified fellowship-trained radiologists (19 years of experience). Most of FNs were fracture lines paralleling in close proximity to vertebral end plates and to degenerative joint disease.

The investigators concluded their fully automated computer system detected and anatomically localized thoracic and lumbar VFs on CT with a high sensitivity and a low FP rate.[61]

Traumatic cervical Cervical spine injury can be associated with high morbidity and mortality. Multidetector CT has emerged as a critical SOC imaging technique to evaluate cervical spine trauma for rapid diagnosis and intervention.

An FDA-approved CNN by Aidoc (www. aidoc. com) to detect cervical VFs on CT was used to analyze 665 examinations. Ground truth was established by retrospective visualization of VFs on CT using all available CTs, MRIs and CNN output information. The finalized cervical spine CT reports were simultaneously independently reviewed by two fellowship-trained neuroradiologists.

The CNN sensitivity (79%) was lower than the radiologists (93%) and CNN accuracy of 92% compared with 96% for the radiologists. Time from image acquisition to CNN analysis was shorter than time from image acquisition to radiologist report finalization emphasizing the value of the CNN in worklist prioritization. CNN false-negative examinations demonstrated that the locations of CNN misses closely matched those of radiologists, similar by level and location. Fractures the CNN missed included severe fracture–dislocation, distractions, distal spinous processes, and lower cervical spine where fine bony detail was obscured by CT beam attenuation. There were a few instances in which the CNN detected a fracture that the radiologist missed, underscoring the ability of the CNN to function as a useful complementary tool in fracture detection that radiologists would review before report finalization.[62]

Spinal Cord Injury

The degree of abnormal T2 signal on sagittal and axial MR imaging has strongly correlated with diagnostic and prognostic value after SC injury (SCI). The intramedullary lesion length (IMLL) and the Brain and Spinal Injury Center (BASIC) score are two metrics based on single two-dimensional (2D) images that are approximations for true 3D size and distribution of injured SC.

The SCT[63] is an open-source anatomic atlas allowing quantitative volumetric injury analysis. Using a semiautomated image processing pipeline incorporating many tools available freely as part of the open-source SCT, volumetric injury measures were extracted from preoperative MR images in 47 patients who underwent 3T MR imaging within 24 hours of SCI. This customized image analysis and processing pipeline integrated three different novel 2D-CNN architectures for both whole SC and traumatic lesion segmentation. Segmentation results from CNNs were compared with each other and with standard manual segmentation as well as with two current state-of-the-art SC segmentation algorithms (PropSeg; DeepSeg). Compared with manual labeling, the average test set Dice coefficient for the BASIC segmentation model was 0.93 for SC segmentation versus 0.80 for PropSeg and 0.90 for DeepSeg (both SCT components).

These segmented volumetric measures predicted lower extremity motor function at discharge from the hospital more strongly than standard 2D radiographic parameters including BASIC score and IMLL. The investigators concluded that the volume of the T2 lesion after SCI was a more accurate imaging biomarker of injury severity than conventional 2D MR imaging measures of injury[64] (**Fig. 7**).

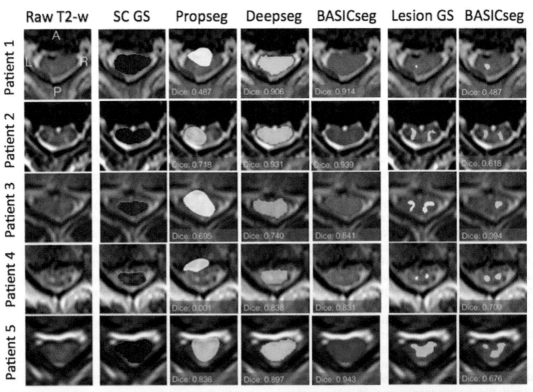

Fig. 7. Whole SC and lesion SC segmentation performance: BASICseg algorithms in five SCI patients at representative axial slices compared with manual ground truth segmentation (GS), PropSeg and DeepSeg models: column 1: conventional axial T2; columns 2 to 5: whole SC segmentation; columns 6 to 7: cord lesion segmentation. (*Courtesy* of JF Talbott, San Francisco, CA.[64])

Spine oncology

Radiomics-based feature analysis and CNNs are two popular ML imaging techniques used in oncology. Radiomics-based techniques extract first and higher order statistical features from radiological images. Interpretability of radiomic features has been a major limitation of radiomics as the features are not standardized and there is difficulty relating them to the underlying biology of the tissue of interest. As the features are limited to the knowledge of the radiologist or clinician, the accuracy of the developed algorithm could be reduced.[65,66]

Differentiating Benign Versus Metastatic Vertebral Fractures

Differentiating benign VFs from pathologic/malignant VFs is critically important for treatment decisions. A novel Two-Stream Compare and Contrast Network (TSCCN: three-class classification: normal, benign, and malignant VFs)[67] model was tested on 239 VFs on median sagittal T1W, T2WFS, and a combination T1W/T2WFS sequences.

Three radiologists (11, 15, and 8 year experience) assessed the same MR images twice at different times within 1 month and were blinded to patient history, treatment details for fair comparison with the TSCCN.

The model achieved average sensitivity, specificity, and accuracy of 92.6%, 96.3%, and 95.2%, respectively. The sensitivity of the model overlapped or was less than the sensitivity of the most experienced radiologist; the accuracy and specificity of the model was higher than achieved by the radiologists. The investigators concluded that the model had the potential to enhance VF diagnostic accuracy, sensitivity, and specificity.[68]

Deformity

ML has also analyzed spinal deformity. Spinal parameters are time-consuming to manually annotate and inter-rater reliability can vary. Research has focused on automated quantitative spinal parameters localizing various landmarks: endplates, hip joints, S1 angle, T4–T12 kyphosis, L1–L5 lordosis, Cobb angle, pelvic incidence, sacral slope, and pelvic tilt. Although model-generated parameters can show good correlation to radiologist-derived values, the standard errors of the estimated parameters can range from 2.7 for pelvic tilt to 11.5 for L1–5 lordosis.[69,70]

Landmark annotations are not feasible within the clinical workflow as they require significant user input and are vulnerable to user error. Severe spinal deformity, overlapping soft tissues, lead shields, body habitus, osteoporosis, transitional anatomy, and variable skeletal maturities are several factors reducing visibility and reliable manual identification. Iriondo and colleagues developed a new method for automatic extraction of vertebral midline from biplanar radiographs and 3D spine shape models. The developed landmark extraction algorithms demonstrated robust performance across the tested data sets, are fully automatic, and may integrate into the clinical workflow, allowing temporal evaluation of deformity progression (**Figs. 8** and **9**).

A surprising finding was the range in actual sagittal and coronal imbalance among images linked to radiology reports stating "no imbalance" with true measurements of approximately ±2.5 cm of coronal imbalance and ±5 cm sagittal imbalance. This has important implications, when no exact measurement was provided, qualitative descriptions of spinal alignment were subjective.[71]

CLINICAL IMPLEMENTATION

Many AI models discussed can be integrated into automated reading workflow. Reporting individual spinal CC and NF stenoses, disc, and facet degeneration is time-consuming. Clinically deploying DL models could assist in semiautomated reporting under radiologist supervision to provide more consistent, objective, and efficient reporting.

A published DL algorithm, Spine AI, automatically classifies LS CC, lateral recess, and NF stenoses on LS MRIs.[72] Eight radiologists (2–13 year experience), retrospectively reviewed studies with and without DL assistance with a 1-month washout were compared with test data labeled by an external MSK radiologist (32 year experience) as standard. Interpretation time reduced 62% to 74% for DL-assisted radiologists: mean 124-274 to 47-71 seconds (P < .001) with greatest time savings for in-training radiologists: mean 274 (unassisted) to 71 seconds (assisted) (P < .001).

DL-assisted radiologists had superior or equivalent interobserver agreement for all stenosis gradings compared with unassisted radiologists. DL-assisted general and in-training radiologists improved their interobserver agreement for four-class NF stenosis, κ = 0.71 and 0.70 (DL) versus 0.39 without DL, respectively (both P < .001).[73]

DL assistance can streamline report generation, which involves image review and a separate text input into a reporting module. DL assistance can detect regions of interest (ROIs), grade stenosis, and automatically generate a sentence directly into the reporting module. The radiologist can change and control the DL-assisted predictions before a report is generated, important for safety and patient preference.[74] Strategic "one-click" solutions integrated within the normal radiologist workflow will be prerequisite for successful implementation.[75]

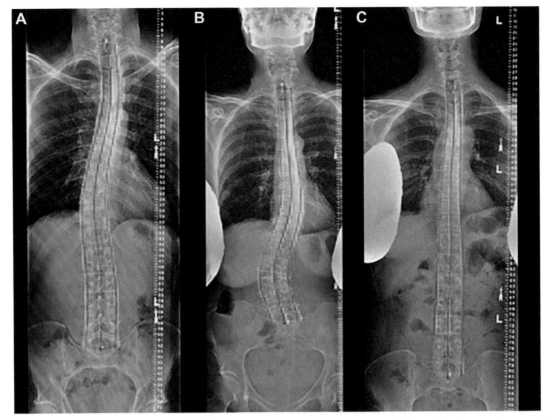

Fig. 8. Frontal spinal radiographs show accurate spine midline identification: model predicted curves (magenta) closely correlate with ground truth curves (blue). Paired dashed lines (—): spine contour curves; Center solid lines (—): midline curves.

CHALLENGES AND FUTURE DIRECTIONS

Most of the AI spine imaging studies are retrospective, single-center with small sample sizes. Randomized, controlled, multicenter studies will be required to validate applications, facilitating clinical practice.[66,73] Future work will test pooled, publicly available data sets from collaborating institutions by multidisciplinary teams, comparing results with published work.[71] Increasing high-quality competitions (ie, 2022 RSNA cervical spine AI fracture challenge) may further research toward novel AI spine algorithms.

Required trained human input limits practical clinical implementation. Manual radiologist image labeling, most accurate for model training, is labor-intensive. Many models also require trained human post-processing (placing ROIs for segmentation).[40] Hardware and innovative data processing developing robust ML models with human-level performance will be needed.[75]

Cultural challenges are also barriers. ML tools requiring large, tens of thousands, annotated data sets face systemic data privacy concerns (storage, transmission, usage) subject to strict regulations despite standard data anonymization.[70]

Another cultural challenge, AI perceived as a "black box," relates to the opaque nature of DL systems. We see the input and output; however, the system's code or logic producing the output is not inherently transparent. Explainable AI is a branch attempting to make the methodology transparent to users.

Medical accountability is another challenge. Would the clinician using the ML system or its manufacturer be responsible for an AI-generated misdiagnosis? This also affects marketing approval and cost of novel AI tools, requiring deeper testing and verification relative to other technologies and longer time to market.[76]

Potential biases are concerning with unintended biases resulting from scarce data sets (rare pathologies, ethnicities) and privileged easier-accessed data sets.[77] Efforts toward governing AI aim to build robust public trust.[78] The European Union's General Data Protection Regulation expanded patient rights considerably with an explicit opt-in policy regarding data processing permission. Open

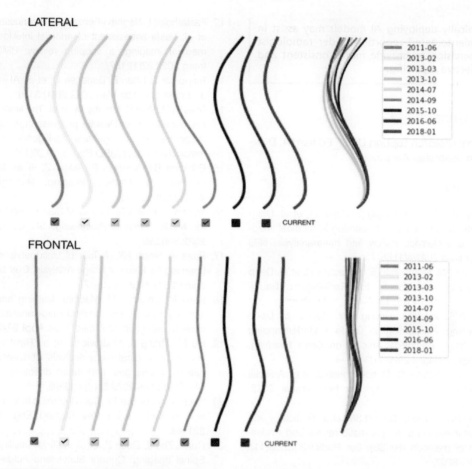

Fig. 9. Sagittal and coronal views of spine midlines in a 12-year-old boy monitored over 6.5 years allow overall comparisons demonstrating progressive levoscoliotic deformity over time.[71]

access to ML models and training data may improve public trust, accountability, and prediction bias. As models improve and clinicians more heavily rely on automated diagnoses, continued multidisciplinary collaboration involving radiologists, clinicians, engineers, data scientists, ethicists, and policy makers is mandatory globally.[76,75]

SUMMARY

AI potentially increases efficiency, reducing time-consuming tasks and assisting radiologists in specific diagnoses with a goal to provide comprehensive automated image analysis. Characterizing lesions and identifying lesions that might be missed are of great benefit, allowing earlier diagnoses, reporting, and treatment.[75] Combining clinical data with image analysis may permit improved and more personalized treatment decision-making. Although challenges remain, AI technology continues to rapidly progress with great potential to improve patient care and outcomes.[70]

CLINICS CARE POINTS

- Artificial intelligence (AI) models can assist in diagnosing spine pathologies such as degenerative disease, tumor, infection, fracture, with increasing sensitivity and specificity when used in parallel with radiologists' input and supervision.

- AI models integrated into automated reading workflow can significantly decrease interpretation time. This is most evident for radiologists in training.

- AI models can improve SNR and reduce artifacts inherent in rapid spine imaging protocols resulting in diagnostic quality imaging with 40-50% reduction in image acquisition time.

- AI models may assist in 'pre-screening' routine imaging examinations and flagging suspicious cases before review by radiologists. This allows added value through worklist prioritization.

- Clinically deploying AI models may assist in semiautomated reporting under radiologist supervision to provide more consistent and objective reporting.

DISCLOSURE

C.T. Chin research support UCSF Edward A. Dickson Professorship Award.

REFERENCES

1. Aggarwal R, Sounderajah V, Martin G, et al. Diagnostic accuracy of deep learning in medical imaging: a systematic review and meta-analysis. NPJ Digit Med 2021;4(1):65.

2. Cheng PM, Montagnon E, Yamashita R, et al. Deep Learning: An Update for Radiologists. Radiographics 2021;41(5):1427–45.

3. Do S, Song KD, Chung JW. Basics of Deep Learning: A Radiologist's Guide to Understanding Published Radiology Articles on Deep Learning. Korean J Radiol 2020;21(1):33–41.

4. Hosny A, Parmar C, Quackenbush J, et al. Artificial intelligence in radiology. Nat Rev Cancer 2018; 18(8):500–10.

5. Kelly BS, Judge C, Bollard SM, et al. Radiology artificial intelligence: a systematic review and evaluation of methods (RAISE). Eur Radiol 2022;32(11): 7998–8007.

6. Montagnon E, Cerny M, Cadrin-Chenevert A, et al. Deep learning workflow in radiology: a primer. Insights Imaging 2020;11(1):22.

7. Bharadwaj UU, Christine M, Li S, et al. Deep learning for automated, interpretable classification of lumbar spinal stenosis and facet arthropathy from axial MRI. Eur Radiol 2023;33(5): 3435–43.

8. Hess M, Allaire B, Gao KT. Deep Learning for Multi-Tissue Segmentation and Fully Automatic Personalized Biomechanical Models from BACPAC Clinical Lumbar Spine MRI. Pain Med 2022. https://doi.org/10.1093/pm/pnac142.

9. Gao KT, Tibrewala R, Hess M, et al. Automatic detection and voxel-wise mapping of lumbar spine Modic changes with deep learning. JOR Spine 2022;5(2):e1204.

10. Almansour H, Herrmann J, Gassenmaier S, et al. Deep Learning Reconstruction for Accelerated Spine MRI: Prospective Analysis of Interchangeability. Radiology 2023;306(3):e212922.

11. Schlaeger S, Drummer K, Husseini ME, et al. Implementation of GAN-Based, Synthetic T2-Weighted Fat Saturated Images in the Routine Radiological Workflow Improves Spinal Pathology Detection. Diagnostics 2023;13(5).

12. Fasterholdt I, Naghavi-Behzad M, Rasmussen BSB, et al. Value assessment of artificial intelligence in medical imaging: a scoping review. BMC Med Imag 2022;22(1):187.

13. Rajpurkar P, Chen E, Banerjee O, et al. AI in health and medicine. Nat Med 2022;28(1):31–8.

14. Shevlin H, Vold K, Crosby M, et al. The limits of machine intelligence: Despite progress in machine intelligence, artificial general intelligence is still a major challenge. EMBO Rep 2019;20(10):e49177.

15. Erickson BJ, Korfiatis P, Akkus Z, et al. Machine Learning for Medical Imaging. Radiographics 2017;37(2):505–15.

16. Aljuaid A, Anwar M. Survey of Supervised Learning for Medical Image Processing. SN Comput Sci 2022;3(4):292.

17. Raza K, Singh NK. A Tour of Unsupervised Deep Learning for Medical Image Analysis. Curr Med Imaging 2021;17(9):1059–77.

18. Rana M, Bhushan M. Machine learning and deep learning approach for medical image analysis: diagnosis to detection. Multimed Tools Appl 2022;1–39.

19. Hu M, Zhang J, Matkovic L, et al. Reinforcement learning in medical image analysis: Concepts, applications, challenges, and future directions. J Appl Clin Med Phys 2023;24(2):e13898.

20. Shen D, Wu G, Suk HI. Deep Learning in Medical Image Analysis. Annu Rev Biomed Eng 2017;19: 221–48.

21. Cui Y, Zhu J, Duan Z, et al. Artificial Intelligence in Spinal Imaging: Current Status and Future Directions. Int J Environ Res Publ Health 2022;19(18).

22. Yamashita R, Nishio M, Do RKG, et al. Convolutional neural networks: an overview and application in radiology. Insights Imaging 2018;9(4):611–29.

23. Soffer S, Ben-Cohen A, Shimon O, et al. Convolutional Neural Networks for Radiologic Images: A Radiologist's Guide. Radiology 2019;290(3): 590–606.

24. Tajbakhsh N, Shin JY, Gurudu SR, et al. Convolutional Neural Networks for Medical Image Analysis: Full Training or Fine Tuning? IEEE Trans Med Imag 2016;35(5):1299–312.

25. Sarvamangala DR, Kulkarni RV. Convolutional neural networks in medical image understanding: a survey. Evol Intell 2022;15(1):1–22.

26. Kiryati N, Landau Y. Dataset Growth in Medical Image Analysis Research. J Imaging 2021;7(8).

27. Kashiwagi N, Tanaka H, Yamashita Y, et al. Applicability of deep learning-based reconstruction trained by brain and knee 3T MRI to lumbar 1.5T MRI. Acta Radiol Open 2021;10(6). 20584601211023939.

28. Sun S, Tan ET, Mintz DN, et al. Evaluation of deep learning reconstructed high-resolution 3D lumbar spine MRI. Eur Radiol 2022;32(9):6167–77.

29. Zochowski KC, Tan ET, Argentieri EC, et al. Improvement of peripheral nerve visualization using a deep

learning-based MR reconstruction algorithm. Magn Reson Imaging 2022;85:186–92.

30. Yeoh H, Hong SH, Ahn C, et al. Deep Learning Algorithm for Simultaneous Noise Reduction and Edge Sharpening in Low-Dose CT Images: A Pilot Study Using Lumbar Spine CT. Korean J Radiol 2021; 22(11):1850–7.

31. Greffier J, Frandon J, Durand Q, et al. Contribution of an artificial intelligence deep-learning reconstruction algorithm for dose optimization in lumbar spine CT examination: A phantom study. Diagn Interv Imaging 2023;104(2):76–83.

32. Chazen JL, Tan ET, Fiore J, et al. Rapid lumbar MRI protocol using 3D imaging and deep learning reconstruction. Skeletal Radiol 2023;52(7):1331–8.

33. Zaharchuk G, Gong E, Wintermark M, et al. Deep Learning in Neuroradiology. AJNR Am J Neuroradiol 2018;39(10):1776–84.

34. Han M, Bahroos E, Hess ME, et al. Technology and Tool Development for BACPAC: Qualitative and Quantitative Analysis of Accelerated Lumbar Spine MRI with Deep-Learning Based Image Reconstruction at 3T. Pain Med 2023;24(Suppl 1):S149–59.

35. Bash S, Johnson B, Gibbs W, et al. Deep Learning Image Processing Enables 40% Faster Spinal MR Scans Which Match or Exceed Quality of Standard of Care : A Prospective Multicenter Multireader Study. Clin Neuroradiol 2022;32(1):197–203.

36. Roberts M, Hinton G, Wells AJ, et al. Imaging evaluation of a proposed 3D generative model for MRI to CT translation in the lumbar spine. Spine J 2023. https://doi.org/10.1016/j.spinee.2023.06.399.

37. Schlaeger S, Drummer K, El Husseini M, et al. Synthetic T2-weighted fat sat based on a generative adversarial network shows potential for scan time reduction in spine imaging in a multicenter test dataset. Eur Radiol 2023;33(8):5882–93.

38. Tanenbaum LN, Bash SC, Zaharchuk G, et al. Deep Learning-Generated Synthetic MR Imaging STIR Spine Images Are Superior in Image Quality and Diagnostically Equivalent to Conventional STIR: A Multicenter, Multireader Trial. AJNR Am J Neuroradiol 2023;44(8):987–93.

39. Cina A, Bassani T, Panico M, et al. 2-step deep learning model for landmarks localization in spine radiographs. Sci Rep 2021;11(1):9482.

40. Hallinan J, Zhu L, Yang K, et al. Deep Learning Model for Automated Detection and Classification of Central Canal, Lateral Recess, and Neural Foraminal Stenosis at Lumbar Spine MRI. Radiology 2021;300(1):130–8.

41. Chen Y, Gao Y, Li K, et al. Vertebrae Identification and Localization Utilizing Fully Convolutional Networks and a Hidden Markov Model. IEEE Trans Med Imag 2020;39(2):387–99.

42. Jamaludin A, Kadir T, Zisserman A. SpineNet: Automated classification and evidence visualization in spinal MRIs. Med Image Anal 2017;41:63–73.

43. Ghosh S, Chaudhary V. Supervised methods for detection and segmentation of tissues in clinical lumbar MRI. Comput Med Imag Graph 2014;38(7): 639–49.

44. Liebl H, Schinz D, Sekuboyina A, et al. A computed tomography vertebral segmentation dataset with anatomical variations and multi-vendor scanner data. Sci Data 2021;8(1):284.

45. Xuan J, Ke B, Ma W, et al. Spinal disease diagnosis assistant based on MRI images using deep transfer learning methods. Front Public Health 2023;11: 1044525.

46. Ronneberger O, Fischer P, Broz T. U-Net: Convolutional Networks for Biomedical Image Segmentation. arXiv. 2015.

47. Chen L-C, Papandreou G, Kokkinow I, Murphy K. DeepLab: Semantic Image Segmentation with Deep Convolutional Nets, Atrous Convolution, and Fully Connected CRFs. arXiv 2017.

48. Wang S, Jiang Z, Yang H, et al. Automatic Segmentation of Lumbar Spine MRI Images Based on Improved Attention U-Net. Comput Intell Neurosci 2022;2022:4259471.

49. Lu J-T, Pedemonte S, Bizzo B, et al. Deep spine: automated lumbar vertebral segmentation, disc-level designation, and spinal stenosis grading using deep learning. Proceedings of Machine Learning Research 2018;85:16.

50. Jamaludin A, Lootus M, Kadir T, et al. ISSLS PRIZE IN BIOENGINEERING SCIENCE 2017: Automation of reading of radiological features from magnetic resonance images (MRIs) of the lumbar spine without human intervention is comparable with an expert radiologist. Eur Spine J 2017;26(5):1374–83.

51. Ishimoto Y, Jamaludin A, Cooper C, et al. Could automated machine-learned MRI grading aid epidemiological studies of lumbar spinal stenosis? Validation within the Wakayama spine study. BMC Muscoskel Disord 2020;21(1):158.

52. Fields AJ, Battie MC, Herzog RJ, et al. Measuring and reporting of vertebral endplate bone marrow lesions as seen on MRI (Modic changes): recommendations from the ISSLS Degenerative Spinal Phenotypes Group. Eur Spine J 2019;28(10):2266–74.

53. Wang Y, Videman T, Niemelainen R, et al. Quantitative measures of modic changes in lumbar spine magnetic resonance imaging: intra- and inter-rater reliability. Spine 2011;36(15):1236–43.

54. Xu L, Chu B, Feng Y, et al. Modic changes in lumbar spine: prevalence and distribution patterns of end plate oedema and end plate sclerosis. Br J Radiol 2016;89(1060):20150650.

55. Jensen TS, Karppinen J, Sorensen JS, et al. Vertebral endplate signal changes (Modic change): a systematic literature review of prevalence and association with non-specific low back pain. Eur Spine J 2008;17(11):1407–22.

56. Mukaihata T, Maki S, Eguchi Y, et al. Differentiating Magnetic Resonance Images of Pyogenic Spondylitis and Spinal Modic Change Using a Convolutional Neural Network. Spine (Phila Pa 1976) 2023;48(4):288–94.

57. Gros C, De Leener B, Badji A, et al. Automatic segmentation of the spinal cord and intramedullary multiple sclerosis lesions with convolutional neural networks. Neuroimage 2019;184:901–15.

58. Tomita N, Cheung YY, Hassanpour S. Deep neural networks for automatic detection of osteoporotic vertebral fractures on CT scans. Comput Biol Med 2018;98:8–15.

59. Burns JE, Yao J, Summers RM. Vertebral Body Compression Fractures and Bone Density: Automated Detection and Classification on CT Images. Radiology 2017;284(3):788–97.

60. Murata K, Endo K, Aihara T, et al. Artificial intelligence for the detection of vertebral fractures on plain spinal radiography. Sci Rep 2020;10(1):20031.

61. Burns JE, Yao J, Munoz H, et al. Automated Detection, Localization, and Classification of Traumatic Vertebral Body Fractures in the Thoracic and Lumbar Spine at CT. Radiology 2016;278(1):64–73.

62. Small JE, Osler P, Paul AB, et al. CT Cervical Spine Fracture Detection Using a Convolutional Neural Network. AJNR Am J Neuroradiol 2021;42(7):1341–7.

63. De Leener B, Levy S, Dupont SM, et al. SCT: Spinal Cord Toolbox, an open-source software for processing spinal cord MRI data. Neuroimage 2017;145(Pt A):24–43.

64. McCoy DB, Dupont SM, Gros C, et al. Convolutional Neural Network-Based Automated Segmentation of the Spinal Cord and Contusion Injury: Deep Learning Biomarker Correlates of Motor Impairment in Acute Spinal Cord Injury. AJNR Am J Neuroradiol 2019;40(4):737–44.

65. Parekh VS, Jacobs MA. Deep learning and radiomics in precision medicine. Expert Rev Precis Med Drug Dev 2019;4(2):59–72.

66. Ong W, Zhu L, Zhang W, et al. Application of Artificial Intelligence Methods for Imaging of Spinal Metastasis. Cancers 2022;14(16).

67. Feng S, Liu B, Zhang Y, et al. Two-Stream Compare and Contrast Network for Vertebral Compression Fracture Diagnosis. IEEE Trans Med Imag 2021;40(9):2496–506.

68. Liu B, Jin Y, Feng S, et al. Benign vs malignant vertebral compression fractures with MRI: a comparison between automatic deep learning network and radiologist's assessment. Eur Radiol 2023;33(7):5060–8.

69. Galbusera F, Niemeyer F, Wilke HJ, et al. Fully automated radiological analysis of spinal disorders and deformities: a deep learning approach. Eur Spine J 2019;28(5):951–60.

70. Merali ZA, Colak E, Wilson JR. Applications of Machine Learning to Imaging of Spinal Disorders: Current Status and Future Directions. Global Spine J 2021;11(1_suppl):23S–9S.

71. Iriondo C, Mehany S, Shah R, et al. Institution-wide shape analysis of 3D spinal curvature and global alignment parameters. J Orthop Res 2022;40(8):1896–908.

72. Ooi BC, Tan KL, Wang S, et al. SINGA: A Distributed Deep Learning Platform. Mm'15: Proceedings of the 2015 Acm Multimedia Conference. 2015;685-688.

73. Lim DSW, Makmur A, Zhu L, et al. Improved Productivity Using Deep Learning-assisted Reporting for Lumbar Spine MRI. Radiology 2022;305(1):160–6.

74. Young AT, Amara D, Bhattacharya A, et al. Patient and general public attitudes towards clinical artificial intelligence: a mixed methods systematic review. Lancet Digit Health 2021;3(9):e599–611.

75. Martin-Noguerol T, Onate Miranda M, Amrhein TJ, et al. The role of Artificial intelligence in the assessment of the spine and spinal cord. Eur J Radiol 2023;161:110726.

76. Galbusera F, Casaroli G, Bassani T. Artificial intelligence and machine learning in spine research. JOR Spine 2019;2(1):e1044.

77. Pesapane F, Volonte C, Codari M, et al. Artificial intelligence as a medical device in radiology: ethical and regulatory issues in Europe and the United States. Insights Imaging 2018;9(5):745–53.

78. Winfield AFT, Jirotka M. Ethical governance is essential to building trust in robotics and artificial intelligence systems. Philos Trans A Math Phys Eng Sci 2018;376(2133).

Printed and bound by CPI Group (UK) Ltd, Croydon, CR0 4YY

08/05/2025

01864747-0017